To my patients
whose patience, strength and perseverance
have taught me much of what is written here.

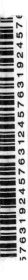

Contents

Presc ... M
Healt. Medi cation

Prescribing Mental Health Medication is a text for medical and nursing practitioners who are learning and refining the prescription of medication in the treatment of mental health problems. The following key issues are highlighted:

- mental health medication – m... and truths
- talking to pa... s about med... on
- starting, stop... ar... monitor... psychotropic medication
- clinical manage... ... ...ifficult medication patients
- modifi...tions ... ...or children/adolescents, pregnant and elderly patient...
- succe... nan... ...ation side effects
- prescr... ...eeping

Icons use... ...ight sample dialogues that can be used to discuss m... ... ...' clinical management tips and special a... ... ...re ...ttings.

Based ... ...al and nursing practition... ...medication manage... ...easily assimilated fo... at. It p... ...escribing, and a comprehensive source of ret... ... ...ioners and teachers.

Dr Christopher Doran is an Associate Clinical Professor of Psychiatry, University of Colorado Health Sciences Center, Consultant to the United States Departments of Health and Human Services, and Veteran's Affairs. He also teaches psychopharmacology nationally and internationally to medical and nursing students, interns, residents and community practitioners.

Prescribing Mental Health Medication
The Practitioner's Guide

Christopher M. Doran MD

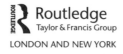

Routledge
Taylor & Francis Group

LONDON AND NEW YORK

First published 2003
by Routledge
29 West 35th Street, New York, NY 10001

Simultaneously published in the UK
by Routledge
11 New Fetter Lane, London EC4P 4EE

Routledge is an imprint of the Taylor & Francis Group

© 2003 Christopher M. Doran

Typeset in Sabon by Wearset Ltd, Boldon, Tyne and Wear
Printed and bound in Great Britain by St Edmundsbury Press, Bury St Edmunds, Suffolk

British Library Cataloguing in Publication Data
A catalogue record for this book is available from the British Library

Library of Congress Cataloging in Publication Data
A catalog record for this book has been requested

ISBN 0-415-28222-5 (pbk)
ISBN 0-415-28209-8 (hbk)

List of tables

Preface

This is a unique book about psychopharmacology. It is written with the intent of teaching clinicians principles and guidelines that will result in successful, rational and evidence-based prescribing. Step by step, it will take the reader from the initial prescriptive evaluation for mental health medication and early follow-up sessions, to the ending of a course of medication. Special populations such as children and adolescents, pregnant and older patients are discussed, noting the adaptations in practice necessary for these populations. Common clinical areas in which psychotropics may be considered, such as in sleep problems, with the cognitively impaired patient and in the treatment of alcohol abuse, are also addressed. Other essentials of prescribing such as measuring serum blood levels, use of generic medications, record keeping, use of the telephone, and interacting with the pharmaceutical industry, are discussed as they apply to the prescription of psychotropics.

Throughout the book there are numerous examples of suggested ways to approach patients verbally, giving the clinician possible scripts and analogies for clinical psychotropic prescription. These suggestions are highlighted under the "Talking to Patients" icon. Specific remedies are detailed for potential problem situations such as side effects and patients who are unusually difficult to treat.

This work is not intended to be a textbook of psychiatry, or to cover in depth the issues of comprehensive psychiatric diagnosis, both of which are available in many texts.[1-5] Although many medication specifics are documented in the text and appendices, this is much more than a compendium of drug facts, dosages or medication side effects, which can be found in other volumes.[6-13]

This book is a necessary precursor and companion to using drug information and mental health textbooks, since it helps the prescriber make sense of the facts. It is a manual for students to learn the essentials of competent clinical practice. The text also serves as an educational tool for current prescribers in helping to refine their clinical practice and to organize the process of prescribing psychotropic medications.

References

1 Gelder M *et al. The New Oxford Textbook of Psychiatry*. Oxford University Press, 2000.

2 Sadock BJ and Sadock VA. *Kaplan and Sadock's Comprehensive Textbook of Psychiatry*, Vol. 7. Lippincott, Williams & Wilkins, 2001.

3 Andreason NC and Black DW. *Introductory Textbook of Psychiatry*, 3rd edn. American Psychiatric Press, 2001.

4 Hales RE *et al.* (eds). *The American Psychiatric Press Textbook of Psychiatry*. American Psychiatric Press, 1999.

5 Henn F *et al. Contemporary Psychiatry*, Vols 1, 2, 3, 4th edn. Springer-Verlag, 2001.

6 *The Maudsley Prescribing Guidelines*, 6th edn. Martin Dunitz, 2002.

7 *The Physician's Desk Reference*. Medical Economics Company Inc., 2002.

8 *U.S.P. Pharmacopia*. Micromedex, 2002.

9 *Drug Facts and Comparisons 2002*, 56th edn. Lippincott, Williams & Wilkins, 2002.

10 Arana GS and Rosenbaum JF. *Handbook of Psychiatric Drugs/Therapy*, 4th edn. Lippincott, Williams & Wilkins, 2000.

11 Fuller MA and Sajatovic M. *Psychotropic Drug Information Handbook*. 3rd edn. Lexi-Comp, 2002.

12 Keltner NL and Folks DG. *Psychotropic Drugs*, 3rd edn. Mosby Press, 2001.

13 *British National Formulary*, 43rd edn. British Medical Association and Royal Pharmaceutical Society, 2002.

Acknowledgments

To:

My wife, Maureen O'Keefe Doran RN MSN, who is an outstanding mental health clinician in her own right and one of the first mental health nurse prescribers in Colorado. I cannot thank you enough for your tireless first-line editing, and your emotional support when I have needed it most.

My daughters, Alison O'Keefe Doran and Meghan Miller Doran. Your generation will see mental health and mental illness treatment with a clarity of vision and freshness of spirit.

My parents, Kenneth and Kathleen Doran. Your reviews of this work brought the wisdom of lifetimes devoted to education and the practical perspective of healthcare consumers.

Ted Levin MD, Yale School of Medicine. Your concise and expert comments on child and adolescent prescribing, arising from your wealth of clinical experience, were invaluable.

Ms Edwina Welham, at Routledge. Thank you for expertly guiding me through the maze of the publishing process. Also, your ability to help me see ways to express my ideas for British readers is a service I could not have done without.

Ms Christine Hackett-Martinez. Thank you for your hours and hours of typing the many revisions of this text. You have a unique perspective on the evolution of these chapters from their roughest beginnings.

A note on the icons used in this book

There are four icons used in this text to highlight special areas of interest to the reader. These are:

 This icon denotes a sample phrasing or dialogue that can be used by the practitioner in discussing a mental health prescribing issue with a patient or family member. Although not intended to be an exclusive way to introduce or discuss an issue, it provides the practitioner with simple, easily remembered concepts and phrases without excessive medical jargon. Novice clinicians will find these suggestions helpful as presented; others may modify them to meet their own style or the clinical situation.

 This icon points out particularly helpful clinical tips, ideas and approaches useful to prescribers.

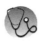 When this icon appears, it denotes a clinical consideration particularly helpful to those prescribing in a general medical/surgical or primary care setting. Mental health providers may find these suggestions useful as well.

 This figure alerts the reader to areas of special risk in the prescription of psychotropics. Most instances of its use are in Chapter 17, on Danger Zones, but others may be found elsewhere in the book.

Part I
The Need for this Book

Chapter 1

General principles of medication management

MENTAL HEALTH MEDICATION IS NOT LIKE OTHER MEDICATION.

Mental health medication is neither chemically different nor necessarily more complicated than other prescription medication. Prescribing a medication for the psyche, however, is a far different process to prescribing antibiotics, pain medications, antihypertensives, cardiac medication, pulmonary medication, or any other group of medications – for the patient and often for the practitioner.

Consider the practice of writing a prescription for penicillin. Once an assessment has been made and a medication selected, there is very little that need be considered beyond writing an accurate prescription and giving appropriate instructions. The patient has an illness, wishes to get better, and comes to the prescriber for medication that will treat the problem. Although patients may wish that they did not need the medication in the first place, prescribing is a relatively simple and straightforward process.

When a patient comes for mental health medication, however, there are many more issues intrinsic to the process that may complicate the prescription. Before patients even set foot in the clinician's office, they may obsessively worry for weeks, months or even years as to whether this is a reasonable, healthy or necessary decision. They may be embarrassed to present to a practitioner, and feel that it reflects badly on them to ask for help. Patients may have strong feelings about whether they wish to have a mental health diagnosis made and recorded in their chart. Even if a correct assessment is made, they may have mixed feelings about whether or not they will allow medication to be part of their treatment.

Once the prescription is written, patients can have fears that the medication will irrevocably change their mind, their behavior or personality. They may be concerned about whether it will be necessary to take the medication for life, and whether or not their lifestyle will be significantly altered or restricted. They worry that the medication may be habit forming, and that they may become addicted to the simple pill they are being offered. They worry about what their family, spouse or friends will think of them for taking a psychiatric medication. They begin to doubt their own abilities and wonder if they are weak for having started the treatment.

These medications – whether we call them mental health medications, psychotropics or psychiatric medications – are unique in the spectrum of medications. Whether an antidepressant medication is prescribed for a diagnosis of depression or in the treatment of irritable bowel syndrome, chronic pain or fibromyalgia (to name a few other common indications), the use of an "antidepressant" has extra meaning to the patient. An anti-anxiety medication carries a similar excess "charge" whether it is specifically for an anxiety disorder or is used as part of an antihypertensive regimen.

Because of their special character and meaning within our culture and practice (see Table 1.1), these medicines require special knowledge, techniques and sensitivity to prescribe effectively. That is what this book is about – describing and teaching the body of knowledge that, when incorporated into everyday practice, will transform a practitioner from someone who merely writes a prescription to a person skilled in mental health medication management.

The special nature of mental health prescription often begins with the practitioner. Many of us, in our personal or family lives, have been exposed to mental illness and/or the varying prejudices about it. On the basis of a family member's experience with medications, shared family beliefs, professional hearsay, or media presentation about psychotropics, many practitioners have mistaken notions of the purpose, therapeutic potential and safety of psychotropic medication. Unfortunately, medical and nursing training is often inadequate in counteracting these misconceptions or mistaken notions. Even when appropriately educated, some practitioners may dismiss the evidence concerning the effectiveness of psychotropic medication and continue to rely on data based on their family or personal experience. More unfortunately, in some areas of the world "mental illness" is still regarded as a function of societal ills without any biological cause. Solutions to emotional problems are thought to lie solely in manipulation of the person's environment, with medications having no part to play in treatment. In parts of the UK, as recently as the early 1990s nursing training had an explicit antipsychiatry content, often leaving nurses highly critical of what they believed to be a malevolent medical model.[1]

Table 1.1 Factors that make mental health medications unique

- Practitioner beliefs
- Media distortion
- Courtroom tactics
- Beliefs about the causes of mental illness
- Artificial separation of the "mind" and the "body"
- Conflicting beliefs about what constitutes treatment for mental health symptoms

Beyond the healthcare community, society at large continues to foster special ideas about mental health medication. Psychotropic medications such as diazepam (Valium), alprazolam (Xanax), and fluoxetine (Prozac) have, at various times, become the most frequently prescribed medications in the world. They also have become cultural icons – the butt of jokes, the material of night-time comedians, and the front-page stories of news magazines. While recent media coverage has tended to be more accurate with regard to psychotropics, in a world of sensationalism and hype where a premium is placed on sales of magazines and on viewership ratings for radio and TV programs, articles designed to grab the public's attention often ignore or distort the true facts. Such presentations reinforce erroneous beliefs, continuing to make these medications uniquely mistrusted.

Courtroom cases that involve psychotropic medications, and the headlines that these cases create, further make these medications "special." An attorney with a defendant who has no other viable defense for a crime can make the taking of a psychotropic medication the focus of the defense case. While few cases have been won on this basis, the fact that psychotropic medications regularly receive headline attention as possibly being the cause of violent, suicidal, abnormal or criminal behavior does little to normalize their prescription and use. Such publicity heightens sensitivity and these medications remain "special" in our repertoire of medicinal treatments.

We cannot discuss the prescription of psychotropics without briefly discussing the evolving (and often confused) beliefs about the causes of mental illness. Within the last century Western civilization has struggled at different times with beliefs that mental illness is caused by demonic possession, willful sloth, religious error, poor social conditions, intemperance, poor parenting, or brain dysfunction. It can be expected, then, that when we talk about medication treatment of mental illness, people's notions of what these medicines are, what their value is and how to prescribe them are also confused and evolving. As we discover more about the underlying biological cause of mental illness, and psychiatry becomes generally seen as a medical science based on objective data, the use of psychotropic medications will be demystified. This is a long and slow process, however. Prejudice dies hard. For the majority of current practitioners' lifetimes, the prescription of these medications will continue to require special skills and sensitivities.

Even medical and nursing practitioners exposed to balanced teaching about mental health are not strangers to misguided notions surrounding mental illness and mental health medication. They may have discussed, learned and believed "facts" that supported the now outdated notion of a split between mind and body. It has often been a standing joke in healthcare training that some practitioners treat the patient from the "neck down," while others treat from the "neck up." For many trainees, it has been an acceptable and routine part of medical treatment to provide medications for illnesses of the heart, kidney, liver, musculature, etc. Neurological and neurosurgical treatment can be comfortably included in this group as "normal," because defined, physical symptoms of a neurobiological disorder can be observed outwardly or on laboratory testing. Brain tumors, degenerative disorders, and seizures are also easily described and documented, and are all considered to be part of the "body." The mind, spirit and emotions, however, have been much more elusive and difficult to define, and this has been reflected in the history of our treatment of mental dysfunction.

Psychiatry's long-standing inability to objectify and make scientific its body of knowledge was particularly complicated in the 1930s and 1940s, with the advent of psychoanalysis. Psychoanalytic teaching suggested that, given enough time and intensity of treatment, talking about one's problems in sufficient depth could remedy most, if not all, symptoms. Even major mental illnesses, which we now know to have strong fundamental biological underpinnings, were seen as being unresolved conflicts from childhood, neuroses, or conflicts of the ego, id and superego. While useful in the treatment of certain neurotic conditions, psychoanalytic concepts only furthered the gulf between treatments for the "mind" and treatments for the "body."

As the new century begins, we now understand much more about brain physiology, genetics, and cellular signaling mechanisms. It is clear that abnormal brain functioning may have substantial effects on major physiological systems including sleep and wakefulness, appetite, energy, concentration, memory, orderly thinking, anxiety regulation, attention, affect regulation, and social relatedness. In many ways, though, we have only scratched the surface of understanding the various aspects of brain function, and how our treatments can remedy brain problems.

The scope of the problem

Mental health problems are a worldwide epidemic. The statistics are staggering, and numbers are increasing rapidly:[2]

- At any time, one in ten adults has a behavioral or mental disorder.
- One in four families will have at least one member with a behavioral or mental disorder.
- 20 percent of all patients seen by primary care professionals have one or more mental disorders.
- Mental and neurological disorders account for almost 31 percent of all years lived with disability.
- Depression is the single largest cause of disability – 12 percent of the total.
- Five of the top ten causes of disability in the 15–44-year old age group are mental health disorders.

Mental health in the spotlight

Mental health medications and treatments have been "discovered." The spotlight of attention has now firmly been fixed on mental health medication by medical research, public opinion, pharmaceutical companies and, gradually, by society at large. Millions of dollars annually are now being poured into mental health research as the major mental illnesses are seen for what they are: public health crises whose incidence is rapidly increasing throughout the world.

There is now a sharply rising exponential curve of knowledge about mental illness, its connection to various areas of brain function, and psychotropic medications that can affect the brain. In the last quarter of the twentieth century, the amount of information available to the practitioner about mental illness and its treatments has grown from a trickle to a river, to the beginnings of a flood. Mental health medications and mental health conditions are now not only confined to books, journals and Internet sites; such topics are regularly discussed in the evening news, newspaper, radio, and magazines. A day does not go by when the informed reader or listener does not hear something about mental health medications or the illnesses that they treat. As medical and nursing professionals, we can expect ever-increasing amounts of information from public health organizations, pharmaceutical companies, and professional societies about mental health medications and psychiatric conditions.

As the use of mental health medication grows and the number of prescribers increases, it is more necessary than ever to learn the prescriptive process well. To do so means being sensitive to the special needs and beliefs of patients, objectively sorting through our own prejudices, and incorporating the growing body of objective, evidence-based data into our work. This book is intended to serve as a manual for professionals to guide their understanding of the prescriptive process. There is little doubt that a gradual movement toward "normalization" of psychiatric conditions is slowly occurring. This will permit and encourage the general medical practitioner to treat a large segment of the growing number of individuals with various mental health conditions. Since the education of most general and family medical practitioners at present remains seriously limited with regard to aspects of mental health, it is hoped that this book will be particularly valuable to this group of professionals.

From the occupational standpoint of the prescriber, the prescription of psychotropic medications can be extremely rewarding. Gaining the ability to use medication to remedy mental health symptoms effectively and promptly reinforces the wish to heal that first attracted us to the healthcare field. The accurate targeting of psychotropics can, in some cases, elicit the response that health professionals desire, when a patient will return and say, "Your treatment has transformed my life." The knowledge that we have increased a patient's ability to work, love, maintain nurturing interpersonal relationships, and enjoy life is truly gratifying.

References

1   Gournay K. Role of the community psychiatric nurses in the management of schizophrenia. *Adv Psychiatr Treatment* 2000;6:243–251.
2   World Health Report 2001, on the Internet at www.who.int/whr/

Chapter 2

Myths and truths about mental health medication

Just as with mental illness itself, there are many beliefs that have evolved about the nature and use of psychotropic medications. Some of these myths are by their very nature untrue, while others may hold some partial validity. Many of these beliefs are so common, however, that at times they form an unchallenged conception of the action and effect of psychotropic medicines. Both well-educated patients and practitioners alike may share portions of these misconceptions. These beliefs are so pervasive and can so strongly affect a practitioner's prescription of psychotropics that it is necessary to devote an early chapter to understanding the facts. Some of the myths apply to all medications, while some relate to specific groups of medications only.

Myth 1: Mental health medication is a placebo

Fact: While far from perfect, mental health medication can make significant differences in patient's lives.

Within both the community at large and, somewhat surprisingly, the medical and nursing communities, there exists a subgroup of people who believe that mental health medications are essentially expensive placebos and have no active value. Often these individuals believe that mental illness itself is not real; the "illness" is just a construct of the person's imagination, or is a result of social circumstance. They further believe there is no underlying chemical abnormality, and that the use of medications to treat this "imaginary" condition must itself be magical, suggestive, hocus pocus, and not scientific.

Individuals with this belief system, even when significantly distressed with mental illness, are reluctant to take medication. Even if they decide to accept medication and experience some benefit, this relief is often attributed to other causes that exclude direct medication effect. Practitioners who partially or fully believe this myth are often minimal prescribers of psychotropics. Inwardly, they may scoff at practitioners who do prescribe mental health medication as being part charlatan, or just uninformed. Even those practitioners who only partially accept this myth and are willing, at times, to prescribe psychotropics may feel inwardly uncomfortable. They wonder what, if anything, they are really doing for patients beyond providing a placebo.

As modern science is better able to demonstrate the physiological changes associated with mental conditions through the use of biological and genetic assays, PET scans, SPECT scans and other imaging techniques, this myth will gradually erode. Such visual demonstrations of biological deficits can be coupled with similar visual images after treatment. These images, showing significant changes in blood flow or in activity of certain cortical areas may convince even recalcitrant individuals of the efficacy of the psychotropic medication.

CLINICAL TIP

It is often useful to have SPECT scan images of individuals with biological mental health conditions, taken before and after treatment, available to show patients in the office, particularly if they are hesitant about trying medications. Such pictures "medicalize" the condition and will often reassure patients sufficiently that they can begin taking medication. Many mental health journals and/or pharmaceutical representatives are sources of such images.

Myth 2: Mental health medication is addictive

Fact: The vast majority of psychotropic medications are not addictive, but may need to be taken regularly.

This myth has multiple roots. In the 1950s and 1960s, a large portion of psychotropic medications were, in fact, habit forming. The widespread use of barbiturates, certain addictive sedative/hypnotics, and eventually benzodiaze-pines, led many practitioners to extrapolate from these classifications of drugs and to assume that all medicines for the mind were habit forming. The fact is that *benzodiazepines, stimulants, and certain hypnotics are the only psychotropic medications on which a patient may become physically dependent.*

While there are individual patients who will overutilize habit-forming medica-tions, practitioners are particularly sensitive to this possibility and often feel that such patients take advantage of them. These instances embarrass and anger the practitioner, and can have an excessive impact on the practitioner's willingness to prescribe psychotropics in the future. These experiences often are generalized such that all psychotropics are seen as habit-forming, even though this is not accurate. As the science of mental health medication has evolved over the past 50 years, a larger and larger percentage of psychotropic medication is not habit forming at all. There is, however, a residual belief that practitioners need to be "on guard" for patients who may try to overuse medication or try to "con" them out of prescriptions for the mind. The facts and specifics of this issue, and tips for the practitioner, are detailed in Chapter 19.

Another important root of this myth is the chronic relapsing nature of mental health conditions. Many patients who stop medication will experience a relapse of symptoms. They request, sometimes strongly, to be placed back on the medica-tion. Practitioners can erroneously interpret this request as indicating that the patient is becoming "addicted" to the medication, when in fact the mental disease re-emerged when the treatment was withdrawn. This is essentially no different to an insulin-dependent diabetic having insulin withdrawn and seeing the symptoms of blood sugar dysregulation recur. The patient is not "addicted" to insulin, but requires it in order to treat the underlying medical condition.

Benzodiazepines, stimulants, and some sedative/hypnotics *are* potentially habit forming, and may be abused by certain individuals. Vigilance on the part of the practitioner is reasonable in the appropriate prescription use of these medica-tions. However, *the vast majority of currently used antidepressants, mood stabi-lizers, antipsychotic and other medications used in a psychotropic practice are in fact not habit forming, are not abused, and have no street value.*

Myth 3: Mental health medication will change personality

Fact: One of the more frequent questions from patients about psychotropics is "Will this medication change me?" The answer to this question is not always simple.
To the extent that we see specific biological symptoms as part of the diagnosed condition (e.g. sleep disorder, appetite disturbance, poor concentration, fluctua-tions in energy, and disordered thinking), these target symptoms *will* hopefully be improved or eliminated with medication. So yes, the patient will be "changed," and that is the therapeutic hope and intent.

It would be misleading, however, to assume that other underlying personality traits – personal likes and dislikes, hobbies, work interests, or many of the ele-ments that comprise personality – are likely to be changed in a direct way. Some patients with long-standing untreated illness may develop new interests, find new employment, or change relationships as a consequence of feeling better, but this is not a direct chemical effect of the medication.

Myth 4: Stop mental health medicine as soon as possible

Fact: One underpinning of this notion is the universally held tenet of good medical prescriptive practice stating that we should prescribe the least amount of medication for the shortest period of time to achieve our medical aim. This is indeed good practice.

While, in general, no one should take any medication longer than needed, the practitioner's good intentions to accomplish this with psychotropics may be clouded by misconceptions. Some roots of these misconceptions have been identified in the previously identified myths that most psychotropic medications are addictive or placebos. Prescribers with this mindset will also subscribe to the corollary that if medication is used it should be used for a very brief period, and that it is inappropriate for a patient to take long-term medication. Clinicians who read statements such as those in the *Physician's Desk Reference* or other sources that "efficacy has not been proven beyond eight weeks" may use this information to support the misconception. Pharmaceutical companies must often make these statements because the initial clinical trials necessary to bring a medication to market were undertaken on a short-term basis and, at the time of initial medication release, longer-term maintenance medication trials had not yet been performed. It is only several years after the introduction of a medication that maintenance trials may be undertaken, and the results may take several more years to be completed and published.

What also reinforces this myth is the notion that many mental health problems are primarily or solely related to life stressors. The assumption is that once these stressors are resolved, the patient should no longer need to be medicated. If symptoms persist significantly after the resolution of a divorce, a job loss, a personal tragedy, or other stressor, the practitioner may assume that any symptoms should disappear, or at least not require medication. Within this belief, the practitioner acts as if the patient should *automatically* be treated with medication for a short period of time following the stressor. The clinician feels that he or she is doing the patient a favor by recommending or insisting that the patient stop medication as soon as possible.

While no ethical practitioner would recommend that anyone be treated longer than needed, we cannot fail to appreciate the chronic nature of many mental conditions. Depression, bipolar disorder, schizophrenia, panic disorder, generalized anxiety disorder and many other mental health conditions are often chronic or relapsing illnesses. It is quite common to have flare-ups of these chronic illnesses triggered by environmental stressors. At times, even when the stressors resolve, symptoms requiring treatment may remain. The treatment of these conditions with medication may be episodic or, in some cases, continuous. *For many patients, it is safe, life enhancing, or even life saving, to remain indefinitely on medication.* Tips for helping the practitioner to make these decisions are outlined in Chapters 8 and 9.

Myth 5: Mental health medication will overcome bad habits

Fact: While medication can help with specific symptoms, personality traits, including undesirable ones, may or may not change.

Many people hope that by taking a pill they can eliminate all unpleasant emotions from their lives – not only diagnostically targeted symptoms such as depressed mood or anxiety, but also elements of life's unpleasantness. They hope that medication will make them "emotionally bulletproof," or compensate for other deficits in their life. There may be a wish on the part of anxious or depressed individuals that once on medication they will automatically overcome procrastination, inattention to detail, abrasive personal traits, social isolation, poor financial budgeting, self-centeredness, psychological resistance to change, or unwillingness to approach difficult personal issues. These traits and behaviors, which fall under the rubric of "personality" and "personal style," are often not affected by psychotropic medications.

Other patients hope that by taking medication their relationship with their parents, their spouse, their children or their neighbors will magically improve. In fact, some patients who take psychotropic medication *may* significantly improve their interpersonal relationships, although it often takes a considerable amount of psychological work. Individual, marital, family or group psychotherapy may help to achieve this goal. Part of our role as clinicians is to help the patient to sort out realistic expectations of medication from wishful fantasies.

Myth 6: If side effects occur, the medication must be working

Fact: Medications, when appropriately tailored and adjusted, usually cause few side effects. *Side effects are not intrinsic to the positive therapeutic mental health benefits of the medication.*

In the past, there was an assumption that the side effects were intrinsically related to the effect of the medication, and that patients must experience them in order to feel better. In today's psychopharmacology, it is a goal to have patients experience minimal or no side effects from their medication. The antidepressant, antipsychotic, mood stabilizing, or anti-anxiety effect is quite independent of unwanted physical or emotional side effects. While this goal cannot always be obtained, there should be no expectation on the part of the clinician or the patient that side effects are necessary in order to feel better.

This myth also relates to the experience of many patients using psychotropic medications from earlier times, who would almost invariably get side effects when they took medication, regardless of dose. Prior to the last decade, this was reinforced when there were few choices or classes of medication to prescribe. Unfortunately, during this time many patients did have to undergo significant side effects in order to remain psychiatrically stable.

Myth 7: Taking medication for depression means weakness

Fact: Depression is an illness. Depressed individuals often have to try harder than most.

This is one of the most common misconceptions about mental illness. For illustration we will use depression, but the principle applies to most emotional illnesses. Because many people with severe emotional illnesses do in fact have some difficulty with day-to-day functioning, job performance and interpersonal relationships, they arrive at the clinician's office already feeling inferior. They may have struggled for months, years or decades, feeling they were unable to "keep up" and perform in the way that they themselves expected. This feeling may be reinforced by critical comments and attitudes from family or friends, or work sanctions from employers. Patients often may have tried a variety of home remedies, self-improvement techniques, or just "trying harder." Now, with trepidation, they are seeking help. We, as clinicians, must understand their struggle and support the efforts they have already made.

When a diagnosis is made and appropriate medication prescribed, most patients are quite capable of increased functioning in their lives. While very ill patients may remain handicapped by their emotional illness, the majority of outpatients can be helped significantly by targeted psychotropic medications. Quality of life can be enriched and the person's level of function improved. Adequate treatment can also help patients to rediscover their strengths and abilities to further grow and prosper.

 TALKING TO PATIENTS

A very powerful and alliance-building message can be conveyed by clinicians in the statement: *"I think I know how difficult it may have been to make the decision to see me about medication today. You may have heard from others (or believed yourself) that all you needed to do was try harder and 'get over it.' After trying many methods that didn't work, you may have even begun to believe that you were just lazy or unmotivated. I believe you have an illness – depression – that has as some of its symptoms, low motivation, decreased energy and an inability to concentrate. You have been using a lot of energy just to get through the day and accomplish tasks that should be routine. One effect I expect from this medication is that it may not be as hard to lead your day-to-day life."*

Myth 8: Antidepressants cause suicidal or homicidal thoughts

Fact: Antidepressant medication is unlikely to create new suicidal or homicidal ideation.

There are several factors leading to this particular myth. A certain number of depressed individuals do attempt or complete suicide. Families and friends of these individuals find it difficult to see their relative "at fault" for this behavior and, in the search for other causes, medication becomes an easy scapegoat. Coroner reports of successful suicides may show antidepressants in the blood of the deceased. This does not necessarily mean that the medication "caused" the suicide; it merely shows that the patient was being treated with medication at the time the suicide occurred. *Many patients have suicidal ideation* before they begin medication therapy *that is part of the underlying illness*. When a depressed person does attempt or succeed with suicide while being medicated, it is often the case that the diagnosis was incorrect, the choice of medication failed, it was given in inadequate doses, or it was taken sporadically by the patient. Several studies[1,2] have revealed that antidepressants do not confer special increased rates of suicidal ideation or attempt.

A second factor that has led people to be concerned about the role of antidepressants in violent or suicidal behavior is that defense attorneys for persons who have committed violent crimes may have only a meager defense for the patient's actions. If the patient was taking a psychotropic medication, it may be very convenient for such an attorney to argue that the medication was to blame for the patient's behavior. Prior to 2002 over 20 such cases had been brought worldwide, in which antidepressants were allegedly blamed for violent acts. Thus far, in only one case did the jury find any significant responsibility caused by the medication. The case was appealed and settled out of court prior to an appeal verdict being rendered. In many situations, when one investigates the past history of persons who have committed violent crimes, they have been found to be aggressive, violent or homicidal prior to the current act, even before they were on medication.

Several truths may also contribute to myth 8:

1 Some, but not most, antidepressants cause akathisia, a very disturbing physical inner restlessness. Patients with akathisia have been noted to have a suicide rate above that of the general population. It is possible that the small percentage of patients who do develop akathisia while on medication could be at some increased risk for self-injury.

2 In general, appropriately treated persons with depression become significantly less suicidal and the likelihood of a suicide attempt drops dramatically. However, we have long known that *the profoundly depressed, suicidal person who has marked psychomotor slowing may be at some measure of increased risk for suicide in the first several days or weeks of treatment*. As the patient first begins to improve, he or she gradually becomes energized. If not carefully monitored or supported during this period, the increase in energy may precede the lessening of the other depressed symptoms, including suicidal thoughts. At this point, the patient may be an increased risk for a self-injury attempt that previously the patient was too anergic to attempt.

3 Mental health medications are more frequently being tried in efforts to address a wide variety of problematic human behaviors, including aggression, violence and suicide. When other treatments have failed, psychotropics may be prescribed as a last resort to seriously violent and suicidal individuals. With the significant gaps in our ability to predict and remedy suicide and violence in general, medications too may fail adequately to correct the underlying factors

that cause these problematic behaviors. With the increased use of psychotropics, it is to be expected that a percentage of people who do act violently or kill themselves may have medication in their bodies at the time of their destructive acts, but it should not be assumed that the medication is the underlying cause.

Myth 9: All antidepressants are alike

Fact: In treating depression alone and measured over large groups, antidepressants have relatively similar statistical effectiveness. They may, however, have quite different therapeutic effects or tolerability for a given individual.

Currently we have over a dozen commonly used antidepressants, and at least an equal number that are less commonly used. Clinical evidence comparing efficacy demonstrates similar statistical short-term effectiveness among antidepressants.[3] In a given clinical trial of 100 patients, approximately 65–70 percent of the group treated with Antidepressant A will obtain some measure of improvement. Approximately one-third of the patients either will not improve or will develop side effects. The same group of 100 patients given Antidepressant B will achieve a similar statistical response. Some patients will have responded to both medications; some to one, but not the other; some to the second and not the first; and some to neither.

Even within the same category, for example Serotonin Specific Reuptake Inhibitors (SSRIs) such as fluoxetine, sertraline, paroxetine, citalopram and fluvoxamine, the individual members of the group are very different medicines even though the purported mechanisms of action are the same. Research suggests that a trial of a second SSRI in a patient who has failed to respond to the first will result in positive response in 50–75 percent of situations.[4]

Myth 10: Alcohol is prohibited while taking psychotropic medicine

Fact: Drinking in moderation can occur safely in most patients taking mental health medications, if alcohol abuse is not a clinical consideration for this patient and the alcohol intake remains moderate.

While the interaction of mental health medications and alcohol may be a problem for certain individuals, particularly those with substance-abuse problems or tendencies to overuse medication, it is not necessary or realistic to expect responsible, compliant outpatients to give up alcohol. On occasion, patients may safely enjoy a cocktail or a glass of wine or beer while they are being treated with medication.

CLINICAL TIP

The rule of thumb is as follows: *no more than one drink in an evening and no more than four drinks in a week*. Patients generally can drink at this level without seriously compromising the effect of their mental health medication or creating a health hazard for themselves. There are exceptions to this general principle, and each situation should be evaluated independently.

Myth 11: Mental health medication will treat alcoholism

Fact: Substance abuse may or may not decrease when a person's mental health condition is treated adequately.

There is a significant overlap between many emotional illnesses and substance abuse, and many mental health patients "self-medicate" with alcohol or recreational drugs. Once they begin feeling better as a result of treatment, which may include psychotropic medication, some of these patients no longer need substances for self-medication. *It is not reasonable, however, to assume that all persons with substance-abuse problems will necessarily decrease their use of substances when they are medicated.* Some may continue to abuse alcohol and/or recreational drugs despite their mental health improvement, and will need separate, independent substance abuse treatment.

Myth 12: A person must be substance-free to be assessed/treated accurately for mental illness

Fact: It depends.

The willingness of practitioners to medicate with psychotropics in those patients abusing alcohol or drugs will vary. There is a group of practitioners who will insist on patients being substance-free before they will medicate. Other practitioners are willing to prescribe for clearly diagnosed mental health conditions despite the presence of mild to moderate drug or alcohol usage. The hope in the latter situation is that when patients are appropriately medicated, they will be better able to give up or cut down their alcohol/drug usage.

Such a premise of reduced substance usage with medication requires constant re-evaluation, and certainly is not universally true. For those patients who, despite adequate medication, continue to abuse alcohol or drugs, continuing medication prescription may not be in their best interest, and may indeed present some medical hazard.

To expect that patients who have been using substances for a long time, particularly for self-medication, will cease their habit prior to being medicated is, in most cases, unlikely and unreasonable. Often such a prerequisite, if strictly and uniformly enforced, will drive such patients from treatment before medication can offer improvement. If, however, as a practitioner, you have a history that a patient is a heavy substance abuser or has abused the combination of medications and alcohol before, it may well be reasonable to insist that the patient be detoxified before medication is prescribed.

References

1   Beasley CM *et al*. Fluoxetine and suicide: a meta-analysis of controlled trials of treatment for depression. *BMJ* 1991;303:685–692.
2   Fava M and Rosenbaum JF. Suicidality and fluoxetine: is there a relationship? *J Clin Psychiatry*, 1991;52(3):108–111.
3   http://www.psych.org/clin_res/Depression2e.book-7.cfm, p. 3.
4   Joffe RT *et al*. Response to an open trial of a second SSRI in major depression. *J Clin Psychiatry*, 1996;57:114–115.

Part II Medication Management Start to Finish

Chapter 3

The initial prescriptive interview

This chapter focuses on the elements of the initial patient contact for the purposes of determining if medication is indicated, and, if so, what kind of medication might be prescribed. Performing an organized, thorough evaluation is crucial to success with psychotropic prescription. Whether conducted in an outpatient office or clinic, an inpatient or institutional setting, the process of this initial evaluation seldom changes. Although each individual is different and each of these initial evaluation sessions may take a slightly different course, it is important to have a general procedural process and goal in mind.

If a clinician is coming to the practice of prescribing psychotropics from a psychotherapy background, the directed, focused interview described in this chapter may seem somewhat foreign and overly structured. Those practitioners who come from a strong medical/surgical background will find this outline very similar to the initial evaluations done for medical problems in a primary care office.

Table 3.1 Framework of a prescriptive interview

- Demographic data
- Chief complaint
- History of present illness
- Past history
- Previous mental health episodes
- Previous mental health treatment
- Medical/substance abuse history
- Mental status exam
- Assessment/diagnosis
- Treatment plan

A useful way to conceptualize the elements necessary in the initial prescriptive interview is to start with the end in mind, and think of *those items that would be included in a written report* following this initial interview. In many cases, in fact, a written report may be necessary, not only as the record of contact but also for the purposes of discussion with a collaborating professional or for distribution to other medical personnel who may be caring for the patient. The overall framework of the elements of such a report is shown in Table 3.1, and is discussed in more detail below.

What to say after "hello"

The first several minutes of a medication interview are often the most important time to an emotionally anxious patient. What is said and done in this initial period can set the stage for a comfortable, helpful experience for the patient, or negatively color the process from the start. After greeting the patient, there are several things a clinician can do in a brief period of time that will facilitate the task and relax the patient.

As simple as it may sound, making sure that the patient knows *who you are* and *why he or she is being seen* is crucially important, and surprisingly is often misunderstood by the patient. Clinicians, therefore, should state not only their name, but also their professional identifier, and why the patient is being seen today.

 TALKING TO PATIENTS

"I am Mary Smith, psychiatric nurse practitioner. Your therapist, Frank Jones, has asked me to see you to determine if medication would be helpful for you as part of your treatment. **How do you feel about coming to see me today?"**

This latter simple question is exceptionally important. Patients coming to see a mental health professional or a primary care doctor about a mental health problem are often very anxious. Their emotions can run the gamut from marked positivity to profound negativity. They may feel relief and eager anticipation ("I'm finally doing something about this"; "I should have done this a long time ago"). They may, however, be openly anxious and fearful about the process of seeing a mental health prescriber, and the possibility of being diagnosed or of being prescribed medications, for all the reasons that are listed in Chapters 1 and 2. Patients may have significant uncertainty or misgivings, or blame themselves unnecessarily ("I never thought it would come to this"; "Just being here means that I couldn't handle things"). Other patients are considerably reluctant and show great resistance. They may be seen under duress, complying with the wishes of others who insist they be evaluated ("I wouldn't be here except my wife said she would leave me"; "My boss said that I needed to do something or I would lose my job").

The discussion regarding how a patient feels about being seen can be relatively simple and brief, or may take some measure of time. The very fact that the clinician is interested in the patient's feelings is a good start. When patients are apprehensive, having an opportunity to say how anxious, reluctant, or fearful they are, often sets them at ease. Sometimes they will say (and genuinely believe) that they do not have a lot of feelings about the evaluation. If so, this should be accepted at face value. Patients who have seen mental health professionals before may be accustomed to such consultations. For some patients, medication and mental health assessments have been conducted on many previous occasions.

If significant affect is revealed regarding the evaluation session, it is worthwhile spending several minutes allowing the patient to vent. The practitioner may also correct any possible misunderstandings or misconceptions. Generally, this will not take more than a few minutes.

TALKING TO PATIENTS

In the rare circumstance where a patient seems to wish to talk for a long period of time about the lead-up to this evaluation, the discussion should be gently curtailed. The practitioner can suggest that; *"We need to move on to specific questions that will help us decide if medicine is for you."*

Following this discussion, another brief but very helpful intervention is to describe the process of the interview.

TALKING TO PATIENTS

If you know beforehand that the visit is specifically for medication evaluation (and not for other mental health services), you can say: *"I will be seeing you today for about [number of minutes]. We will focus on the specific symptoms that are bothering you. We will not be spending as much time talking about the issues in your life even though these are important. For purposes of determining if medication is useful, it is essential that we understand what symptoms you have, and how long you have had them. Our overall plan is to define what the problem is, determine if medication can help, and, if so, what medication would be best for you. How does that sound to you?"*

In the majority of circumstances this brief introduction, which will take as little as one or two minutes, will prepare the clinician to begin specific symptomatic inquiry.

General issues of history taking

Table 3.2 lists some important elements of history taking. It is important in an initial prescriptive interview that this activity is *clinician directed*. The clinician must have an understanding of the information to be covered, and direct the conversation so that the appropriate information is gathered in the time allotted.

This notion opposes tenets taught in schools of psychotherapy about the initial *psychotherapeutic* interview. For therapy evaluations, clinicians are instructed to "let the patient tell his own story in whatever way he needs to." Patients are encouraged to associate freely, telling what is important to them. While this method may be helpful as a basis for psychotherapeutic "talking" therapy, it is an inefficient methodology for gathering necessary data for prescriptive purposes. If patients are allowed to direct the interview, the clinician is often left at the end of the session trying to make decisions with inadequate information.

Most patients are quite familiar with a structured interview. They expect it from the clinician, and fall easily into a question-and-answer format. Other patients expect to tell their life story, or to spend a considerable amount of time talking about a personal crisis. For medication purposes, these latter patients need to be re-directed by the clinician to specific historical elements or specific symptom questions that will lead to the necessary assessment.

Questions should be *asked in a consistent manner* and *framed in an open-ended way*, omitting phrasing that suggests the answer. For example, asking "Have you had any problems with your sleep?" will elicit a more valid answer than "You haven't had any sleep problems, have you?" Similarly, asking "Have you had any difficulty with your concentration and mental focus?" is more helpful than "Given how depressed you've been, I'm sure you've been having trouble concentrating, haven't you?" Particular questions about a patient's symptoms should be phrased in ways that are familiar to the clinician and can be repeated.

An important item in evaluating a patient for medication is the *meaning of the patient's terms or jargon*. Because a patient thinks he is "depressed" or "anxious," has "panic attacks," is "confused" or "doesn't sleep well" does not necessarily mean the clinician's assessment of these problems will be similar.

Table 3.2 Important elements of history taking

- Directed interview
- Ask open-ended questions
- Elicit facts and clarify the patient's words
- Routinized
- End product is a chronological symptom history, hopefully leading to a diagnosis

---

Essential to performing a good medication evaluation is asking patients questions to elucidate what they mean by the terminology that they use. *The clinician needs to elicit and record behavioral facts, not the patient's assessment of the facts.*

For example, when someone comes in saying "I'm depressed," elucidate specifics with questions such as:

■   What do *you* mean when you say you are depressed?
■   How do you recognize when you are depressed compared to when you are not?
■   What changes indicate to you that you are depressed?

If a person complains of "problems sleeping," ask:

■   When do you go to bed?
■   When do you fall asleep?
■   How many times do you awaken?
■   How long do you stay awake?
■   When do you arise for the day?
■   Do you nap? How often? For how long?
■   Do you work different shifts or have a markedly varying sleep/wake cycle?

Similarly, with eating and appetite, if a patient complains of a poor appetite or of "not eating well," clarify using the following:

■   How many meals do you eat in a day?
■   What does a typical meal consist of?
■   Does food taste normal? Has it lost its taste?
■   Is your weight changing? By how much?
■   If you do not measure your weight, do your clothes fit differently?
■   Over what period of time has this change occurred?
■   Are there periods of increased appetite?
■   Have there been any food binges?
■   Have you intentionally vomited food? How often?

The medication interview should be routinized. There should be a framework that the clinician is familiar with and has practiced over time, and that can be repeated with limited variations as necessitated by the patient. It is often helpful for clinicians to use a written outline of those elements to be included in the evaluation.

A checklist can be helpful, particularly for less experienced clinicians. Many clinicians with limited experience assume that using a written checklist indicates their inexperience to the patient, or that they will be seen as novices. They assume that experienced clinicians have all the needed information "in their head." This, in fact, is not true, and many patients see the use of a written format as thoroughness on the part of the clinician, not inexperience. Several examples of such checklists to guide clinicians in an initial interview are provided in Tables 3.5–3.7 at the end of this chapter.

Essentials that must be obtained for medication prescription

Demographic data include age, sex, ethnicity, marital status, and occupation. The *chief complaint* (CC) is the patient's statement of the reason for seeking assessment. It is very useful, if possible, actually to quote the patient's words. The *history of present illness* (HPI) is a specific history of those complaints or symptoms that occurred with or led up to the chief complaint. The time period covered by this HPI may be weeks, months, years or much of the patient's life, depending on how long the symptoms have been present. *Past history* (PH) for a psychotropic medication evaluation specifically focuses on previous episodes of symptoms, previous mental health treatment episodes including hospitalization, psychotropic medications previously used and response or non-response to medication (see Table 3.3). Elements of childhood developmental history, education, military service, marital history and chronological occupational history, while interesting and useful in other contexts, may not be crucial initially to assessing the patient for mental health medication.

The elements of the *medical history* portion should include:

■   Current medical problems for which the patient is being treated
■   Current medications taken, dosage and frequency (both prescription and over-the-counter medications should be included)
■   Any history of medication/food/substance allergies
■   Use of caffeine/nicotine.

If the patient is female, a specific assessment of pregnancy status is essential.

■   Are you sexually active?
■   Is there a possibility you could be pregnant now?
■   If not, how do you know?
■   Is any form of birth control being used?
■   When was the date of your last menstrual period?

The patient's substance use should be evaluated, not only currently, but also regarding any previous history of overuse of alcohol or drugs.

Table 3.3 Essentials to be obtained for medication prescription

■   Symptom-focused psychiatric present illness
■   History of past symptoms and episodes
■   Previous treatment response to psychotropics
■   Medical history
■   Current medications used (prescription and OTC)
■   Assessment of suicidal and homicidal risk
■   Substance use – current and past
■   Pregnancy status

- Do you drink alcohol? How much? How often?
- Do you use recreational drugs? Which ones? How much? How often? Orally, intravenously or by other means?

If the patient does drink or use drugs, two useful screening questions can often detect a possible substance abuse problem:[1]

1 In the last year, have you ever drunk alcohol or used drugs more than you meant to?
2 Have you felt you wanted to, or needed to cut down on your drinking or drug use in the past year?

If either of these questions is answered positively, follow up with:

- Have you ever drunk alcohol or used drugs to deal with your feelings, stress or frustration?
- As a result of your drinking or drug use, did anything happen to you that you wish hadn't?
- Does anyone else think you have a problem with substances?

Mental status exam

Most outpatients undergoing a medication evaluation for mild to moderate anxiety or mood disorders do not require formal mental status testing unless:

1 There are *signs of memory loss, poor concentration, confusion or disorientation*
2 *Psychotic signs* or symptoms are present
3 It is *required by the clinic or institution*, in which the evaluation occurs or, in the US, it is requested by a third-party payer.

Patients with severe psychiatric symptoms and any patient admitted to an inpatient or custodial setting should have a full mental status exam on admission. Even if a full mental status exam is not performed, a behavioral descriptive summary of the patient during the evaluation, including any outstanding elements of appearance, behavior, speech or thought pattern, is often useful.

The format for elements of a mental status exam is detailed in Appendix 1.

As part of the mental status assessment, evaluation of the patient's suicidal and homicidal risk must be included. If the patient has had suicidal ideation, estimation must be made of the frequency, intensity and lethality of these thoughts:

- Have you ever had *thoughts* of hurting or killing yourself?
- If suicidal thoughts have been present, how often?
- How easy/difficult has it been for you to deal with these thoughts?
- If there have been thoughts, do you have a *plan* for killing yourself?
- How would you commit suicide, if you were to attempt it?

■ Do you have access to the *means/weapon* needed to carry out the plan?

■ Have you tried to kill yourself in the past? When? How was the attempt discovered?

■ Was any medical or psychiatric intervention required?

■ Were there any medical sequelae to the attempt?

■ Is there anything that would prevent you from following through with such an attempt now?

If homicidal ideation or thoughts of direct self-harm to others are present:

■ How often have they occurred?

■ Toward whom are the thoughts directed?

■ Have you made any specific plans?

■ Is there any direct plan to harm someone now?

■ Is there anything that would prevent this from happening, now or in the future?

Useful but optional information

There is information that may be helpful, but is not essential for evaluation (see Table 3.4). If possible, it is reasonable for the clinician to ask about these items, knowing that in some cases there will be insufficient time to do so.

A *history of psychiatric illness in the patient's blood relatives*, particularly first-degree relatives, can be diagnostically helpful. For example, a child brought for evaluation of attention and behavior problems who has several relatives with a history of bipolar disorder raises the clinician's suspicion that this patient may have a bipolar diagnosis, rather than Attention Deficit Disorder. In this case, more detailed questions about hypomanic behavior would be warranted. Whenever a family history is positive for psychiatric illness in blood relatives, it is useful to learn if any medications have been prescribed, and the effect of such medication.

Additionally, it is helpful to ask what the patient thinks about the use of psychotropic medications. What have you read? What have you heard from friends or relatives? Do you have any particular overriding concerns about how medication may affect you? Do you have any particular side effects or risks about which they are concerned? These questions, when asked before recommending a particular medication, can be very helpful in assisting the clinician in choosing a medication. If the patient, for example, is very concerned about weight gain, then

---

Table 3.4 Other information that may be useful

■ Family psychiatric history
■ Use of psychotropics by family members and results
■ Patient's thoughts about using medication
■ Knowledge of/or concerns about medication
■ Sexual history

---

perhaps a medication can be chosen in which weight gain is a minimal side effect. If a blood relative has done well on a particular medication, the patient may be positively predisposed to that medication.

Target symptoms

As the chronological symptom history is being obtained, the clinician can begin to identify target symptoms to be treated with medication. Items such as sleep disturbance, appetite dysregulation, concentration difficulties, diminished energy, thought disorganization, hallucinations, delusions, anxiety, panic attacks, excessive ruminations, social avoidance, confusion, suicidal ideation/behavior, homicidal ideation/behavior, irritability and rage attacks are examples of possible target symptoms. When the information gathered leads the clinician to make a diagnosis, this should be made and recorded. When a positive diagnosis cannot be determined, a list of possible diagnoses or "rule outs" should be created.

Historical information from others

Input from other sources can be very helpful to the clinician in making decisions about medication, particularly when patients are:

- Poor observers of their own behavior
- Having trouble with memory or concentration
- Having trouble verbalizing their symptoms
- Frankly confused or psychotic
- Intoxicated.

It can be assumed that anyone who accompanies a patient to an initial prescriptive interview is there for a reason, and should be at least offered the opportunity to provide input. This person may be a family member or spouse, a therapist, social worker, home health visitor, probation officer, friend or neighbor. If the patient has not asked to have the visitor come into the consultation room, the clinician should ask the patient's permission to speak with the accompanying party before completing the assessment. If, in the initial portion of the interview, it becomes clear that the patient is having significant concentration or memory problems, it is generally most efficient to bring any accompanying visitor in during the early portions of the interview.

Identify other important sources of information that need to be collected, including:

- Psychotherapists
- Medical colleagues
- Psychological testing
- Family input
- Laboratory tests
- Physical exam or assessments.

When another clinician is to be contacted, obtain a signed release of information and consent.

The medical work-up

Prior to prescribing a psychotropic, a recent full physical examination is not mandatory for a healthy patient without medical problems. If, however, there are uncompensated medical issues or the patient has significant somatic complaints, a physical exam should be performed as part of the initial evaluation or soon thereafter. Attention should be paid to the organ systems about which the patient complains (e.g. back, headache, bowels, fatigue), with follow-up of any abnormal findings. If the screening physical exam is negative, emotional causes are often hypothesized, at least initially, to be the cause of the somatic symptoms. In such situations, further physical diagnostic work-up is not warranted unless new symptoms emerge or mental health treatment does not improve the symptoms.

If there are signs, symptoms or a history suggestive of liver disease, a *liver function panel* should be obtained because almost all medications are hepatically metabolized. *Pregnancy testing* should be performed on any menstruating female who cannot give a reliable history of consistent use of birth control measures or sexual abstinence for the previous menstrual cycle. In any depressed patient the work-up should include a *TSH* (thyroid stimulating hormone) level, since up to 15 percent of depressed patients will have abnormal thyroid tests without any other symptoms of thyroid dysfunction. Prior to instituting a *mood stabilizer* such as lithium, valproic acid or carbamazepine, a *full chemical panel, including liver functions, electrolytes, kidney functions, blood sugar, a CBC and TSH* level, is recommended. If there is a history of kidney disease, a urinalysis should also be obtained.

The next decision

Following information-gathering, the next decision for the clinician is whether or not medications are indicated. Obviously, if the clinician decides that medications would not help the target symptoms or chief complaint, this should be stated and any other treatments that might be helpful discussed with the patient. Referral can be made to another clinician who might be consulted for the patient's particular complaint.

If medication is deemed appropriate, the first question is, what *category* of medication is useful for this patient: antidepressants, anti-anxiety medicine, antipsychotics, a mood stabilizer, another category, or a combination? Once decided, a single category may have *several classes* from which to choose. For example, within the antidepressants the clinician may choose an SSRI, a non-SSRI new generation antidepressant, a tricyclic antidepressant, or a monoamine oxidase inhibitor. Within the antipsychotic category, the clinician may prescribe a traditional or atypical antipsychotic. Once the class is identified, the clinician must choose a *specific medication* within that class.

Although it is clearly desirable to use monotherapy whenever possible, in some cases it may be necessary to use more than one medication simultaneously or to prescribe one medication on a regular basis while providing another medication on a PRN (as needed) basis. Further information on selecting an initial medication is specified in Chapter 5.

Assessment and formulation

Having responded to the clinician's questions and having revealed significant personal information, the patient will eagerly, and often anxiously, await the practitioner's reaction. Many patients remain uncertain about presenting for medication evaluation, and are concerned as to how the clinician will react. A brief preface to your assessment and formulation can often set the patient further at ease.

TALKING TO PATIENTS
"Making an appointment for mental health medication is not always easy. Having heard what you have been experiencing, I think you have made a good decision to come today. Here is my assessment and what I think will help."

Summarizing the information, the clinician should then provide the patient with an assessment in layman's terms. For clarity, it is important that long diagnostic or medically complicated terms be avoided. When such language must be used, simple definitions are helpful.

The clinician can then make pharmacological and non-pharmacological recommendations to the patient. Non-pharmacological interventions may include psychotherapy, cognitive/behavioral therapy, relaxation training, biofeedback light therapy, or social skills training. Pharmacological recommendations should include the name of the medication, its classification, which target symptoms the medication is likely to improve, and the probable timetable for results.

A discussion of side effects is appropriate at this time. There is a delicate balance involved in any discussion of side effects. On one hand, the patient must have enough information to be truly informed. However, overloading the patient with data will likely produce increased fear, anxiety, and non-compliance. In general, mentioning the three or four most commonly experienced side effects with the medication chosen will suffice. A detailed explanation of all possible side effects will only confuse the patient, and not be helpful to the prescriptive process. If there are any serious risks (for example, hypertensive crisis with MAO inhibitors, and/or alcohol/antabuse reaction with disulfiram), specific risks should be discussed in more detail. If there are particular medications to avoid because of possible medication interactions, they should be mentioned and included in written information given to the patient. (See Chapter 16 for a more in-depth discussion of side effects.)

A crucial point, often overlooked, particularly if the clinician is busy or new to the prescriptive process, is patient feedback and consent. It is critical to be sure that patients understand what the assessment is and what role medication may play, and, most importantly, whether the patient concurs with the medication recommendations. A thorough examination, culminating in an accurate diagnosis followed by appropriate treatment recommendations will be futile if the patient deposits the carefully written prescription into the trash!

Non-compliance with a prescription medication often results from:

- *Ignorance* (the patient did not understand or hear what was said)
- *Disagreement* (the patient disagreed) with the use of medication at all
- *Fear* (the patient has not been adequately reassured about the safety of medication)
- *Denial* (the patient does not want to believe, or disagrees with, the diagnosis).

Completing the patient feedback loop is essential. Does the patient understand? Are there any fears? And is the patient willing, with your support, to try medication?

TALKING TO PATIENTS

Following your statement of diagnosis and treatment: *"That is my assessment of the problem and what I think will help. Does that sound reasonable? Do you have any concerns about what I said? Can you follow through with these recommendations?"*

Purely verbal instructions to patients are often misheard, misunderstood, or totally forgotten in the midst of the probable anxiety present in the prescriptive interview. If the clinician verbally describes a quick set of instructions and asks "Do you understand?" or "Any questions?" patients will often nod "yes," even when they are quite unsure. Therefore, *written instructions are extremely helpful*.

If there is agreement, the prescription is written, dosages and directions for use are reviewed, and the patient should be given the opportunity to ask questions. If the clinician has done a solid, thorough job in the previous steps, questions are usually minimal. In some cases, though, the patient may have several questions held in abeyance for just this opportunity. Once the questions are answered, an appointment for a *follow-up evaluation* is made. A written appointment card given to the patient is beneficial. It is seldom appropriate to have the patient leave the office without a definite time agreed upon for follow-up.

Immediately after the interview, the patient's *written record* should be completed. This will document the above mentioned steps, including the chief complaint, present illness and target symptoms; negative responses to important questions within the assessment; mental status examination; medical history; medication history; alcohol and drug history; clinician assessment and recommendations; and a record of the specific medication and prescription data.

Although there are time pressures on all clinicians, it is crucial that the record be completed as soon as possible. Even an hour or two later, if the clinician has seen more patients, it will be difficult to remember details from an earlier evaluation. Whether the clinician handwrites, dictates or types the record is immaterial, as long as the information is documented quickly and substantively. (See Chapter 21 for further details about record keeping.)

Within 24–72 hours, with a signed release of information completed, the clinician should *telephone the patient's referral source* and also *contact any other treaters* who will be involved in the patient's medical care. Some clinicians prefer to dictate an evaluation and send/fax a copy to the referring clinician. In the US, some third-party payers require the mental health prescriber to have contact with the primary care provider.

Length of an initial prescriptive interview

In reality, the initial prescriptive interview is of varying length depending on the complexity of the patient and the time that the clinician has to spend with the patient. Ideally, an experienced clinician can conduct a full, thorough evaluative interview, provide patient education, prescribe medication and devise an initial treatment plan in a 60-minute time period. There are some patients for whom this can be realistically compressed into a 45-minute time slot. In general, those clinicians who have less than 45 minutes to spend in an initial evaluation will almost certainly have to eliminate certain elements from the evaluation.

When time is short

PRIMARY CARE

The timeframes described above are realistically necessary and appropriate for thorough mental health prescription. While primary care practitioners should strive to allow for sufficient time to perform a complete exam, busy primary care clinics may need to streamline the amount of clinician–patient contact. There is an ongoing concern about the length of time that primary care clinicians may make available for an initial psychotropic evaluation. *If the time is pared too greatly, important elements of effective prescription will be omitted or overlooked.* A reasonable assessment for mental health medications simply cannot be performed in five or ten minutes.

There are several ways that busy clinicians can maximize their efficiency, however. One is to have the patient complete a symptom screen or checklist prior to entering the consultation room. There are many such screens that have shown validity and have been used consistently worldwide. By focusing on the elements identified by the patient, clinicians can maximize their diagnostic skills and available time. These screening tools include:

■ *The Prime-MD*, developed in 1994 by Robert Spitzer *et al.*, is a very complete clinician tool for evaluation of mental conditions in a primary care office, but the original format was time-consuming to fill out. A shorter version, the Patient Health Questionnaire,[2] is an abbreviated three-page version that is self-completed, and can be reviewed by the clinician in three minutes.[3]

■   *The Mini International Neuropsychiatric Interview*, by David Sheehan *et al.*,[4,5] is a useful clinician-administered set of questions that lead the clinician to a specific mental health diagnosis. It has been tested and validated around the world and translated into a number of languages.

■   The Beck Depression Inventory (BDI) is one of the most widely used and simple screens for depression. It consists of 21 multiple-choice questions that can be completed by the patient quickly. Repeated administration of the test can also reflect the extent of progress and symptom improvement. The original version was published in 1961,[6] and has been validated on multiple occasions. It was revised and copyrighted in 1978. The copyrighted version and many other office screening tests are available for purchase at www.psychcorp.com.

■   Descriptions of a number of screening tests used by primary care practitioners for mood, anxiety, sleep, psychosis, and substance abuse are available on the Internet at www.fpnotebook.com.

The most commonly used screens are copyrighted proprietary tests, and further sources are listed at the end of the chapter. Many pharmaceutical firms also have access to office screening questionnaires and evaluation tools.

The primary care practitioner may also choose to retain in-house specialists, such as specially-trained psychiatric nurses, physician's assistants, psychologists or social workers, to do all or part of an initial patient screening. In a situation where there is a prescriber such as a psychiatric nurse with prescriptive authority in the office, the nurse may be able to conduct the initial evaluation and write the prescription either independently or under the collaboration/supervision of the primary care physician.

A primary care provider may also choose to schedule patients with mental health concerns into a longer initial time slot. Sometimes an interview before the lunch hour or just before the day's end will allow extra time for a more thorough interview. The extra time spent in this initial interview will often pay off in better patient communication, better treatment of the mental health problem and, ultimately, a diminished use of medical/surgical services and fewer demands on the professional's time in later months.

While most professionals like to complete an initial evaluation in a single session, it can sometimes be useful to complete the evaluation in two closely-spaced separate appointments. A busy primary care physician can see a patient, gather initial information, order appropriate laboratory tests, and see the patient again in several days to complete the diagnostic work-up. If the patient is particularly symptomatic, the prescription of a sleeping medication or an anti-anxiety medication can sustain the patient until seen for the second evaluation interview.

Written or multi-media education materials are abundantly available and can accomplish the patient education portion of the interview, which is critical to compliance. Educational organizations and pharmaceutical companies have produced many pamphlets, videotapes, audiotapes, and CD-ROMs that can help the busy clinician avoid having to repeat baseline instructions. Some clinicians may choose to devise their own instruction sheets that include educational information about common medications they prescribe. Preferably, the clinician will review such education sheets in the office personally with the patient; however, when this is not possible, the patient can read the information at a later time. At times in a busy primary care office, the physician or the prescribing nurse will write the prescription and then have the patient seen by another professional (another nurse, a physician's assistant or mental health technician), who will answer questions, review educational materials, or perform other patient education tasks.

Sample clinician guidelines

The following are examples of formats for checklist reminder outlines that could be used by a clinician during an initial evaluation interview. Some prefer to use brief phrases on a single sheet to serve as an outline and prompt for thoroughness (e.g. the depression issues checklist in Table 3.5). Other prescribers prefer to devise multi-page sheets with spaces after each question to write in the patient's responses. This document is then included as part of the patient's record (e.g. the mania/bipolar issues shown in Table 3.6). Others may prefer to write out exact phrasing for questions so they can be asked in a routine way (e.g. the anxiety issues checklist in Table 3.7). Each format is useful, and each clinician will benefit from customizing a personal list of questions in a format and sequence.

Table 3.5 Depression issues checklist

- When were you last well?
- Describe your current symptoms:
    - Depressed mood – crying spells, feelings of worthlessness
    - Sleep
    - Appetite, weight change, food not tasting good, binges, excessive concerns with eating or weight
    - Concentration – school, work, reading, TV
    - Any change in the way your mind works?
    - Change in speed of thoughts
    - Mental confusion, indecisiveness
    - Inappropriate anger, irritability, violent feelings
    - Excessive anxiety, agitation
    - Change in activity level or energy
    - Headache, head pains
    - Mood reactivity – do positive events cheer you up?
    - Sensitivity to rejection – "leaden paralysis"
    - Loss of pleasure in activities
    - Suicidal ideation – plan – attempts
    - Social isolation
    - Change in sexual interest, drive or performance

Table 3.5 cont.

- Known life precipitants
- Rating of mood on scale of 1 to 10 – now, 1 month ago, 6 months ago, 1 year ago
- Age of first episode – what were the symptoms? Similar or different to current episode?
- Subsequent episodes – length and timing
- Return to normal between episodes?
- Psychiatric hospitalizations? ECT?
- Previous treatments
    - Medications – duration, response, side effects, dose
    - Psychotherapy – issues, results, who was therapist?
    - Technique?
- Current medications
- Ongoing medical problems
- Medical hospitalizations/surgeries
- Allergies
- Possibility of pregnancy
- Using any form of pregnancy prevention?
- When was last physical exam?
- Drug/alcohol usage
- Family history of substance abuse
- History of thyroid problems in self or family
- Family history of depression or psychiatric problems
- Is there a pattern to the onset or remission of depression (seasonal, with the menstrual cycle, postpartum)?
- Psychiatric medications used by family members – response
- Hallucinations?
- Paranoia?
- Manic episodes? Describe length, frequency and intensity
- What have you read about treatments for depression?
- Preferences for treatment?
- Concerns about treatment?

Table 3.6 Mania/bipolar issues symptoms checklist

- Lack of need for sleep without loss of energy
- Unusual activity in the middle of the night (cleaning, writing, shopping)
- Speeded/racing thoughts, rapid speech
- Too many thoughts at once
- Impulsive decisions
- Increased spending/buying/generosity
- Start many projects, but finish few

Table 3.6 cont.

- Rapid mood shifts, with or without precipitant

- Marked fluctuations in emotions/behavior

- Excess irritability, rages

- Unusual endurance when fatigue would be expected

- Inability to slow thoughts or behavior

- Family history of bipolar disorder

- Previous excessive/agitated accelerated response to antidepressants

- Any pattern to these symptoms

Table 3.7 Anxiety issues checklist (panic disorder/generalized anxiety disorder (GAD)/obsessive–compulsive disorder (OCD)/social anxiety disorder)

- Have you had problems with anxiety or nervousness?
- Is the anxiety present almost all the time, or does it come in sudden bursts or attacks?
- What are these attacks like? Do you have any physical signs that go along with the anxiety (e.g. rapid heart beat, shortness of breath, sweating) (panic disorder)
- Are there any places or activities that you avoid because of these attacks? (phobias)
- Have you had to alter your daily routine because of them? (panic disorder)
- Does the anxiety affect your eating or sleeping? (all)
- Do you have recurrent, repetitive worries, such that you are worrying about something almost all the time? (GAD)
- Do you have repetitive thoughts that you can't get out of your head (similar to getting a song "stuck in your head")? (OCD)
- What are these thoughts about? (OCD)
  Dirt/contamination
  Diseases
  Fear of harming self/others/pets
  Violent scenes/images
- Do you have repetitive behaviors that you do over and over, even if they are unnecessary or seem silly? (OCD)
  What kind of behaviors?
  Washing/showering/cleaning
  Collecting/hoarding
  Checking locks/appliances/for mistakes in writing or papers
  Excessive doubt or indecision
- How much time per day do you spend thinking of these thoughts or performing these behaviors? (OCD)

Table 3.7 cont.

- Do you have mental rituals or sequences that must be repeated in an exact way? (OCD)
- Do you regularly count items? (OCD)
- Do numbers have special meanings? (OCD)
- Do you pull or remove any hair on your head or body unnecessarily? (trichotillomania)
- Has anyone told you about or have you noticed recurrent facial movements that are hard to control? (tics – OCD)
- Are you fearful of speaking in large or small groups? (social anxiety disorder)
- Do you avoid social gatherings? (social anxiety disorder)
- Do you fear being watched closely by others when doing an activity? (social anxiety disorder)
- Which activity?
    Talking
    Eating
    Writing
    Voiding or bathroom issues
- Do you blush or sweat easily? Does this bother you? (social anxiety disorder)
- Do you use alcohol to "loosen up" before a social gathering? (social anxiety disorder)
- What treatment, if any, have you had for these problems? (all)
- Have you ever taken medication for this?
    What medication? For how long?
    Did it help? How did it help?
    What were the side effects, if any?
- Have you ever used alcohol or recreational drugs to deal with these problems?

References

1 Brown RL *et al*. A two-item conjoint screen for alcohol and other drug problems. *J Am Board Fam Pract* 2001;14(2):95–106.

2 Spitzer JP, Datto CJ, Weinrieb RM *et al*. Detection and diagnosis of psychiatric disorders in primary medical care settings. *Med Clin North Am* (in press).

3 Staab JP and Evans DL. A streamlined method for diagnosing common psychiatric disorders in primary care. *Clinical Cornerstone* 2001;3(3):1–9.

4 Lecrubier Y, Sheehan D, Weiller E *et al*. The MINI International Neuropsychiatric Interview (M.I.N.I.). A short diagnostic structured interview: reliability and validity according to the CIDI. *Eur Psychiatry* 1997;12:224–231.

5 Sheehan DV, Lecrubier Y, Harnett-Sheehan K *et al*. The Mini International Neuropsychiatric Interview (M.I.N.I.): the development and validation of a structured diagnostic psychiatric interview. *J Clin Psychiatry* 1998;59(suppl. 20):22–33.

6 Beck AT, Ward CH, Mendelson M *et al*. An inventory for measuring depression. *Arch Gen Psychiatry* 1961;4:561–571.

Chapter 4

Helping a patient decide to try medication

There are multiple resistances and obstacles to a patient's beginning psychotropic medication. Specific concerns regarding this class of medication typically exceeds concerns regarding medical/surgical medications. Some of these worries are enmeshed in the myths described in Chapter 2; others are based on other beliefs about how medication might affect personality.

When the clinician raises the concept of beginning psychotropic medication and there is resistance from the patient, there are several common issues that are likely to be present, alone or in combination. A brief discussion can often allay concerns or fears.

Patient issues

The following issues should be addressed, even if the patient does not raise them directly:

1 Is this medicine for life?
2 Is this medication addictive?
3 Will I be different?
4 Will I get side effects?
5 Can I drink alcohol while taking this medicine?

Is this medicine for life?

Many patients know of relatives or friends who have been on medication indefinitely. Their fear is that if a medication is started, it means a life-long commitment. In fact, while some patients may need long-term medication, many patients will take medication intermittently or for an isolated period. Explaining that virtually all patients will be given a trial period without medication at some point is reassuring to the patient. The approximate timeframe for when this trial will occur should be defined, and should be part of the treatment plan that the clinician describes. More detail on this issue is described in Chapter 8.

Is this addictive?

Many patients (and some clinicians) consider all mental health medications to be addictive or habit-forming. There may be an assumption that patients will need (or want) to take more of the medication than prescribed. While this is true for some addictive personalities, as well as some people with substance-abuse problems, the vast majority of patients will not only *not* abuse medication; they will also not feel the need to. They will also not develop any physical dependence on the medication. It is often very useful to define specifically that antidepressants, mood stabilizers, antipsychotic medications and many other psychotropics have no potential whatever for physical tolerance or addiction. Benzodiazepines and stimulants are the primary medications that can have habit-forming potential, and should be differentiated from other types of medication for the patient.

Will I be different?

This is often a difficult question to answer, since both clinician and patient obviously want the patient to be different, at least in terms of symptom relief. Usually this question actually overlies the concern, "Will my personality be altered? Will I be a different person?" This, too, is not easily answered, since many mood, psychotic and anxiety disorders, when properly treated, can lead to significant differences in behavior, attitude and interrelatedness. No evidence exists, however, to suggest that antidepressants, antipsychotics, or anti-anxiety medication will alter a person's fundamental personality.

TALKING TO PATIENTS

When a patient asks "Will I be different?", a possible response is: *"You will be the same person, but I am hopeful that you will not be experiencing these troublesome symptoms that you are now having."* Then list the target symptoms that have been identified earlier in the interview.

Will I get side effects?

The details of this issue and the approaches to discussing side effects with patients are covered in Chapter 16. As indicated there, the clinician needs to address several common side effects that occur with the medication selected. Examples might be drowsiness, dizziness, nausea, or interference with sexual arousal. Fortunately, although the vast majority of these side effects are annoying, they are physiologically not life-threatening. In the initial interview, clinicians should ask patients what they have read or heard about specific side effects, and if there are side effects that would be of particular concern to this patient. If so, then these concerns can be addressed specifically.

Can I drink alcohol while taking this medication?

As discussed in more depth in Chapter 14, the answer is that usually it is not desirable to drink during the first several weeks of medication so that the patient can adjust to the medications' effects and any side effects without the confounding effect of alcohol. Thereafter, most patients without a history of substance abuse can drink in moderation. "Moderation" must be specifically defined by the clinician, since people have distinctly different ideas of what it means to be "moderate" in their drinking. For a majority of patients, this is no more than one drink in an evening and no more than four drinks in a week. Patients should be cautioned about the possibility of increased reaction/intoxication when drinking while taking medication, and the risks of exceeding recommended limits. Chapter 14 contains a specific *Talking to Patients* dialogue for covering this issue.

Other resistances to psychotropic medication

Some other common resistances are:

1 Medication will change my personality
2 You should not tinker with "Mother Nature"
3 "Natural" remedies are always best
4 The cure (with its side effects) will be worse than the illness
5 I mistrust doctors, nurses and hospitals in general
6 On medication, my life will not be the same
7 Medication will control me
8 Medication is only for "crazy" people.

Other more "psychological" reasons for resisting psychotropic medication are not always conscious, or verbalized by the patient, but are nonetheless powerful roadblocks to beginning a course of medication treatment. Some examples of intrapsychic reasons include:

1 Because of my past behavior or my lack of self-confidence, I do not deserve to feel better

2 If I take medication and get better, I will have to confront . . . [some element of my life]. Such as:

- I will have to deal with the lack of intimacy in my marriage
- I will have to confront the fact that my job is repetitive, boring, stressful or inappropriate to my skills
- I will have to confront the fact that my social acquaintances and social behaviors may be contributing to my problem
- To solidify my recovery, I may have to make substantial lifestyle changes
- If I feel better, I may have to reassess the nature of, and with whom I have, interpersonal relationships.

While these issues are not often overtly brought up, it is important that the clinician be aware of some of these common resistances and be alert to cues that resistance may be occurring in a particular patient. When patients resist trying or continuing medication, it is worth asking whether any of these reasons may be present.

The use of levers

Even when the above five issues have been addressed and discussed, and some of the more psychological reasons considered, some patients may remain resistant to the concept of using medication for emotional illness. In these situations, the clinician who has obtained a history of symptoms and (more importantly) the activities, behaviors or lifestyle alterations that have occurred because of the symptoms, can utilize this information to help convince the patient to try medication. Simply put, *what has the patient given up, and what does he or she avoid or no longer enjoy because of the symptoms of the illness?* When clinicians know which significant parts of the patient's life are being affected, they can use these "levers" as reasons to try medication.

This process involves determining what behaviors are important to *this* patient. These factors may be very different from patient to patient. It may be far less important to patients that a diagnosis is made, than how the illness specifically impacts their life. At other times, the patient's symptoms may be of far greater concern to someone other than the patient. Understanding how the condition impacts the relationships within the person's family may also lead to powerful tools for encouraging appropriate treatment.

 TALKING TO PATIENTS

A 60-year-old grandmother may resist the concept of taking a medication for her anxiety disorder; however, she may be quite upset that her anxiety is keeping her from being able to cook the holiday meal that she has traditionally been proud to prepare for her family. Therefore, proposing the medication to such a person could include: *"I want you to feel less anxious so you can do the good job of cooking your usual Christmas dinner."* This can be much more powerful than "I think we need to treat your anxiety disorder."

Similarly, a 35-year-old man who has no belief that he has bipolar disorder, but is on probation at work and on the verge of losing his job, may be willing to try medication solely for the purpose of maintaining his employment and livelihood despite the fact that, if pressed, he would say he doesn't have a psychiatric condition. The clinician may say: *"I know how important it is for you to be a good provider for your wife and children. I would like to help you do that. I know that medication for this problem is probably not your first choice, but I strongly suspect that, if we start medication now, it may help you feel well enough to stay on the job."*

A third example is a 27-year-old single mother with depression who presents only at the insistence of her boyfriend, Mark, who is considering breaking up with her because she is so lethargic, has repeated crying spells, and "is no fun any more." Although she does not recognize her depression, she does worry that, at times, she is so tired she cannot manage to play with her three-year-old son, Bobby. The clinician may say: *"I know you want to be the best Mom for your son that you can be. Right now, this fatigue and crying is keeping you from being the kind of parent you always imagined yourself to be. I am suggesting this medication to help reduce these crying spells and increase your energy so you can be a bigger part in Bobby's life. If you can feel more like your old self, and I think the medicine will help, perhaps you and Mark can get out more and you will enjoy it."*

Reasons that patients take psychotropic medication

Clinicians usually assume that patients take medications to resolve their symptoms. While this may be true for many patients taking psychotropics, there may be many other reasons as well. Some of these include:

- To please their spouse
- To save their marriage
- To keep their children happy
- To allow them to interact with their children in a way that they find appropriate
- To save their job
- To please the clinician
- To prove someone else wrong (e.g. I'll try this medication to show my girlfriend that it is not going to work)
- To have a longer life
- For "general improvement"
- To satisfy the courts or the law
- To help in a lawsuit, claim for disability or child custody

■ Because someone else they respect has already tried medication and found it helpful (a friend, relative or celebrity)

■ Because they are totally desperate and must do *something*.

Although it is desirable that the clinician and patient agree on the reason for the patient taking the medication, it is not critical. *At times, the patient's reason for taking the medication may, in fact, be very different from the clinician's.* If the clinician has made a thorough assessment and supports the use of psychotropic medication for a patient, any reason may be a good enough reason to start. Ultimately it is not essential that the patient and the clinician have the *same* rationale for taking the medication, but it is essential that there must be *a* rationale for taking the medication.

TALKING TO PATIENTS

The practitioner may believe that an overweight female patient is depressed and assumes that she concurs. She may be willing to take antidepressant medication in part because she feels badly, but inwardly she may hope it will make her lose weight, and then she will be more attractive. If asked if the medicine will help her to lose weight, the clinician can reply, *"It may or may not have a direct effect on your weight, but I do expect that, if you are feeling less down and more in control, you will be better able to stick with a healthy diet and exercise plan that would help control your weight."*

Lastly, there may be some non-reality (psychotic) reasons for taking medication that develop in patients with true psychotic conditions. Even when their rationale appears delusional, if medication is needed, there may be no need to correct the delusion in order for medication to be taken and to be effective. What is important is to have a workable relationship between clinician and patient.

An interesting example of this latter scenario comes from an English psychiatrist[1] who was treating a patient who was obviously delusional. She felt her neighbors were talking about her and saying derogatory things about her behind her back. When she eventually came into the psychiatrist's office, he persuaded her to start antipsychotic medication, hoping that it would diminish her hallucinations and delusions. The patient did not believe she had delusions, but did have confidence in this psychiatrist. She agreed to take the medications on a trial basis, and in fact came back in several weeks with the report that people were no longer talking about her. Although the psychiatrist believed this was because of the antipsychotic effect of the medication, the patient verbalized this improvement as having occurred because the psychiatrist was secretly talking to the neighbors and advising them to stop the malicious gossip. Although not true, it was not crucial that the psychiatrist correct this mistaken belief. As long as there was a consensus that coming to see the psychiatrist and taking the medication was helpful, they could agree on a medication treatment plan.

The use of metaphor

Many of the concepts of mental health and illness as well as the use of psychotropic drugs in treatment are often mysterious for many patients, and, as discussed earlier, are filled with prejudice. A very useful way for practitioners to discuss with patients the process of using psychotropics to treat their emotional illness is to use common metaphors. By analogizing mental health conditions and the effects psychotropic medication can bring, as in the following examples, the clinician can often enlighten the patient in a way that promotes compliance and agreement.

In depression

The clinician can discuss the effects of depression as being like looking at life through very dark sunglasses. Everything looks dim, indistinct, ominous and, at times, scary. When the glasses are dark enough, patients may have difficulty in finding their way and making decisions, and may feel lost and apprehensive. Antidepressant medications will help them gradually to remove the dark glasses so that life may be seen in the light, showing its clarity and joy.

For patients with dysthymic disorder, a chronic low-grade depression, the clinician can discuss how they are living life at "snorkel depth." They are expending great energy to tread water to keep them from sinking. They do not sink to the bottom and drown, but feel they are working very hard just to minimally stay afloat. They are often just below the surface of the water, unable to see the clouds and the sunshine that life has to offer. Medication can provide support analogous to a boat on which they can sit; without having to work so hard to keep from sinking, they will be able to see the clouds, sunshine and the beauty above the surface of the water.

In bipolar disorder

Bipolar disorder can be analogized to being on a raft in the middle of the ocean during a furious storm. Giant waves will raise patients to great heights, then send them crashing down. They are often hanging on for dear life, afraid of being overturned and swamped. They may often have very little energy left for doing anything but pure survival. Mood stabilizing medication can help calm the waves so that patients can sit comfortably on the raft and begin to observe their surroundings. Things that may not have been apparent before will emerge, and new choices will be present. They can now see a pier to which they may wish to paddle or swim, or a new island that they may wish to explore. Once the sea is calmer, they may be able to even start out on a distant journey to places they previously could only imagine.

In panic attacks

Following the concept that a panic attack is a "biological false alarm," the clinician can use the analogy to a smoke detector. A smoke detector on the wall of an office has a useful purpose; it is there to warn of danger. If there were a fire, it would emit loud sounds and light to warn people that they need to take action. If the clinician were to light a fire in a wastebasket, it would set off the smoke detector, telling people to leave the building. A panic attack is like a smoke detector with an electrical short circuit. It will trigger and sound alarm when there is no fire or minimal danger. It will be just as loud and, perhaps, even more scary than usual, since it comes on suddenly when no danger is apparent. Typically, when a smoke detector goes off, people exit the building very quickly and call for professional help. This is similar to patients going for emergency medical care because of the alarm that their body is sending them during a panic attack, even when no obvious danger is present. If the smoke detector continues to be triggered, patients may continue to seek reassurance or medical care when there is no fire. Use of medication to treat panic attacks is analogous to fixing the electrical problem so that the alarm triggers only when true danger is apparent. In the initial stages, however, patients may be considerably anxious and be on guard for any alarm, even if the circuitry has been fixed (analogous to the anticipatory anxiety of panic disorder).

Reference

1   John Doran, MD, Stratford on Avon Conference on Nurse Prescribing, July 2001.

Chapter 5

Starting medication

There are multiple factors for the clinician to consider in choosing and starting medication. Ideally, medication should be selected using evidence-based data, confirmed efficacy, documented safety, known dosage range, and likely response rates. Also, it would be helpful if all data, including studies with negative results, were available. Particularly useful would be head-to-head comparisons of medications used to treat the same illness.

The gold standard for such data is the double-blind, placebo-controlled study of effectiveness. While such studies are available for some mental health medications and some clinical conditions, there are many situations in which well-defined, double-blind placebo-controlled studies do not exist, or give contradictory results. In other cases, studies of newer medicines are compared to outdated treatments and not to other more popular, currently used medications.

Data used in support of using medications are often confounded by a number of other issues:

- Placebo response rates in psychotropic medication trials are very high; therefore many patients in these studies would improve without the presence of active medication and this makes the exact amount of positive change difficult to assess.
- Many studies documenting medication effectiveness are open-label studies, in which both clinicians and patients know whether or not the patients are receiving active medication or placebo. Such studies are notoriously inaccurate, and may show a positive bias toward the medication being utilized.
- Many medications are used for broad indications, including non-FDA approved indications. Their usage is supported by word-of-mouth, "curbstone consultations," or non-evidence based beliefs.
- Pharmaceutical companies fund much of the research on medications. They have a vested interest in manufacturing and selling their products. Studies with a positive result, showing that the active medication is beneficial, will almost certainly be published and promoted to the practitioner. Negative studies, or ones in which the active ingredient is shown to be less effective than other medications, may or may not reach publication. This is sometimes referred to as the "file drawer effect."

While clinicians study scientific data and constantly strive to obtain further information, prescribing decisions must be made daily when definitive, evidence-based studies are unavailable or conflicting. There are useful general strategies in helping a clinician to move ahead when scientific data are unavailable. These principles become part of the art of mental health prescribing, and are summarized in the sections below.

Monotherapy

For any condition, the use of a single medication, monotherapy, is always the simplest and safest treatment. When effective, it is the treatment of choice. In many mental health conditions, however, medication monotherapy is unsuccessful or only partially successful. While successive trials of monotherapy may ultimately identify one medication that satisfactorily controls most or all target symptoms, it is increasingly common to use polypharmacy in mental health prescribing. Multiple medications from one category, or medications from different categories, may be necessary to treat the patient's condition satisfactorily.

Overlap and "indications"

Over the last decade, one of the most dramatic changes in day-to-day practice has been a broadening range of usage for many medications and classes. While the names of medication categories have persisted (e.g. "antidepressants," "antipsy-chotics," and "mood stabilizers"), many medications within each category are used for much broader symptom profiles or other diagnoses. Antidepressants are used not only for depression, but also for anxiety disorders, bulimia, impulse control disorders, and a long list of other conditions. Similarly, both traditional and atypical antipsychotic medications are used for bipolar disorder in addition to psychosis. Newer atypical antipsychotics are also now used in treatment resistant depression, obsessive–compulsive disorder (OCD) and eating disorders. Although not a complete list, the spectrum of mental health uses of various commonly used mental health medications as of 2002 is summarized in Table 5.1.

What is the target of the medication?

While the presence of a diagnosis is helpful and desirable, precise diagnosis in mental health may be elusive and there may be multiple co-morbid diagnoses. Although every effort should be made to arrive at a precise diagnosis, the generation of a differential diagnosis may be the optimal level of specificity possible for a particular patient. It is quite permissible to treat target symptoms without a precise diagnosis. As noted in Chapter 3, identification of these target symptoms is an important part of the initial evaluation. It is possible to modulate or correct certain symptoms while an ultimate diagnosis is being considered and evaluated. Sometimes a more precise diagnosis emerges with time and more targeted medication treatment can follow; in other cases, diagnosis remains elusive indefinitely. If the prescription of psychotropic medications adequately treats significant symptoms, and is tolerated by the patient without adverse consequences, ongoing medication treatment is justified even if an exact diagnostic label is not discovered.

Choosing a starting dose

Overall, initial dosing strategies may be summarized in the following statements:

1 Standard dosing is useful for many patients
2 Start with half-doses for several days, when possible
3 Use high-level dosing only if necessary, in cases of intense or incapacitating symptoms.

The Physicians' Desk Reference, *The Maudsley Prescribing Guidelines*, individual drug package inserts, pharmacological textbooks and Appendices 2, 3, 4 and 5 of this text list typical starting doses for various psychotropics. In the uncomplicated non-hospitalized patient with moderate symptoms, the doses found in these sources are reasonable initial doses. For the mild to moderately symptomatic outpatient, however, there is little to lose, and potentially something to gain, by starting with half the standard dose for the first day or two. By using less than a usual starting dose for the first several days, patients are often spared significant side effects, if they are particularly sensitive to the medication. Although rare, in the event of acute drug allergy, half dosage also minimizes the

Table 5.1 Other common mental health uses of FDA-approved drugs*

Medication	Common non-approved use
Antidepressants	
Bupropion	Depression, attention deficit disorder (ADD), smoking cessation
Citalopram	Depression, obsessive–compulsive disorder (OCD)
Fluoxetine	Adult, adolescent, and pediatric depression, bulimia, autistic disorder, panic disorder, OCD, premenstrual dysphoric disorder (PMDD), bulimia
Fluvoxamine	OCD, pediatric OCD, depression
Mirtazapine	Depression
Nefazodone	Depression, post-traumatic stress disorder (PTSD)
Paroxetine	Depression, OCD, PTSD, panic disorder, social anxiety disorder, generalized anxiety disorder (GAD)
Sertraline	Depression, OCD, PTSD, PMDD, panic disorder
Venlafaxine	Depression, GAD
Mood stabilizers	
Carbamazepine	Bipolar disorder, organic psychosis, borderline personality disorder, aggression, alcohol withdrawal, schizophrenia, restless legs syndrome, PTSD
Lithium	Bipolar disorder in children, rage reactions, PMDD, treatment refractory depression
Valproic acid	Bipolar disorder, schizophrenia, panic disorder, hypnotic sedation, agitation in dementia, PTSD
Anti-seizure medications	
Clonazepam	Bipolar disorder, panic disorder, OCD
Gabapentin	Bipolar disorder, social anxiety disorder, panic disorder
Lamotrigine	Bipolar disorder, treatment refractory depression
Oxcarbazepine	Mania, bipolar disorder, aggression disorder
Topiramate	Bipolar disorder, appetite suppression/weight control when using other psychotropics
Antipsychotics	
Atypical antipsychotics	Psychosis, schizophrenia, bipolar disorder, treatment resistant depression, OCD, bulimia
Traditional antipsychotics	Bipolar disorder, schizophrenia
Other medications	
Clonidine	PTSD, ADD, sedative/hypnotic
Verapamil	Bipolar disorder
Cholinestrase inhibitors	
Donepezil	Dementia, memory difficulties secondary to psychotropic usage, remedy for anticholinergic side effects
Galantamine	Dementia, memory difficulties secondary to psychotropic usage, remedy for anticholinergic side effects
Rivastigmine	Dementia, memory difficulties secondary to psychotropic usage, remedy for anticholinergic side effects
Anti-anxiety agents	
Benzodiazepines	Anxiety, panic disorder, GAD, OCD, sedative/hypnotic, phobias, treatment-resistant bipolar disorder, adjunctive treatment for psychosis, social anxiety disorder, PMDD
Buspirone	GAD, OCD

*Collated from:
Pharmaceutical company product labelling
The Maudsley Prescribing Guidelines, 6th edn. Martin Dunitz, 2002.
Jamcak PG *et al. Principles and Practice of Psychopharmacotherapy*, 2nd edn. Williams & Wilkins, 1997.

allergic response. If patients are started on a half dosage, the full typical starting dose should be attained rapidly – no later than by day three.

Other situations when initial half dosing is recommended include:

1 Geriatric patients
2 Anxious "medication averse" patients
3 Patients who perceive themselves as "medication sensitive."

When treating *outpatients* with mild to moderate symptoms, increase medication dose by 25–50 percent every 4 days as tolerated by the patient. For *inpatients* and/or those with severe symptoms, increase medication by 50–100 percent every 2–4 days depending on symptom severity and side-effect tolerance.

In an *inpatient setting*, with a patient who has intense symptomatology, larger initial doses may be necessary. The possibility of increased side-effects is counterbalanced by the need for rapid symptom control. Psychotic patients, deeply depressed and suicidal patients, patients with intense mood swings and extremely anxious patients usually need higher initial doses in an inpatient setting where their status can be monitored continuously.

If rapid dosage titration is attempted, ensure there is frequent oversight, support and monitoring by inpatient staff or, when outside the hospital, by the family. With larger dosing, more frequent direct observation and/or telephone contact with the patient is necessary. When using larger doses of medication with an outpatient, follow-up should be no less than every 2–4 days as the patient's clinical condition warrants.

Always use blood levels to adjust dosage (see Chapter 19) for TCAs, lithium, valproic acid, carbamazepine and clozapine.

Loading doses

The vast majority of psychotropic medications are taken orally as pills, capsules or liquid concentrates. As described earlier, gradually increasing doses of psychotropic medication is generally the preferred dosing strategy to minimize side effects and allow the patient to accommodate to the medication. There has been limited research into giving patients larger than normal amounts of medication as a "loading dose" in order to facilitate behavioral management and rapid symptom control of agitated, psychotic or manic patients in an emergency room setting or on an inpatient unit. The majority of evidence relating to loading doses of medication refers to the use of valproic acid for manic patients, or of intramuscular antipsychotics and benzodiazepines (alone or in combination).

Over the last 20 years there has been a number of studies looking at the use of intramuscular antipsychotic medications alone, intramuscular benzodiazepines alone, and the combination of these medications for the rapid tranquilization of severely agitated patients. Obviously, when a patient is willing to take oral medications, the use of pills and liquid concentrate is desirable. However, when an agitated, psychotic patient is unable or unwilling to take oral medications, some form of intramuscular medication is necessary. A commonly used combination of medication in this clinical scenario is 5–10 mg of intramuscular haloperidol plus 2 mg of intramuscular lorazepam.[1,2]

Since intramuscular preparations of atypical antipsychotics are relatively recent phenomena, there currently are few controlled studies of usage of these agents, alone or in combination with benzodiazepines, in a large population of agitated, psychotic patients. (Intramuscular ziprasidone and olanzapine have been approved by the American Food and Drug Administration (FDA). Intramuscular preparations of risperidone and aripiprazole are likely to be approved soon.) As more such preparations become available, and as the atypical antipsychotics continue to replace typical antipsychotics in general psychiatric practice, it is expected that evidence will emerge that evaluates various combinations. Currently, however, data supporting the use of atypicals are primarily anecdotal or related to oral doses of medication.[1,3–5]

The other compound that has evidence to support the use of rapid loading doses is valproic acid. There have been several studies showing oral valproic acid in doses of 30 mg/kg of body weight per day for the first 2 days of treatment of acute mania followed by 20 mg/kg per day to be effective and well tolerated.[6–8]

Loading dose strategies for lithium have been attempted where a single dose of 600–1200 mg is given initially and then the stabilization dose of lithium is calculated based on a serum lithium level drawn 24 hours later.[9] Although possible, this strategy is little used and has not been studied extensively, particularly regarding whether this method achieves more rapid clinical outcomes than standard lithium dosing. Carbamazepine has been loaded in patients at risk for seizures, but has generally not been used in loading strategies for psychiatric purposes. Oral olanzapine loading has been reported in which a loading dose of 40 mg per day is given for 2 days, followed by 20–30 mg per day for the ensuing 2 days, then reducing to 15 mg per day.[10] This small sample tolerated the procedure well, although the number of patients was minimal. In general, other psychotropics (including all antidepressants, stimulants, anticholinergics, and anti-anxiety medications) have not been studied with loading dose strategies.

The art of choosing a medication

For purposes of example, this section discusses choosing an antidepressant. Similar logic, however, applies to mood stabilizers, antipsychotics, and other medication groups.

Since overall efficacy is approximately equal among antidepressants,[11] there are several good medicines from which to choose without one clear, consistent first choice for all patients. For a patient who has never taken antidepressants, and for whom there is no previous treatment history, several factors may be of use, and these are summarized in Table 5.2. Any or all of these indicators may be important to a clinician in choosing a particular medication.

Table 5.2 The art of choosing a medication

In a patient who has not previously been treated, you may choose a medication because it:

- Will also treat comorbid conditions present
- Avoids a particular side effect
- Avoids complicating a medical condition
- Avoids an interaction with another medication
- Has side effects that may be to the patient's advantage
- Is preferred by the patient
- Has been helpful to a close blood relative of the patient
- Is affordable for this patient

The presence of a *co-morbid condition* may dictate the optimum first medication choice. A medication used successfully for several conditions can "kill two birds with one stone." For example:

- A patient with panic disorder and episodes of depression may get relief for both conditions from using an antidepressant rather than a benzodiazepine. The benzodiazepine could work well for the panic, but is likely to do little for the depressive component.
- A person with schizophrenia who has a strong component of depressive affect is likely to receive more benefit from an atypical antipsychotic (which often has antidepressant activity) than from a traditional antipsychotic (which is likely to have little).
- A person suffering from attention deficit disorder and depression could have both illnesses improved by the use of bupropion.

In choosing a medication, a clinician may try to *avoid a particular side effect* that would be of significant concern or risk to the patient. Ziprasidone may create less weight gain than olanzapine for an already obese psychotic patient. Bupropion, nefazodone or mirtazapine will likely cause less sexual interference than an SSRI for a depressed patient who is significantly concerned about sexual performance. (See Chapter 16 for a more detailed and referenced discussion of these issues.)

Concurrent medical conditions, if any, may affect the choice of medication. A clinician will want to use medications that minimally affect the stability of concurrent medical illnesses. For example, patients with a seizure disorder would preferentially not be started on bupropion, which has a somewhat higher incidence of seizures than other antidepressants. It is also possible to use medications that may have a positive beneficial effect on the concurrent medical condition. A depressed patient with migraine headaches might benefit from an SSRI, a class of medication that has been shown to be useful in the treatment of migraine.[12,13]

Medications currently used by a patient can also point toward one psychotropic medication rather than another. If, for example, the addition of an antidepressant will result in an altered blood level of a currently taken medication (perhaps via a P-450 interaction), medical management becomes more complicated. An example of this is a patient who is being treated with cyclosporine for rheumatoid arthritis. Such a patient will have any cyclosporine levels altered by the addition of nefazodone or fluvoxamine, both of which alter the P-450 enzymes 3A/3 and 3A/4 that metabolize cyclosporine. Therefore, these drugs may not be the first choice antidepressant for this patient. A patient who is taking a TCA for pain control could have the blood level of the TCA changed if fluoxetine or paroxetine was added because of P-450 enzyme 2D6 blockade. Therefore, an initial choice of antidepressant such as venlafaxine or mirtazapine without this potential interaction would be simpler. Such interactions seldom rule out choosing a particular antidepressant medication. Even if an interaction could occur, this medication can be an effective, safe choice if the interaction is known, the dosage of the substrate is altered and, when possible, serum blood levels followed. (See Chapter 17 for further detailed directions for handling P-450 interactions.)

Utilizing the intrinsic side effects of a particular medication may incline a clinician toward a particular choice. For example, a depressed patient with a sleep disorder might be started on a more sedating antidepressant such as mirtazapine or nefazodone, where the sedative effect would be useful in improving sleep problems. Likewise, a patient who has psychomotor retardation and is oversleeping might benefit from an activating medication such as desipramine, bupropion or reboxetine. A depressed patient with low appetite might benefit from a medication that potentially stimulates appetite such as mirtazapine or a TCA, whereas a patient with excessive appetite might benefit from a medication that, as a side effect, has the potential to lower appetite, such as any of the SSRIs, bupropion or venlafaxine.

Patient preference is another possible factor in medication choice. While a clinician should not choose a particular medicine solely on the basis of patient preference (unless it is clinically reasonable and appropriate), it is often much easier to convince patients to try a particular medication toward which they are favorably predisposed. Patients may have heard positive reports about a specific medication from friends, relatives or co-workers. They may have read positive aspects about a particular drug in the media or on the Internet, which inclines them favorably to a medication choice.

The reverse is also true. A patient may be negatively predisposed to one particular medication for exactly the same reasons. The clinician can have a difficult time prescribing a medication if a patient has heard significant negative feedback regarding the drug. If the patient's beliefs are based on misinformation, corrective education may be helpful and necessary. If there are two equally effective choices, however, and the patient feels strongly for or against one of them, the clinician will have more success prescribing that medication which the patient already believes will help.

Of some value is a history of *positive response in a close blood relative*. When there has been a positive medication response in a first-degree relative, the identified patient may also benefit from this medication. The current patient may also be favorably predisposed to trying a particular medication if a family member has responded well to it. This method, however, is far from an absolute predictor, and the clinician should not hesitate to try other medications. Clinical lore is replete with family trees in which various family members have responded to different medications.

Lastly, *cost* must always be considered. No matter how elegant a clinician's thinking, a prescription for a medication is useless if the patient cannot afford to fill it. Knowing (or asking about) the patient's financial resources, insurance coverage and/or willingness to pay out-of-pocket are important issues when there are equally effective medication choices that vary in cost. If a generic medication is cheaper and, in the clinician's mind, a reasonable choice, there is little reason not to use it. Even when a particular medication is a decided second choice, a clinician may choose a less expensive medication if a patient cannot afford the first choice. Being able to purchase and comply with a second choice is much better for the patient than offering a first-choice prescription that never gets filled.

Selecting medication in the previously treated patient

Again using depression for purposes of illustration, when a patient presents having had previous trials on antidepressants, it is useful to ponder several other clinical factors in addition to the issues in the above section. Clearly, the most important and overriding factor is a *previous positive response* to a particular medication. If a patient has had a good response to a particular medication, completed treatment and stopped medication, a strong first choice to treat recurrence would be to use the same medication.[14] *Patients who have episodic illness with symptom-free intervals will often respond to the same medication during a recurrence.* It is neither necessary nor prudent for the clinician to prescribe a newer medication just because it is new, or because it happens to be one of the clinician's current favorites. Additionally, patients are positively predisposed to retrying a medicine that they know from experience is effective and tolerable.

This general principle can be modified in two ways:

1   The patient did respond to medication, but had considerable side effects while taking it
2   The patient has relapsed despite taking the medication.

The first principle is illustrated by the use of tricyclic antidepressants. While shown to be no less effective than newer antidepressants, TCAs have a side effect profile that, for most patients, is much more burdensome than that of newer antidepressants. If a patient suffered significant side effects while taking a TCA, a trial of a newer medication would be indicated. Another example would be a depressed patient who responded well to an SSRI, but had significant sexual dysfunction. Such a patient might benefit from the use of a medication with less propensity for sexual dysfunction, such as bupropion, mirtazapine, or nefazodone.

The second exception to retrying a previously used medication involves the patient who has relapsed while on the medication. An example would be a patient who initially did well on a medication, but lost the antidepressant effect quickly thereafter. Such a patient does not usually respond to the reinstitution of the same medication, and a change to another medication within the class or to another class of antidepressants is much more likely to be helpful. (See Chapter 9 for more information about this issue.)

The liver-impaired patient

Patients with impaired hepatic functioning, from whatever cause, create special issues for the mental health clinician when prescribing psychotropic medication. Because of their impaired hepatic function these patients may be more susceptible to side effects from hepatically metabolized medications, and serum blood concentrations may be altered significantly. In general, it is the *severity of the liver disease rather than its cause* that most directly affects serum blood concentrations. Therefore, assessment of the severity of liver function should be undertaken with a panel of liver function tests before beginning psychotropic medication in liver-impaired patients. In general, the more abnormal the liver function test, the more severe the impairment and the lower the initial psychotropic dose should be. Unfortunately, the test values do not always precisely correlate with the level of impairment of drug metabolism.

Other considerations for hepatically compromised patients include the following:

1 Whenever possible, *consider using medications* that have minimal liver metabolism and/or are *excreted primarily through the kidney*.

CLINICAL TIP
Almost all psychotropics are primarily metabolized by the liver. The notable exceptions are lithium, gabapentin, topirimate, amisulpride (UK only) and sulpiride (UK only), which undergo minimal hepatic metabolism and are primarily excreted through the kidney.

2 Patients with hepatic dysfunction are more sensitive to the routine side effects of hepatically metabolized drugs, even at technically "therapeutic" levels.
3 When using a hepatically metabolized medication in a hepatically compromised patient, the following strategies should be employed:
   ■ Start at a lower than normal dosage
   ■ Make any dosage increase slowly
   ■ Watch for side effects from medication build-up
   ■ If a medication has valid serum blood level testing, monitor these levels frequently.
4 The ultimate target dose of the medication will generally be lower than in non-hepatically impaired patients.

Table 5.3 Preferred choices of psychotropics in hepatically-impaired patients*

Psychotropic classification	Recommended drugs
Antidepressants	Paroxetine or imipramine (in low dose)
Antipsychotics	Olanzapine Haloperidol (in low dose) Sulpiride (UK only)
Mood stabilizers	Lithium and gabapentin
Anxiolytics	Lorazepam and oxazepam (in small doses)

*Adapted from *The Maudsley Prescribing Guidelines*, 6th edn. Martin Dunitz, 2002, p. 124.

5 Severe liver disease, which may be characterized by marked elevation of liver function tests, jaundice, ascites, and encephalopathy, can require particularly delicate clinical management. For patients with severe liver disease:

■ Begin any psychotropic at the lowest possible dose.

■ Avoid compounds with a long half-life.

■ Observe carefully for sedation and cognitive interference.

■ Psychotropics with a strong history of possible hepatic dysfunction are contraindicated. Therefore, avoid nefazodone, MAOIs, carbamazepine, valproate, lamotrigine, and sertindole (UK only).

■ Sedatives or anxiolytics should be used with great caution, at a low dose, because of the potential of precipitating further encephalopathy or falls.

■ *The Maudsley Prescribing Guidelines*[15] should be seen for a summary of current research on individual psychotropics and parameters of use in hepatically compromised patients

Preferred medications to be used in the hepatically impaired patient are listed in Table 5.3.

The kidney-impaired patient

A parallel situation occurs for patients who have renal impairment. Whenever possible with these patients, psychotropics that have primary *hepatic* metabolism should be considered as first-line drugs. When possible, the renally-excreted medications mentioned above, including lithium, gabapentin, topirimate, amisulpride (UK only), and sulpiride (UK only), should be avoided. Prior to beginning psychotropic medications with a renally impaired patient, an assessment of the severity of renal impairment should be undertaken, remembering that renal function will decline with age and that some level of renal impairment will occur even if serum creatinine is not elevated. Principles of medicating the renally impaired patient include:

■ Start any medication at the lowest tolerable dose. It may be necessary to divide doses to maintain tolerability.

■ Make any dosage increases slowly.

Table 5.4 Recommended medications for the renally impaired patient*	
Psychotropic classification	Recommended drugs
Antidepressants	SSRIs (most experience is with fluoxetine and paroxetine)
Antipsychotics	Atypical antipsychotics, including olanzapine and ziprasidone. Quetiapine and risperidone may be started in smaller than usual doses. Haloperidol
Mood stabilizers	Carbamazepine and valproic acid

*Adapted from *The Maudsley Prescribing Guidelines*, 6th edn. Martin Dunitz, 2002, p. 130.

■ Watch for side effects from medication build-up.
■ If the medication has valid serum blood levels, monitor them frequently.
■ Observe for side effects of sedation, postural hypotension and confusion.

Information on specific recommendations for individual psychotropics is, again, documented in *The Maudsley Prescribing Guidelines*.

Preferred psychotropic medications for the renally impaired patient are shown in Table 5.4.

How many pills to prescribe?

The general rule of thumb for how many pills to prescribe to a patient is enough to last until their next scheduled follow-up visit plus a few more. At the initial evaluation this principle should be adhered to firmly, such that the patient has enough medication to last only until he or she can be seen again, but not significantly in excess of that. At this first visit, the clinician does not know the patient well and cannot be sure about the patient's ability to take the medication in a safe and responsible manner as prescribed. By prescribing only sufficient medication to reach the next visit, one also emphasizes the necessity of the follow-up visit for reassessment in order to obtain further medication. As the clinician gets to know a patient better, and finds that he or she is responsible, more latitude can be given regarding how many pills are dispensed. It is particularly important to avoid giving large quantities of pills to suicidal or medication-abusing patients. If there is concern about the patient's suicidal ideation and the possibility of overdose, it may be reasonable to prescribe only 3 or 4 days' worth of medication, requiring frequent refills, so that the patient does not have access to a large number of pills until he or she is more stable. While this is inconvenient for the patient, it is safer, particularly if prescribed medications are ones that are dangerous in overdose (e.g. tricyclic antidepressants, lithium, and MAO inhibitors). Another strategy at an initial interview of a potentially suicidal patient is to give a 10-day or 2-week supply of medication, but insist that the prescription be handed to, filled by, and administered by a family member or other responsible party. It is always unwise and poor practicing habit to prescribe a large number of pills and/or multiple refills to a patient whom the clinician does not know well. Long-term patients on a stable medication regimen, well known to the clinician, can be prescribed a 30-day supply of medications with an appropriate number of refills to reach the next visit, or even a 90-day supply.

The five points of education about psychotropics

There are five principles that should be emphasized to every patient who is beginning a psychotropic medication. They are simple and may, for some clinicians, seem obvious. Patients, however, are not intuitively aware of these principles, and they should always be presented directly to any patient during the first session when medication is prescribed.

1 *Take the medication as prescribed every day.* Patients need to understand that regular dosing is central to obtaining and maintaining response. Antidepressants, antipsychotics and mood stabilizers are generally not to be taken on an "as needed" basis (often abbreviated in medical orders as "PRN" from the Latin *pro re nata*). With medication for mood, taking more medication when feeling worse on a particular day is also of relatively little use. If patients are not consistently doing well on a particular regimen, it may be necessary to increase the dose; however, this is a decision that should be made on the advice of the clinician. The patient must understand that missing doses, or changing the dose day-to-day depending on one's mood, is contraindicated.

2 *It may take time to see a response.* Many patients, anticipating instant relief, expect a response quickly and, if this does not occur, will stop the medication.

 TALKING TO PATIENTS
To present this issue to patients in a valid but optimistic way, a clinician can say: *"You may notice some positive benefit within a few days, but it often takes several weeks for medication levels to rise in your system and for you to begin noticing feeling better."*

---

3 *Don't stop the medication without contacting me.* Particularly early in treatment, patients who are not immediately responding, or who may be experiencing side effects, need to be cautioned against stopping medication without the clinician's input. Often a simple dosage adjustment or medication change can rectify a problem. In other cases, the clinician may decide to encourage the patient to continue to take the medication for a longer period to adapt. It is important to instruct the patient to call before deciding that the current situation is intolerable.

4 *Don't stop the medication just because you're starting to feel better.* Patients are often prone to discontinuing their medication after starting to feel better, unless they are given specific instructions to continue medication for the purposes of maintaining response.

TALKING TO PATIENTS

"As you begin to feel better, I want you to continue the medication until, together, we decide to stop. If you stop too quickly, there is a good chance your symptoms will return. By continuing the medication, even after you begin to respond, we give you a better chance to stay well. In time, we can discuss a plan to discontinue your medication successfully."

5 *Call with any concerns or questions.* Patients should not only be given permission, but also encouraged, to contact the clinician if they are not doing well or have questions. Patients should be advised to stay in contact with the clinician, particularly over the early stages of treatment.

Other issues to be discussed

Whenever a new medication is started, other specific areas must be discussed with the patient, including:

- Medication interactions and/or medications to be avoided
- Activity restrictions
- Dietary restrictions
- Laboratory screening tests, including serum blood levels, when necessary
- Common side effects

With most psychotropics, there are minimal activity restrictions. Particularly if medications are begun at a low dosage and increased gradually, patients can drive a vehicle, operate machinery and engage in other physical activity, including vigorous exercise. If a medication is particularly sedative or causes symptoms of hypotension or dizziness, patients should be advised temporarily to avoid the above activities until they are adjusted to the medicine. Most patients, even when taking significant medication doses, can resume normal activities. On rare occasions, patients who are excessively sedated or dizzy may be advised not to drive a car or perform activities requiring significant coordination. The need for this restriction is generally apparent from the clinical presentation of the patient at a follow-up evaluation. If there is doubt about a patient's ability to perform these activities safely, it is best to recommend a temporary cessation and ask for family/caretaker input about the patient's level of alertness and coordination at the first follow-up visit.

With the exception of lithium (salt and fluid considerations) and MAO inhibitors (significant dietary restrictions), there are virtually no psychotropics that require dietary restrictions. In general, patients may eat a normal balanced diet without constraints. If weight gain becomes an issue, however, calorie restriction may be necessary. (See Chapter 16 for issues on weight gain, and Chapter 17 for further information on lithium toxicity and MAO inhibitor diets.)

Informed consent

For years lawyers, legal scholars, and health-care professionals have debated the issue of what constitutes informed consent for taking medication. There is no single agreed-upon assessment of what constitutes a patient being fully informed and what constitutes true "consent." When working in an institutional setting, rules may be established by the institution for written, informed consent prior to use of any medications. In an outpatient office, there is wide variability as to how clinicians implement informed consent.

Some clinicians do obtain written, informed consent for each medication prescribed in an outpatient office, particularly if it is for a non-FDA approved indication. While this may have some benefit, it is not uniformly deemed medicolegally necessary. A significant number of clinicians will document a discussion of expected benefits of the medication, possible side effects, possible alternatives to this medication, and overall risks. This is then documented in the written record with a phrase such as "outcomes, side effects, alternatives, and risks discussed."

At the first session, clinicians should obtain a written general "Consent to Treatment" that may include the use of recommended medication. This document should remain a permanent document within the patient's record. Such consent could be worded:

> I consent for [*name of clinician*] to assess and treat me. This treatment may include psychotherapy, medication, and/or other recommended therapy for mental health problems which is administered within current community standards.
>
> Signature _____
>
> Date _____

The issue of informed consent becomes more complicated for the incompetent patient and for non-emancipated minors. Patients declared legally incompetent, and for whom a guardian has been appointed, should have consent for medications signed by the legal guardian. Except in emergency situations, no medication should be started until this consent is obtained. Minors under the age of 18, unless fully emancipated from their families, should also have written informed consent from the parent or legal guardian prior to beginning medication.

Emergency situations (usually present in an emergency department or on an inpatient unit) can supersede the necessity of obtaining of written informed consent for both incompetent patients and minors. In such cases, the clinician should document the nature of the emergency, the medication prescribed, and dosage. Every attempt should be made to obtain consent from the appropriate party as soon as possible. If repeated emergency dosing is necessary, the necessity of continued emergency medication should be noted and documented in the chart.

Involuntary medication

Involuntary medication (medicating patients against their will) of an adult patient is a totally distinct issue, and is different from medicating the *incompetent patient or minor* as discussed above. Adult patients who are being treated involuntarily retain their right to accept or refuse medication unless they are deemed legally incompetent. It is generally necessary for a court or judge to determine that an involuntary patient can be medicated against his or her will. *Except in emergency circumstances*, which should be documented as such, *a written court order must generally be obtained prior to medicating an involuntary patient*. There are variations of law from state to state, and country to country, regarding involuntary medication procedures. These should be consulted to determine the appropriate procedure in any given locale.

Involuntary medication is an area of law that is fraught with complications and medicolegal pitfalls. Except in emergency situations, clinicians will frequently find it helpful to consult knowledgeable colleagues, legal counsel or administrators within an institution in which they practice, prior to medicating an involuntary patient.

Education as treatment

When starting medication, do not underestimate the power and therapeutic benefit of patient education. Instructing the patient on why the medication is being prescribed, how it is being prescribed, its method of action and its intended effects, and describing any possible side effects, has powerful therapeutic benefit. Informed, knowledgeable patients are, in general, more compliant with treatment and more likely to follow through with their treatment plan.

The use of placebo

Some clinicians, and/or patient's families, believe that a patient's mental health symptoms are "all in their head," implying that the symptoms are a mental construct created, used by or wished for by the patient. Under this assumption, these clinicians advocate administering a placebo to "prove" that the symptoms are "imaginary" or fool the patient into getting better. Unless patients are enrolled in a documented research study in which they are clearly informed that they may be taking a placebo, *there is no place for the use of placebo in general medication management*. Even if some short-term benefits might occur, they are rarely long lasting. Symptoms of underlying biological illness almost always quickly recur, and little has been gained by the use of the placebo. Any use of a placebo also creates a "secret" between the clinician, the patient's family, and/or the unit staff, which becomes an increasing burden to all concerned. If the patient becomes aware of the deception, all trust with the clinician is lost and the therapeutic alliance is broken, usually irrevocably.

References

1 Currier GW and Simpson GS. Respiridone liquid concentrate and oral lorazepam versus intramuscular haliperidol and intramuscular lorazepam for treatment of psychotic agitation. *J Clin Psychiatry* 2001;62:153–157.

2 Hillard JR. Choosing antipsychotics for rapid tranquilization in the ER. *Curr Psychiatry* 2002;1(4):22–29.

3 Tohen M *et al*. Efficacy of olanzapine in acute bipolar mania: a double-blind placebo-controlled study. *Arch Gen Psychiatry* 2000;57:841–849.

4 Zarate CA *et al*. Clinical predictors of acute response with quetiapine in psychotic mood disorders. *J Clin Psychiatry* 2000;61:185–189.

5 Fukutaki K and Allen M. Rapid stabilization of acute mania. *Primary Psychiatry* 2002;9(1):60–62.

6 Martinez JM *et al*. Tolerability of oral loading of divalproic sodium in the treatment of acute mania. *Depress Anxiety* 1998;7:83–86.

7 Hirschfeld RM *et al*. Safety and tolerability of oral loading divalproic sodium in acutely manic bipolar patients. *J Clin Psychiatry* 1999;60:815–818.

8 McElroy SL and Keck PE. A randomized comparison of divalproex oral loading versus haliperidol in the initial treatment of acute psychotic mania. *J Clin Psychiatry* 1996;57:142–146.

9 Carroll BT *et al*. Loading strategies in acute mania. *CNS Spectrums* 2001;6(11):919–930.

10 Glazer W *et al*. Rethinking strategies for managing the acutely psychotic patient. Available at http://www.psychlink.pwpl.com

11 American Psychiatric Association, Treatment Recommendation for Patients with Major Depressive Disorder, http://www.psych.org/clin_res/Depression, 2e.book-7.cfm, p. 3.

12 Marcus D. Serotonin and its role in headache pathogenesis and treatment. *Clinician J Pain* 1993;9:159–167.

13 O'Carroll P. Serotonin and the mind–body dilemma. *TEN* 2001;3(3):56–59.

14 Fava M *et al*. Treatment approaches major depressive disorder relapse, Pt 2. *Psychother Psychometrics* 2002;71(4):195–199.

15 *The Maudsley Prescribing Guidelines*, 6th edition. Martin Dunitz, 2002, pp. 120–124.

Chapter 6

Follow-up appointments and strategies

After the initial evaluation, the next most important element of medication management is the follow-up session. Having a structure in mind for this meeting is crucial to successful management. Follow-up sessions are likely to be repeated many times, and it is wise to spend time early in one's prescribing career defining and refining what is essential to a thorough, medically complete and efficient session. This chapter sets out the key elements of an effective follow-up session, and highlights some exceptions to the general rules.

When do I schedule follow-up?

The timeframe for a follow-up session will be determined by the severity of the patient's condition and whether the patient is in the hospital or seen as an outpatient.

In an outpatient setting, the first follow-up session usually takes place from 1 to 2 weeks after the initial evaluation. This 7- to 14-day interval allows for medication to begin taking effect, for the patient to accommodate to minor side effects, and for you, the clinician, to have valid information about whether the medication is working. At the initial evaluation session, the patient was encouraged to contact you by telephone if significant problems emerged, and usually, if no call has been made, the medicine has been tolerated without major complication. You would probably choose to schedule a follow-up sooner than 1 week if one of the following conditions is present:

1 If the patient is in a serious mental health crisis, it may be important to schedule follow-up at any point within the first 7 days, depending on how worried you are about the patient's clinical condition.
2 If the patient has serious medical problems that may be affected by the use of psychotropic medication, or if you are concerned about the medical status of the patient, likewise it may be useful to see the patient sooner.
3 Anxious, needy patients may wish to be seen sooner because they are uncomfortable with the concept of not having professional contact. Beginning what they perceive as a medicine that may be problematic for them, they will perhaps need reassurance and support to remain compliant.

Unfortunately, at times the practitioner's schedule, availability, or the mandate of the clinic may solely determine the timing of a follow-up visit.

PRIMARY CARE

In some primary care offices, it is not uncommon to schedule follow-up medication appointments many weeks after the initial appointment or, in some cases, not to schedule a follow-up appointment at all – advising the patient to *"call if you have any problems."* When dealing with mental health medication, *this model is inappropriate, dangerous, and will lead to frequent non-response or non-compliance.* Lack of timely follow-up visits can lead many patients to stop medications prematurely because of minor side effects, or not to understand how or when the medication is supposed to work. When an initial prescription runs out and the patient is not seen, medication may not be renewed appropriately. *Schedule a face-to-face follow-up evaluation 10–14 days after the initial visit.*

How long does it take?

Ideally, the length of time devoted to a follow-up medication visit would be dictated by the needs of the patient. For primary mental health practitioners, a 30-minute follow-up exam will allow adequate time to evaluate the effectiveness of medication, adjust dosage, remedy side effects, make any medication changes, *and* review significant issues in the patient's life. Primary care providers and mental health practitioners whose time is tightly managed can usually complete the medication portion alone in 15 to 20 minutes.

Inpatient medication follow-up

In inpatient settings, monitoring of medication will often occur at an entirely different frequency and level of intensity. It is not unusual for patients to be seen by their prescribers every day, particularly just after arrival at the hospital. It is not, however, unreasonable to evaluate medications every second or third day, if the patient is improving without significant side effects and is not labile. Once a patient is stable on medication, weekly follow-up visits are typical. For a long-term chronically hospitalized patient, monthly visits for the first year followed by a visit every 3 months is usual. The elements of the evaluation in the hospital are essentially similar to those of the outpatient follow-up visit, with the addition of feedback from the unit staff concerning the patient's condition.

Preparing for a follow-up

Detailed, lengthy preparation is generally not needed prior to meeting with a patient for a follow-up visit. However, some brief re-familiarization with the patient's chart, clinical course, current medications and any occurrences that have transpired since the last visit can be done quickly. Whenever possible, a similar brief review should be done prior to returning a patient's clinically related telephone call.

Just prior to seeing the patient, take a minute to look at the patient's medical record, and specifically at the following three items:

1 The last progress note of face-to-face contact, noting any intervening telephone calls, crises, or input from other sources
2 The patient's current medication list
3 *The laboratory results/physical exam/allergy sections* of the chart, noting any needed laboratory tests, current allergies, changing physical condition or reports/data from other healthcare providers (see Chapter 27).

This review usually takes no more than a minute or two but accomplishes several crucial tasks, especially for the busy clinician seeing many patients. It clears the clinician's mind from any previous patient activity and focuses him or her on the patient at hand. It prepares the clinician to present to the patient refreshed, refocused and knowledgeable about the current patient's issues, strengths, dilemmas, progress, and medication issues. It also minimizes the likelihood that the practitioner will commit any of a series of embarrassing or potentially careless errors that could occur when past history, treatment or medical issues are not noted or remembered. *The prepared practitioner is viewed by the patient as professional, unhurried and attentive to their needs, and as someone in whom they can have confidence.*

Conversely, the unprepared clinician comes across to the patient as disorganized, rushed, and less likely to be focused on a patient's individual needs. Busy practitioners are tempted to rush in to meet the patient as they open the medical record, trying to save time by talking to the patient, thinking, evaluating, and trying to read the chart at the same time. This is to be discouraged, since it inevitably leads to spotty performance on the five most important tasks that the clinician must accomplish during the follow-up:

1 Know accurately what has transpired with this patient up to this point
2 Evaluate the patient's current state
3 Logically think through the data gathered to make clinical decisions
4 Modify the treatment plan
5 Communicate directly and clearly to the patient.

No matter how organized, intelligent or knowledgeable a clinician is, these five tasks simply cannot be accomplished simultaneously.

Goals of a follow-up

Specific goals in a follow-up session are to:

■ Check target symptoms
■ Quantify response
■ Underscore progress
■ Address side effects
■ Assess any pertinent medical changes
■ Use the input of significant others
■ Encourage phone contact.

The key questions to be answered with respect to medication are:

■ Is the medication effective?
■ Is the dose appropriate?
■ Is the patient complying with treatment?
■ Is the patient experiencing side effects that might interfere with compliance?
■ Is any addition or change to medication necessary?

The assessment of medication effectiveness has two principal elements:

■ Evaluation of the target symptoms identified in the initial evaluation
■ Quantification of response.

Target symptom assessment

In a follow-up session, the target symptoms that were identified and highlighted in the initial evaluation should be inquired about specifically and individually. For example:

- Has the patient's sleep pattern changed?
- How is the patient's concentration in settings where mental focus may be needed?
- Has the patient's eating, appetite, or weight changed?
- Have there been any panic attacks?
- How often has the patient heard voices?
- What is the frequency and/or intensity of any other identified target symptoms?

It is useful to ask if any new symptoms have emerged since the initial visit. At the first follow-up, it is also important to check if there were any specific items of history or symptomatology that the patient did not discuss in the initial evaluation.

Quantification of response

A crucial part of the follow-up session is helping patients to quantify their symptom response to medication. This quantification will help clarify the subjective nature of their responses to questions such as "How are you feeling?" The patient will often respond "good," "fair," "okay," "not very good," "better," or something similar. Different patients use these words quite differently. In order to make precise decisions about medication dosage, it is necessary to probe the meaning of these responses. If a patient's words are taken at face value, without the assessment of specific data, inherent inaccuracies will occur in clinical decisions made about dose, or this may result in an unnecessary change of regimen.

When patients say they are "good" or "better," they should be asked, "What specifically is improved since the last time I saw you?" This will usually lead into a discussion of target symptoms. The clinician should also ask about any target symptoms the patient does not spontaneously report as different. Because patients are almost always interested in pleasing the clinician, many will say that things are "going better" or they are "well" just because they think it is what the clinician wants to hear. When the target symptoms are probed, it can turn out that there have been minimal changes in the symptoms you have targeted to treat.

Patients who say "there is no change," "I'm no better," or "this stuff isn't working" can, when their target symptoms are evaluated, discover that some symptoms have improved, but they failed to notice the improvement. In some cases, target symptoms are better but the patient has attributed the reason for the improvement to other causes.

Similarly, when patients say a medication is working "fair" or "so-so," the clinician is often left in a quandary as to what to do with the dosage unless he or she pursues the meaning of those words. Quantification of the patient's response is essential to decisions about the dosage.

Two simple, powerful questions

Two simple questions allow the clinician to quantify the patient's response and provide significant data that will help decide whether or not the medication dose needs to be changed.

TALKING TO PATIENTS

1   *"Rate yourself on a scale from 0 to 100 – with 0 being the worst you've ever felt with your [depression, anxiety, etc.] and 95–100 as feeling comfortable, well, and balanced. No one is at 100 all the time. Give me two numbers. Where were you before starting medication, and where are you now?"*

2   After the patient gives you the two numbers, take the second of these responses and ask: *"What would need to be different for you to get from this number to 95?"*

Beyond the information it provides to the clinician, many patients find this brief exercise engaging and useful. It helps them to think more precisely about how they are responding to medication. Some patients will say that it is hard to quantify, although most can, and do, make this assessment quite readily. Interpretation of these numbers also gives you a clear framework on how to proceed with medication dosage.

Generally, there are two types of answers that emerge from the second question (what needs to change to get to 95?) that provide perspective. Some patients refer to target symptoms that have not improved, or have improved only partially. A second type of response will describe environmental issues, for example:

- Now I need to change jobs
- All I need now is a new boss
- Now if my wife and I would stop fighting
- If only I had time for a vacation
- If my parents would stop criticizing me.

If the patient refers to target symptoms and is not close to the target figure of 95, it is clear that the illness is only partially treated and generally an increase in dosage is indicated. On the other hand, the second type of response, referring to the patient's environment or lifestyle, is unlikely to be affected by medication changes and it may be that a dosage change is not indicated. These questions can, and should, be asked at each succeeding follow-up session until patients consistently rate themselves at 90 or above.

Know what is changing medically

Prescription of psychotropic medication is a process that cannot be taken out of the context of the patient's overall health and medical treatment. *It is imperative that, at every follow-up session, the clinician inquires about other medical changes, including medication additions that may have occurred since the last session.*

While some illnesses, medications or treatment may have little impact on the mental health prescription, others may have a critical or life-threatening impact. Knowledge of other medical treatment is essential. Illnesses or non-psychotropic medication changes can:

■ Worsen or improve the mental health condition
■ Affect the blood levels of the psychotropic via P-450 interactions or by other mechanisms (e.g. decreased GI absorption), requiring dosage adjustment
■ Account for new or intensified side effects that might otherwise be attributed to the psychotropic
■ Lead to changes in compliance with the psychotropic.

Inquiry into what medications are being prescribed by other providers may also uncover circumstances in which two or more practitioners are providing the same or multiple psychotropics. If the practitioner is not aware, this can lead to possible medication interaction or undiscovered abuse.

Inquiry about medical problems and medications does not imply that the prescriber should treat these medical problems, unless trained and credentialled to do so. In general, except for primary care providers, most mental health prescribers will not treat the patient's medical conditions. (See Chapter 9 for further information about this issue.)

Side effects at follow-up

Further goals of the follow-up session include side-effect assessment and management. The key point to remember here is that the patient should be asked specifically "*Are you having any side effects or unwanted symptoms from the medication?*" The patient should assess the frequency, intensity, and amount of interference with functioning caused by these side effects. When they are minor, reassurance may be all that is needed. If they are more significant, the clinician must decide whether to modify dosage, reassure and wait, add a remediative factor, or change medication. This topic is so important that it is discussed in detail separately in Chapter 16.

Maintaining the bond with the patient

Another (often unspoken) goal of the follow-up session is to maintain and strengthen the alliance between clinician and patient. *The relationship you maintain with the patient can be as important as the prescription you write.* In some clinical situations, it is more important. A solid alliance with a patient will not overcome medication that is ineffective or poorly tolerated, but it will foster the trust necessary to keep the patient compliant with your prescription. When patients feel listened to, respected, empathized with, and made partners in medication decisions, they will often gather the courage to try a medication about which they are anxious, and to persist even if they are uncomfortable. Although serious adverse consequences of psychotropics are uncommon (see Chapter 17), when they do occur, the quality of the relationship with the prescriber will often significantly influence the patient's response.

The very fact that the follow-up session is scheduled and carried out indicates that the clinician is interested in how the patient is progressing, and what role the medication is taking in that progress. It also indicates willingness to answer questions about the medication, and to help the patient manage any bothersome side effects. At follow-up sessions, the clinician has an opportunity to reinforce the treatment plan outlined in the initial session and to identify the patient's position on the timeline toward recovery. If the patient is not fully recovered at the first session – which he often is not – it is important to state that full recovery is not expected immediately. If there are promising signs and improvement in some symptoms, this indicates that the medication and therapy programs are "on the right track" and this should be underscored. At this session, it is also possible to see if the patient has followed through with any talking therapy that may have been suggested during the initial treatment plan.

The power of positive comments

Patients taking mental health medication are anxious, depressed, confused, and demoralized, and some have lost hope of ever feeling better. As part of their illness, often they have received negative comments, disparaging remarks and overt criticism from family and friends, as well as poor work evaluations. They may have perceived that others think little of them or look down on them. Many patients, in fact, look negatively on themselves. It is crucially important that the clinician remains upbeat, positive, and enthusiastic, and shows measured hopefulness about the potential benefits of psychotropic medication treatment. This cannot be stressed strongly enough. *There can never be too many encouraging statements or compliments, or too much praise for the patient's behavior and improvement.*

Use phrases such as:

- You did well to . . .
- I am impressed by . . .
- I can see all the effort you put into . . .
- You showed good judgment when . . .
- Wow, it is impressive that . . .
- You obviously gave a lot of thought in coming up with that decision
- You showed a lot of strength to endure . . .
- That must have taken a lot of strength to . . .

- Your lab tests look great
- I appreciate that you stayed with our plan despite . . .
- Given what you have had to face, you have done better than a lot of people would have
- You have been really patient with . . .
- You did just what I would have wanted you to do
- I see why you did what you did, and I think you did the best you could with the situation you faced
- Well done!
- Great job!
- Congratulations!
- Very nice!
- Keep up the good work!

Finding positive ways to discuss the patient's actions, decision-making and compliance provides powerful reinforcers to the treatment plan. The alliance with the clinician is greatly strengthened by these brief but meaningful statements, which can often mean continuation and success with your recommendations in the face of medication non-response, side effects, or a stressful personal life crisis.

If the clinician has a mind set to consciously support and reinforce the patient in some way at each visit, it is usually not hard to find an area of discussion around which to make these affirmations, even in the most regressed, negativistic or non-compliant patient.

What is an adequate trial?

The length of time that you keep a patient on a specific medication is a clinical decision based on the assessment of several factors, including:

- Is the patient showing any response? Is the response increasing with time?
- How intense are the patient's symptoms? Is the patient's condition deteriorating during the current trial of medication?
- How well is the patient tolerating the medication (severity of side effects)? Are the side effects lessening or intensifying with time?
- Has the patient reached (or come close to reaching) a therapeutic dose of the drug, and maintained the therapeutic dose for a period of time?
- What other promising medication alternatives do you have if you switch?
- How willing is the patient to pursue a continuation of the current trial?

Although some patients will only respond fully to a drug at 60 to 90 days after beginning medication, most patients will have begun to show some initial sign of response by 30 days. Further gradual improvement can appear later. It is unlikely that a patient who shows absolutely no change in symptoms at 30 days will suddenly (or gradually) show significant improvement at a later date. Therefore, clinically useful timeframes for medication trials of an individual medication are as follows:

- For a *mildly to moderately symptomatic outpatient*, continue a medication for 30 days before switching. During this period the dose of the drug is likely to be increased using the quantification of response data noted earlier in this chapter.

- For an *inpatient or severely symptomatic outpatient*, continue a medication for 15 days before switching. With these individuals, particularly on an inpatient unit, the use of multiple medications on a daily or an as-needed basis is common and often necessary for acute behavioral control and management during this first 2 weeks.

These general time guidelines can be modified by several circumstances. For example, a patient's medication trial may be shortened owing to significant medication side effects or intolerance. It does not, however, usually make clinical sense to change a patient's antidepressant, mood stabilizer, or antipsychotic every several days for "non-response," since a valid, expectable response simply is unlikely to occur in that period.

Conversely, a patient's medication trial may be lengthened if partial response is occurring, or if full therapeutic dosing has not been reached. An outpatient who has shown some improvement but has not achieved full response may become substantially asymptomatic with a longer period on medication. A patient who has required low initial dosages with very gradual increases (because of side effects, concurrent medical condition or advanced age, for example) may not have reached full therapeutic levels in 30 days. If the patient is tolerating the drug, continuation of a medication may extend for 60 to 90 days before a valid assessment of its usefulness can be made. Therapeutic blood levels, when appropriate, can also guide this process. *Maintain a drug for at least 30 days after adequate therapeutic blood levels have been reached to assess response.*

CLINICAL TIP

Significant drug effect is unlikely unless at least modest gains have been seen in the first months. Continuing a medication for 6–12 months with an expectation (and message to the patient) that *"you will feel better in a while – just keep taking it"* is not good medicine, and is seldom true. Either decide that medication is not useful for this patient or change medications, but do not simply continue the drug and wait for response. This practice occurs most frequently in primary care offices or institutional settings.

Switching and side effects

Table 6.1 gives some practical advice about switching medication, based on the amount of response and the intensity of side effects.

A measure of experience helps in knowing whether a certain side effect is likely to pass with time or, once present, is unlikely to go away. If side effects are serious, interfering with functioning and/or increasing in intensity, it is usually

Table 6.1 When to change antidepressants

Side effects	Level of improvement		
	Little or none	*Partial*	*Significant or full*
None or mild	Change	Increase dose	Maintain dose
Moderate but tolerable	Increase dose slowly	Increase dose slowly	Maintain dose
Significant or serious	Change	Change	Decrease dose or change

necessary to change medications, sometimes as soon as the initial follow-up visit. If side effects are lessening and have minimal interference with the patient's day-to-day life, it may be quite appropriate to wait until at least the second follow-up visit to see if symptoms pass fully or become more tolerable. Chapter 16 gives detailed advice on strategies for managing side effects without necessarily needing to change drugs.

When changing, gradual is best

With most psychotropics, once a decision has been made to change medications, there should be a gradual cross-taper from one medication to the other – that is, the first medication can be gradually decreased in dosage *at the same time as* the second medication is being started. In general, if dosage is moderate or high, this is a better strategy than stopping the first medication totally before starting a second medication. Stopping totally can leave the patient "uncovered" and symptomatic for a period before the second medication begins to take effect. This principle applies to virtually all medicines in all classes, including antidepressants, antipsychotics, mood stabilizers and anti-anxiety medications. If the patient takes a small dose of medicine, no taper is necessary.

CLINICAL TIP
When changing medication, a cross-taper of medications is almost always safer and less bothersome to the patient than stopping one medication totally before starting another.

A notable exception to the principle of cross-tapering is when the medication to be stopped or started is a monoamine oxidase inhibitor (MAOI). *If the MAOI is being stopped, the patient must be totally off it for at least 2 weeks prior to starting another antidepressant. If the medicine to be started is an MAOI, the safe starting point is determined by the time to full elimination of any current medication with which the MAOI could interact.* Generally it is safe to begin an MAOI 1 week after stopping the previous medication. (The commonly used psychotropic that needs a much longer interval before starting an MAOI is fluoxetine, which has a long-acting metabolite, norfluoxetine, that is not excreted for up to 4 weeks.)

During a cross-taper the clinician may see that the patient is beginning to feel better with the addition of a second medication, and decide to continue with both medications. By assuming that both medications are necessary to the patient's response, however, the clinician may get "caught in the middle." In general, in the change from medicine A to medicine B, it is best to continue a cross-taper until medicine A is fully stopped, and maintain the patient solely on medicine B before deciding that both medications are necessary. If the patient begins to back-slide on medicine B alone, it is simple to return to the combination. Using two medications can at times be beneficial, but this should only be decided in hindsight, rather than stopping in the middle and assuming it to be so.

When changing medications, especially via a gradual taper, a written instruction sheet is crucial. Patients can easily mishear, misunderstand or forget orally given schedules under the best of clinical circumstances. As shown in Table 6.2, a "changeover sheet" with blanks to be filled in by the clinician with specific dosage amounts is a valuable educational office tool.

An example of such a sheet filled in by the clinician is shown in Table 6.3.

Some clinicians may prefer to use numbers of pills rather than milligrams, as in Table 6.4.

Table 6.2 Changeover sheet

Day	(Medication A)	(Medication B)
1		
2		
3		
4		
5		
6		
7		
8		
9		
10		
11		
12		
13		
14		

Table 6.3 Completed changeover sheet (dosage)

Day	(Medication A)	(Medication B)
1	300 mg	10 mg
2	300 mg	10 mg
3	250 mg	10 mg
4	250 mg	10 mg
5	200 mg	20 mg
6	200 mg	20 mg
7	150 mg	20 mg
8	150 mg	30 mg
9	100 mg	30 mg
10	100 mg	30 mg
11	50 mg	30 mg
12	50 mg	30 mg
13		Call me

Polypharmacy – from the doghouse to the penthouse

Polypharmacy of psychotropic medication is an area in which there has been a major shift in philosophy over the past 10 years. As recently as the early 1990s, it was believed by most prescribers that one medication was preferable to a combination of medications. Within the medical community there was an implicit or expressed assumption that a patient taking several medications was being inappropriately treated with polypharmacy. This was particularly the case when two medications from the same class were used. This practice was generally regarded as being representative of sloppy prescribing, potentially harmful to the patient, and poor clinical practice. As the knowledge of psychotropics has progressed, and patient expectations of full relief have increased, it is clear that many patients not only benefit from multiple medications, but also that a multiple medication regimen may be essential to achieving and maintaining their recovery.

It is now not uncommon[1] to have a patient on several antidepressants simultaneously, particularly if they have different mechanisms of action. Similarly with mood stabilizers; some bipolar patients simply cannot be stabilized on one medication alone, but improve considerably on a combination of mood stabilizers from different medication families.[2]

For example, a patient may experience panic attacks and depression. On an antidepressant alone the patient may be overstimulated, or have partial control over anxiety symptoms, while on a benzodiazepine alone the patient may have

Table 6.4 Completed changeover sheet (number of pills)		
Day	Medication A (100 mg)	Medication B (10 mg)
1	3 pills	1 pill
2	3 pills	1 pill
3	2½ pills	1 pill
4	2½ pills	1 pill
5	2 pills	2 pills
6	2 pills	2 pills
7	1½ pills	2 pills
8	1½ pills	3 pills
9	1 pill	3 pills
10	1 pill	3 pills
11	½ pill	3 pills
12	½ pill	3 pills
13	—	Call me
14		

breakthrough depressive symptoms or breakthrough panic attacks. On the two classes of medications together, the patient feels in control – neither depressed nor anxious.

Another common example of the patient helped by polypharmacy is the bipolar, depressed patient who when on a mood stabilizer alone has breakthrough depressions, but when on an antidepressant alone has lack of response, hypomanic overstimulation or erratic, unpredictable response. When the two medicines are given together, however, the patient remains mood-stable and free from depression.

Polypharmacy is also becoming more common in treatment-resistant psychosis and schizophrenia.

Synergy

Another factor supporting polypharmacy is the additive response of patients taking two medications from the same class simultaneously. There can be an additive, synergistic effect between two medicines such that the overall benefit is greater than that achieved by either of the medicines alone – in common terms, "one plus one equals three."

The use of combined mood stabilizers in treatment of bipolar patients demonstrates this principle. On lithium or valproic acid alone, the patient may have a partial but limited response. When lithium and valproic acid are used together, the patient is significantly improved and has fewer relapses.[3] If the "two powerful questions" mentioned earlier in this chapter were put to such patients, they might rate themselves at 35 on lithium alone, 40 on valproic acid alone, but 90 on the combination.

The best clinicians – those sought out as tertiary referral sources, or experts used for consultation – often practice polypharmacy. Those who do it expertly are leaders in their field. Polypharmacy has gone from the "doghouse" to the "penthouse."

Inadvertent polypharmacy

While planned, rational polypharmacy can be quite helpful to patients, there are several circumstances that result in inadvertent, non-therapeutic polypharmacy. Such polypharmacy is not helpful, may reflect clinician inexperience, and may lead to increased side effects, drug interaction and cost. The first circumstance has already been mentioned, when the clinician gets "caught in the middle" during a cross-taper of two medications. In this scenario the patient takes two medications, one of which may not be needed.

A second common scenario leading to unintentional and unwise polypharmacy involves a patient who has been stable over a long period of time on medication A alone. A symptom flare-up or breakthrough occurs. To deal with breakthrough symptoms (e.g. psychotic symptoms in a schizophrenic patient, manic symptoms in a bipolar patient, panic symptoms in a panic disorder patient), a second medication B is added. If the patient responds, the clinician may fail to assess whether the second medication (B) can be stopped once the crisis has passed. Even if the addition of medicine B was necessary and beneficial during the crisis, can the patient be managed on medicine A alone after the crisis remits? If medication B makes a substantial improvement, could medication A now be eliminated? Newly-added medicine B alone may be sufficient.

Some patients who experience multiple relapses over time may develop a very complicated medication regimen and inadvertent polypharmacy. The group most vulnerable to non-therapeutic polypharmacy is the elderly population. Older patients who have been treated over much of their lives for mental health conditions may be taking an impressively large number of various medications in different classes. It is not uncommon to be confronted with a new elderly patient who has been taking four, five, six, or more psychotropics for many years. This accumulation of medications may lead to excessive complexity of regimen, increased side effects and interactions with other non-psychotropic medications, and unnecessary cost. Since geriatric patients are particularly sensitive to medication side effects and dosages, it is very important to reevaluate their regimen frequently and to check to see whether all medications are still necessary (see Chapter 12).

Feedback from others

Input from a caretaker, child, parent, or other person who may be knowledgeable about the patient's condition is especially helpful in making appropriate assessments at the follow-up session. This is particularly so if patients are not good observers of their own behavior. *If a caretaker, relative, or friend accompanies the patient to the office, it is generally helpful to briefly ask this person about his or her perception of the patient's response.* Early in treatment, severely ill patients, geriatric patients, or persons who are not good self-observers will often return to the clinician saying that nothing has changed or nothing is better. When input from the family member is obtained, it reveals that significant benefits have started to occur. While the patient may not be fully responsive, many times family members will begin to see positive changes before patients themselves identify progress.

Helping a patient stay on medication – the compliance dilemma

As with medications in general, non-compliance with psychotropic medication is a major public health problem.[4,5] Patients often do not take all their prescribed medication, or frequently miss doses. Some patients cut down on their medication doses because they are concerned about side effects or cost. Others, for a variety of reasons, stop medication altogether without informing the clinician. Unbeknownst to the clinician, some patients throw the prescription away and never start the medication. How then can the clinician raise the odds for successful compliance? Some factors are listed in Table 6.5.

Forming a *strong initial contract* with patients is the cornerstone to compliance. This contract should include the clinician's assessment or diagnosis, why the medication is indicated, what symptoms the medication is intended to help, and an outline for duration of usage. *It is important to make sure patients understand the plan and agree to it.* Such an approach ensures that the patient becomes an active participant in the process, and raises the likelihood of compliance.

One of the most important elements to eliminating missed medication doses is to establish a *simple regimen with the fewest daily doses possible.*[6] Repeated

---

Table 6.5 Factors that can increase compliance with psychotropic medication

- An openly discussed and reinforced agreement with the patient as to why the medication is to be taken, in what doses, and for how long
- A simple medication regimen with the fewest daily doses possible
- Written directions for taking the medication
- Regular follow-up visits
- Assessing compliance at follow-up visits
- Evaluating and remediating side effects of the medication
- Assessing patient resistance to taking medication
- Prompt telephone availability between office sessions

medication studies have shown that the higher the number of doses per day, the more likely it is that patients will miss one or more doses. Many psychotropics can be dosed once daily, and do not require multiple doses to be effective. Simplicity of dosing (e.g. the same strength and number of pills at each dose) also helps. Avoid every other day, twice weekly, or otherwise complicated schedules unless a patient's clinical situation and response demands it.

Early, frequent contact with patients will also increase the odds of compliance. The longer the time until the first follow-up session, the more likely it is that patients will not comply or will have taken the medication in an inappropriate way. Over the first 4–6 weeks at least two follow-up sessions should be undertaken, to reinforce the medications and the treatment plan, as well as to assess for any side effects.

Availability of the clinician by telephone will also improve compliance. If patients know that they can call the clinician, simple issues can be clarified immediately, allowing them to continue the medication appropriately until the next visit. Telephone reassurance and education about what they are experiencing can prevent patients from discontinuing medication prematurely.

Another extremely important item in improving compliance is to *ask about, listen for, and remediate side effects*. While there are many explanations for patient discontinuation of medication, the single largest reason is that the medication produces a side effect that patients find intolerable.[7] Because of their discomfort, patients do not comply. (See Chapter 16 for an in-depth discussion of side effect management.)

The clinician should also, in the first several follow-up sessions, ask about and evaluate *signs of resistance*. If patients are hesitant about increasing a dose or continuing on the medication, the clinician needs to inquire specifically about the hesitation. Often it is an issue that can be handled quickly and expediently. If a patient has serious resistance, it may be better to halt the medication trial or delay the dosage increase and deal with the resistance first. In a mildly/moderately symptomatic patient, if the resistance is addressed the medication can be retried when the patient is more cooperative and understands the rationale for the treatment plan.

It is also useful for the clinician to *assess how many pills a patient has been taking daily*. How much medication does the patient have left? Does that match the patient's records? If the patient has far too much medication left over it is a clear sign that the medication has not been taken consistently, and the reason for this needs to be evaluated.

If patients do improve, but stop medication prematurely or intermittently, encourage them to step back and look at the "big picture." *Use specific dates, holidays, and life events* as markers or identifiers to reinforce your assessment of the positive results that the patient has experienced.

TALKING TO PATIENTS

"Let's remember where you were last Christmas. You weren't working and you were living at your parents' home. You were feeling so anxious that you were fearful of going to the store by yourself. After you had taken the medication for 3 months, you were able to go out to the mall alone and to apply for a job, and were thinking about moving into your own apartment. After you stopped medication in March, you felt too anxious to go to the job interview and spent most of the day watching television because you didn't want to leave the house. When you started medication in May, you started to look forward to getting out again. Remember, that's when you went to the neighborhood picnic that you enjoyed so much. You even began to think about wanting to visit your cousin in Springfield. When you stopped medication in August, that's when you cancelled the trip to see your cousin and started lying on the couch again for hours each day. I think there is a direct connection between your taking the medication and being able to do many of the things you want to do."

A final factor that will help to increase compliance is *flexibility about the decision as to when and how to discontinue medication.* If patients have the clear understanding that the clinician will not maintain a rigid, inflexible approach to discontinuation, they are usually more willing to tolerate medication for a period of time until a mutually agreed discontinuation date can be determined. Stopping medication will be discussed in more detail in Chapter 8.

How and when to refer to a mental health specialist

As with other specialty providers, the primary care provider (PCP) will benefit from cultivating contacts with specialists in psychotropic prescribing. This may be an adult or child psychiatrist, or a mental health nurse practitioner with specialty training. Having a tertiary referral source (a university-based psychopharmacologist or an especially knowledgeable practitioner in the community) available is also helpful, but is not always possible in all communities. The reality of medical practice in many areas is that mental health prescribing specialists are in short supply, and often have a long waiting period for appointments. Emergency, same-day evaluations for psychotropics are often only available through an emergency department or psychiatric hospital. Because of these realities, a PCP will often have to make urgent decisions about psychotropic medication with a limited comfort level.

In general, a patient is appropriate for referral to an available mental health specialist when:

- The patient is acutely and highly suicidal
- The patient is psychotic

- Bipolar symptoms are present, or emerge during treatment
- The patient has been minimally responsive to the PCP's prescriptions
- The patient experiences multiple disabling side effects from psychotropics
- The diagnosis is uncertain and the appropriate course of medication is unclear
- The PCP needs assistance with a "difficult" patient (see Chapter 25 for more on this topic)
- The PCP wants clarification/confirmation of the need for ongoing habit-forming psychotropic medications
- The patient's medical condition is seriously adversely affected by a mental health problem requiring medication
- The patient has a complex psychopharmacological combination of medications
- The PCP is uncomfortable managing this particular patient or a specific class of medications
- Repeated relapse occurs when medication is withdrawn
- There is patient frustration with the process of repeated medication trials.

TALKING TO PATIENTS

Making the referral to a mental health specialist is not always simple. Some patients resist the referral, and never follow through. There is no single way to ensure that the patient will accept the referral, although some strategies are helpful:

- Emphasize that it is you, the PCP, who needs assistance, not the patient: *"Mrs Gordon, I have tried several antidepressants with you for your depression and I need some consultation and help. I would like you to see Gloria Boyle. She works regularly with these types of medications and can help me decide what is best for you."*
- If the referral is for medication, specifically using the term "psychopharmacologist" or "practitioner with expertise in mental health medication" may carry less stigma than referral to a "psychiatrist" or "therapist."
- Describe the initial visit as a "consultation," with the possibility of return to your care when the situation is appropriate: *"Miss Porter, I would like to get a consultation from Dr Pindar. He is a specialist in this area of medication. Once he has evaluated your situation, he, you, and I can decide how best to follow-up. Regardless, I would like to stay involved, and if it is appropriate for me to continue to prescribe I will do so. Most of all, I want to ensure that you get the help you need."*
- If you are not willing to continue to prescribe a particular medication without a confirmatory evaluation, say so clearly but not punitively: *"Mr Edwards, we have been prescribing* [name of medication] *for your anxiety. When we stopped the medica-*

tion your anxiety returned, and recently you have requested additional refills at increasing frequency. Before I am willing to continue prescribing, I want a second opinion about your condition and if we are on the right track. Greg Boyle is a nurse practitioner who deals with anxiety medications regularly, and I would like you to see him."

■ If the patient has expressed reluctance regarding the referral, recognize the patient's ambivalence and your inability to provide what he or she needs. Focus on these needs: *"Mr Vincent, I can see that you are not pleased with the idea of my referring you to a mental health specialist. I am concerned about the intensity of your depressive symptoms. You have been "hanging on by your fingernails," sleeping poorly, losing weight, and you have begun thinking that the world would be better off without you around. We have tried several antidepressants. You have been very diligent in taking the medication as I have asked, but have minimally improved and gotten side effects that really bother you. Despite your strength in following through with my recommendation, I see you wearing down and tiring out. The most important thing is to get you well as quickly as possible. I know you would prefer to do this another way, but I am worried about you. I need some assistance, and I want you to see Dr Wong. I have worked with her several times before, and she has been extremely helpful. Will you keep an appointment if my staff helps to set it up?"*

■ Involve the family. For example, in any of the above dialogues, if the patient still refuses referral you could request to talk to the patient's family. *"Mrs Donovan, I believe you are at serious risk for worsening of your depression. Things are not better despite both our best efforts. I need to talk with your daughter to discuss my concerns, since I cannot continue to prescribe for you when your condition is worsening as it is. I feel I need some assistance."* If the patient agrees, call a responsible family member.

■ Utilize one of the individualized "patient levers" discussed in Chapter 4.

Missed doses

No matter how conscientious a patient may be, missing an occasional dose of medication is understandable and a fact of clinical practice.

The instruction given here regarding missed doses is generally applicable for most patients and most mental health medications.

TALKING TO PATIENTS

"If you miss a dose of medication, take it when you remember, unless it is 4 or less hours until your next scheduled dose. If your regular dose will occur within 4 hours, skip the missed dose and resume your normal dose at the regularly scheduled time. Do not double up on your medication to 'make up' for the missed dose."

Exceptions to this principle include:

1 *Short half-life serotonergic antidepressants* such as paroxetine and venlafaxine that are particularly sensitive to serotonergic rebound withdrawal (see Chapter 8). Because of the propensity of such short half-life medications to produce unpleasant rebound symptoms (including dizziness, nausea, agitation, and sleeplessness) when a dose is missed, patients should take the missed dose *whenever* they remember it, particularly if they are experiencing some measure of serotonergic rebound withdrawal.
2 *Sedative medicines taken once daily at bedtime.* If patients remember such a medication in the morning, they may or may not find this medication too sedative for daytime activities. For those who cannot risk any sedation, it may be safer to wait until their next bedtime dose before taking any further medication. A second alternative is for the patient to take a smaller amount (one-fourth to one-half of their regular dose) in the morning and then take a full dose at bedtime as prescribed.

How patients respond to missed doses

The clinical results of missing a dose vary markedly from patient to patient. Some patients are significantly sensitive to even a single missed dose of their psychotropic, and will notice symptoms within hours of missing it. Other patients seem impervious to such missed doses and, unless there are frequent missed doses resulting in significantly lower serum blood levels, they note very little difference in their clinical condition.

The clinical reaction to missing a dose of medication is composed of two elements:

1 Any physiological reaction caused by the sudden absence of the medication
2 The return of target symptoms that the medication is attempting to treat (e.g. anxiety, depression, psychosis, etc.).

Our level of scientific understanding of what happens when a dose is missed is almost solely related to the first of these factors. We do understand clearly the serotonergic withdrawal syndrome that occurs with strongly serotonergic antidepressants, and the withdrawal syndrome from benzodiazepines. Our clinical experience supports our knowledge that patients taking short half-life compounds are much more vulnerable to withdrawal phenomena than those taking long half-life compounds. Short half-life antidepressants such as paroxetine and venlafaxine cause many more serotonergic withdrawal symptoms than long half-life compounds such as fluoxetine. When stopped quickly, short half-life benzodiazepines such as alprazolam cause more withdrawal symptomatology than longer half-life compounds such as chlordiazepoxide or chlorazepate. This scientific evidence is solid, and knowledge of a compound's half-life is necessary in order to assess whether a patient's reaction to a missed dose is likely to be withdrawal-related.

Where our science is limited is in the second element – the propensity for a particular patient to have a return of symptoms quickly when a medication is missed. Some patients are quite vulnerable to symptomatic return, and will become anxious, depressed, or psychotic quickly, beginning even after just one missed dose. Other patients can go several days or even weeks without obvious reaction to missing regular dosing. What biological (or psychological) underpinnings cause one patient to react this way and another not, is unclear. Only past clinical experience with a particular patient can help the clinician to decide how vulnerable that patient is likely to be. While each clinician should encourage patients to be conscientious and diligent about taking their medication regularly, what happens in reality with a specific patient is quite variable.

Parenteral medications

The vast majority of psychotropic medications are dispensed in oral form, pills, capsules, liquid preparations, or, for some medication, as dissolving lozenges. Intramuscular dispensing of medication is used in the following circumstances:

1   For immediate behavioral control in acutely psychotic or manic patients. This usually involves the use of an antipsychotic, a benzodiazepine, or both.
2   For the acute treatment of extrapyramidal side effects (usually from traditional antipsychotics), anticholinergic medication such as benzotropine, an antihistamine such as dyphenhydramine, or a benzodiazepine may be used intramuscularly.
3   As long-acting, depot preparations of traditional antipsychotic medications used to increase compliance for psychotic patients. At the time of this writing, only ziprasidone of the atypical antipsychotics has an approved intramuscular preparation, although several other pharmaceutical firms are developing intramuscular preparations for other atypical antipsychotics.

CLINICAL TIP
When stabilizing a patient on antipsychotic medication, it is always preferable to do so with an oral dose of medication or regular preparation intramuscular injections. *It is very difficult to achieve good therapeutic benefit and avoid significant side effects if the stabilization is attempted using long-acting depot preparations.* Important considerations in using long-acting depot preparation traditional neuroleptics are listed in Table 6.6.

Table 6.6 Using long-acting depot preparations of traditional neuroleptics

1   Preferably stabilize the patient on the oral medication first
2   Approximate conversion factors when switching: 10 mg/day oral haloperidol =
    100–200 mg of haloperidol decanoate every 4 weeks
    10 mg/day oral fluphenazine = 12.5–25 mg fluphenazine decanoate every 2 weeks
3   When switching to depot preparations, use the lowest effective dose
4   Use the longest possible recommended dosing intervals between injections
5   Allow adequate time (at least 1 month) to assess adequacy of symptom response
6   For breakthrough symptoms, which may occur when depot preparations are first
    used, supplement the depot preparation with oral doses of medication and adjust
    depot dosage at next injection. Do not attempt to manage breakthrough symptoms
    initially with further injections of depot medication

At this time, there are no intramuscular or intravenous preparations of antidepressants or stimulants. Intramuscular dosing is seldom used in an outpatient setting, except for the depot antipsychotics. The practical use of intravenous medication in mental health treatment is rare, since those patients who are agitated enough theoretically to benefit from the direct intravenous injection are often physically too disruptive to permit an intravenous access to be established.

Pill facts

Knowledge about size, expiration dates and other pill facts can often allay patient's fears or answer questions during follow-up sessions.

Pill size

The amount of medication in a typical pill or capsule will fit on the head of a pin. Most of the substance of a pill or capsule is composed of inactive elements, including filler and the capsule used to contain the granules or powder. The manufacturer can, therefore, determine the size of the pill rather arbitrarily. The size of the pill has no relationship to its potency or the amount of medication contained within. Larger pills or capsules are larger so that they are easier to handle; their size does not necessarily reflect strength or the number of milligrams in the dose.

Milligrams of medicine

Patients often confuse the number of milligrams in a pill with its potency, assuming that a 500-mg pill is considerably stronger than a 1-mg pill. The clinician may wish to explain that with psychotropics, as with many other medications, the number of milligrams in two different medicines is not usually comparable. Many psychotropics have a dosage range that is a fraction of 1 mg to several mg, while other medications have typical therapeutic dosages measured in thousands of milligrams. The effective range of dosage is unique to each medication, and has no bearing on its strength.

Expiration dates

Patients often ask how long their medications will stay "good," particularly if they use a medication only infrequently, and may have it on hand for a lengthy period of time. A drug's expiration date is generally 2 years after it has been sealed in the container by the manufacturer. The projection of continued stability to this date is based on a closed and protected environment, and no longer applies once the original container is opened. As long as the medication has not come into contact with water, been partially dissolved, or been exposed to excessive heat or the sun (for example left on a car dashboard or in a glove compartment for a prolonged period), medications remain active. Most medications, however, will become less potent with time. The rate of declining activity correlates with many factors, but most tablets or capsules retain most of their potency for at least 1 year after the expiration date, even after the container has been opened. The clinician can reassure patients that office samples or prescription pills will retain the majority of their potency for at least 1 year beyond the expiration date. However, any pills exposed to water or excessive sunlight, or not kept in brown-shaded pharmacy pill containers, run the risk of earlier deterioration. Pills that have become wet have extremely variable potencies. When exposed to water or other liquids, it often becomes impossible to know how much of the active medication ingredient remains in a partially dissolved pill, and such items should generally be thrown away. Psychotropic medications do not "go bad," transform into other chemicals, or become toxic with time.

Traveling when on psychotropic medications

Patients traveling away from home, particularly if they are at a distance or in developing countries, benefit from a simple precaution: tell them to pack two separate stores of medication, each containing enough medication to last for the entire trip. One set is to be packed in the luggage, and one to be kept on the person. In the event that the personal supply is lost, there is a second supply in the luggage; in the event the luggage does not reach the intended destination, the patient has a full supply on their person. Having a second supply drastically simplifies the situation when the patient's supply of medicine is lost, stolen, knocked into the toilet by the hotel maid, or meets some other fate.

While many psychotropic medications are commonly available in most parts of the developed world, there are some countries where specific medications will not be available or will be significantly difficult to obtain. Since patients can have significant symptom breakthrough or rebound physical symptomatology when they stop their medication abruptly, the simple double-packing precaution virtually ensures that they will not need to undergo needless discomfort while traveling. This precaution will turn out to be unnecessary 98 percent of the time, but, in the event it does become necessary, it can be extremely helpful.

Traveling with psychotropic medications, even in less developed countries, is generally not a problem at customs or immigration. It may be helpful, however, to carry psychotropic medications in the original, pharmacy-labeled containers, rather than putting a large number of pills in an unmarked container with no identification. This is a simple precaution that further reinforces that the medication is a validly prescribed medication rather than some other substance.

References

1   Nichol MB *et al.* Factors predicting the use of multiple psychotropic medications. *J Clin Psychiatry* 1997;56(2):60–66.

2   Kirk DD *et al.* Comparative prophylactic efficacy of lithium carbamazepine and the combination in bipolar disorder. *J Clin Psychiatry* 1997;58:470–478.

3   Solomon DA *et al.* A pilot study of lithium carbonate plus divalproex sodium for the continuation and maintenance treatment of patients with bipolar I disorder. *J Clin Psychiatry* 1997;58:95–99.

4   Murphy J and Coaster G. Issues in patient compliance. *Drugs* 1997;54:797–800.

5   Cramer JA and Spiker B. *Patient Compliance in Medical Practice and Clinical Trials.* Raven Press, 1998.

6   Maddox JC *et al.* The compliance with antidepressants in general practice. *J Psychopharmacology* 1994;8(1):48–53.

Chapter 7

Medication and psychotherapy

With the introduction of psychoactive medications in the 1950s, and with their increasing usage over the subsequent decades, several issues have emerged regarding the interrelationship of psychotropic medications and psychotherapy ("talking" therapy with any of a variety of formats and orientations). These include theoretical issues about the value of medication in the overall treatment of a patient, as well as the practical issues of whether a psychotherapist can also be a medication provider.

During the 1960s and 1970s a battle raged between the "talking therapy" supporters and the "biological" school as to which method would best treat a person with psychological problems. Psychotherapists in the "therapy only" camp saw medications as intrusive, unnecessary, and even harmful. Their belief was that relief was provided by talking with patients, understanding their problems, and assisting in resolving developmental conflicts and early life traumas. Within this view, medications were at best marginally tolerated band-aids that missed the true nature of treatment and cure.

Some biologically oriented mental health professionals, on the other hand, began to assume that medication was the way to change brain functioning and that biological change was the only method leading to symptom relief. If the right combination of medication and/or medications could be found, the patient could eventually be "cured." In this framework, verbal therapy was superfluous and of relatively little value. Such clinicians also began to discount the importance of the prescriber/patient relationship, feeling that the only important mechanism was the chemical effect of the medication.

While vestiges of this debate remain, most clinicians now see value for both medication and psychotherapy. Both have importance, and both can result in symptom relief. Often the combination of medication and verbal therapy is the most efficient route to rapid symptom relief.[1,2]

It is a fundamental premise of this book that a combination of both forms of treatment, *psychotropic medication and psychotherapy* of various kinds, *will not only be helpful, but also* should *be prescribed for many patients*. While not all patients will opt for both therapies, it is the task of the clinician to reinforce that a combination of verbal and medication therapy is the preferred treatment.

The first session dilemma

Even if a patient is first screened over the telephone, an initial evaluative sessions can present the mental health clinician with a clinical decision. Is this to be a psychotherapy or medication evaluation? In general, this dilemma should be resolved in favor of evaluating for and prescribing medication at the earliest opportunity. While there is always a possibility that initial psychotherapeutic interventions may have a significant impact, even targeted verbal psychotherapy typically takes several sessions or longer to be significantly useful. On the other hand, medication can, for many patients, make significant and rapid inroads into symptomatology. Anti-anxiety, mood-stabilizing and antipsychotic medications can often be effective within a matter of days. While medication levels are slowly raised, psychotherapeutic interventions can then also be undertaken.

Another factor favoring early medication intervention is that psychological distress is often accompanied by (or has as an intrinsic feature) difficulty with concentration, attention and other cognitive functions. Full cognitive focus is often necessary to participate in and profit fully from verbal interventions. Therefore, if medication can positively affect the patient's cognitive focus, attention and energy level, patients can better utilize psychotherapy and be more involved in their own treatment.

In the course of the initial evaluation, if it appears that the patient is suffering from a condition that is likely to respond to medication and the patient is agreeable, the evaluation session should be structured as described in Chapter 3 to obtain the necessary information that can lead to medication prescription. If the clinician is in doubt or senses resistance on the patient's part regarding medication, it may be helpful to engage the patient in the decision and together negotiate how the process should proceed.

 TALKING TO PATIENTS

After you begin to hear the patient's initial complaints, one way to engage the patient in being an active part of this medication/psychotherapy decision is to say: "*I am hearing that you are experiencing ... [list the target symptoms] and having trouble with your [job, marriage, friendships, etc.]. I believe your symptoms may be helped with medication. In order to safely choose medication and begin it today, I need to gather some medical information. This will*

mean we won't be able to spend as much time talking about the problematic environmental issues in your life today. I know these issues are important to you, but we will not have time to focus on both. What do you think would be most helpful?"

If the patient agrees to evaluation for medication, proceed with the elements described in Chapter 3. If the patient opts for discussing family/environmental/interpersonal issues, it is seldom helpful to insist on medication until the patient has had the opportunity to deal with these concerns even if it requires several visits to do so. If you feel strongly about the probable positive benefit of medication, an agreement can be made to follow the patient's preference during this visit. At the end of the session, state that you would like to discuss the medication issue at the next session and mention the reasons why you believe this might be helpful. This allows the patient to have an opportunity to mull over the idea in the interim.

Patient's preference

At times, patients come to the clinician with a clear agenda in mind for the type of treatment they desire – medication alone or psychotherapy alone. In this case, it is not unreasonable initially to accede to the patient's wishes, even if combination therapy may ultimately be seen as desirable. Patients who have verbal therapy as a goal may show considerable resistance to starting medication. If the clinician automatically launches into the medication evaluation and prescription, the patient will feel that important issues are being ignored or overlooked. Once psychotherapy has begun and a trusting relationship has been established, and if symptoms persist, the suggestion of medication may be better received.

Likewise, patients who present requesting medication may be reluctant to undertake psychotherapy until they have evaluated the benefit of medication alone. Patients who believe in the primary value of medication are often resistant to, and apprehensive about, entering into a verbal therapy relationship and revealing personal history. If the medication management relationship with the prescribing clinician proceeds well, patients may be open to entering into a more in-depth psychotherapy. When the clinician is non-judgmental, accepting, and supportive, patients begin to trust and confide.

While it is the duty of the clinician to recommend combined therapy when appropriate, little is lost in the treatment of most outpatients with mild to moderate symptoms by taking a "wait and re-evaluate" approach while beginning the type of therapy the patient prefers.

Introducing medication therapy may become necessary for a patient involved in ongoing psychotherapy who experiences a sudden life crisis. Crises such as a death, job change, serious illness, financial reversal, separation, or divorce can significantly upset the equilibrium of the patient's life, and verbal therapy alone may be insufficient. The introduction of medication at that time may be a useful and welcome intervention. The reverse can also be true. A successfully treated "medication only" patient may find, in the face of a crisis, that more frequent active verbal intervention and support is needed. Individual, couple's, or family therapy can provide the necessary help to stabilize the crisis situation.

What can medication do?

A continuing and evolving area of research is the question of what can, and what cannot, be treated with medication. While illness symptoms involving behavior, affect, anxiety and mood can be positively modified by medication, there are many aspects of what we label as "personality" that cannot be changed or modified significantly with medication. Even among psychopharmacologists, there is significant debate as to whether it would be useful or desirable to alter personality structure. It is the premise of this book that the major mental illnesses – depression, bipolar disorder, anxiety disorders, and psychosis – involve symptoms that profoundly and negatively affect the way people feel and function. As practitioners, we can and should treat the symptoms of these illnesses in an attempt to help the patient. The borderline between treating these symptoms and treating underlying personality remains blurred. Although some may fear that we have already crossed (or will soon cross) the line into areas of the human mind that we should not be modifying, we are still far from being able satisfactorily to treat many of the symptoms that are clearly disabling to our patients. To fail to continue to treat illness as we refine the borderline between illness and personality ignores our calling, as healthcare professionals, to heal.

Who prescribes psychotropic medication?

When psychotropic medication emerged into clinical practice during the 1950s and 1960s, it was the province of the psychiatrist to prescribe. Many changes in the medical and mental health landscape have occurred to change the way psychotropic medication is provided. These include:

■ Growing demand for mental health prescription
■ Fewer psychiatrists to meet this demand, particularly in underserved locations and populations
■ Increasing safety and ease of prescribing newer psychotropics
■ Emerging comfort of primary care providers in prescribing psychotropics
■ Growth in the number of advanced practice nurse prescribers, both in primary care and in mental health
■ Financial pressure to provide mental health care in the most cost-effective manner.

There are now three common delivery systems for provision of psychotropic medication and mental health therapies:

1 A single person (psychiatrist or advanced practice mental health nurse with prescriptive authority) who provides both mental health therapy and medication

2 A non-medical psychotherapist (psychologist, social worker, psychiatric nurse, counselor, or other mental health professional) who provides mental health counseling and therapy, with medication provided by a mental health specialist (psychiatrist or advanced practice mental health nurse)

3 A non-medical psychotherapist providing psychotherapy with the primary care provider (family practice physician/advanced practice nurse, internist, OB/GYN, or other medical specialist) prescribing the psychotropic medication.

Each modality has advantages and disadvantages, and these are listed in Tables 7.1–7.3.

While much philosophical debate remains as to the desirability of who should prescribe, some communities simply do not have sufficient numbers of mental health prescribers to provide a service, even if that is desired. In other communities, multiple variations of the above three delivery systems co-exist.

Table 7.1 One-stop shopping – psychiatrist or advanced practice mental health nurse only

Advantages	Disadvantages
Simple, efficient for patient	Most expensive method of delivering medication and psychotherapy
Unified treatment approach	
Works well for patients with complicated psychotropic medication regimens	Mental health specialists may be less expert in the evaluation/treatment of other medical conditions

Table 7.2 Non-medical psychotherapist with mental health specialist prescribing (psychiatrist or advanced practitioner nurse)

Advantages	Disadvantages
Less expensive than "one-stop shopping"	Requires good communication between two parties, or mixed messages to the patient may result
Allows specialists to do what they do best	May be inconvenient for patient to see two different practitioners
Better than psychotherapist plus primary care provider (PCP) for complicated mental health problems, poorly responding patients, or a frequently changing medication regimen	

Table 7.3 Non-medical psychotherapist with primary care provider (PCP) prescribing psychotropics

Advantages	Disadvantages
Allows for smoother integration of mental health care in a patient with multiple medical complaints	Requires frequent communication to ensure unified treatment
Less costly method of prescription of psychotropic (compared to a mental health specialist)	PCP may not have most expert knowledge about complicated mental health conditions, combination treatments, unresponsive patients, or a regimen that requires frequent adjustment
Useful for patients on a stable medication regimen with minimal side effects	
Easy access to serum levels/laboratory tests	
Can permit simpler access to insurance formularies	May be inconvenient for the patient to see two different practitioners

References

1   Lenze E *et al*. Combined pharmacotherapy and psychotherapy as maintenance treatment for late-life depression: effects on social adjustment. *Am J Psychiatry* 2002;159:466–468.
2   Barlow DH *et al*. Cognitive-behavioral therapy, Imipramine, or their combination for panic disorder: a randomized controlled trial. *JAMA* 2000;283:2529–2536.

Chapter 8

Stopping medication

One of the first questions patients ask, often before they even begin medication, is "How long do I have to take this?" Beyond a straightforward request for information, the patient may be asking what the clinician's viewpoint is on the commonly held myth that once a person starts on a psychotropic medication it must be continued for life. At other times, the question may be based on the assumption that there will be a number of side effects to "bear with," and the patient wants to know how long the period of discomfort will be. These questions are an opportunity for the prescriber to begin to discuss the "game plan" for medication treatment.

There are relatively few patients who are started on medication and continue indefinitely without at least one medication-free trial to observe for relapse. While in fact a percentage of patients do need medication on a chronic or life-long basis, this is recommended only when the clinician is armed with the results of at least one trial off the medication. During a first trial starting medication, there are almost no historical or response data that will accurately predict whether or not a patient will need to stay on medication indefinitely. Severity of illness, length of symptoms prior to treatment, length of time needed for response to medication or family history of emotional illness cannot accurately foretell whether a patient will require long-term medication. However, *during a first medication trial it is not sound clinical practice to automatically assume that chronic, long-term medication will be necessary.* The number of previously documented illness episodes may suggest that relapse is likely at some point, but not always *when* this will occur.

The one useful predictor available to the clinician during a second or subsequent trial of medication is the result of previous trials off medication. If a patient has been on medication for this condition, tried off medication on several occasions, and relapsed quickly into similar symptomatology, there is a strong likelihood that it will happen again.

TALKING TO PATIENTS

When a patient, during a first medicine trial, asks "Will I be on this forever?" the answer is invariably:

"We do not know yet and I assume not. Here is how we will find out ..." followed by discussing the regimen outlined here and in Chapter 5. Knowing that he or she will be taken off medicine at a certain time in the future will usually satisfy the patient so that the trial can be started.

The clinician can and should *involve the patient in the decision of when discontinuation of medication is attempted.* Some measure of knowledge that the clinician has flexibility as to when this trial will occur goes a long way toward initially securing the patient's compliance.

A significant number of patients who come to the treatment setting resistant and skeptical about medication may change their mind when they notice the positive results that the medicine achieves. When the issue of stopping the medication is raised, they may actually be quite apprehensive and hesitant about stopping. In such patients, the principle of a medication discontinuation is not abandoned, but a short delay is not unreasonable, if necessary, to accommodate and help them deal with their apprehension.

When to stop

If possible, do not try the patient off medication in the midst of a major life event (see Table 8.1). Stopping at the same time as a job change, final exams, marriage, divorce, changing residences, moving to a different town, taking a promotion, or undergoing other significant life stress leaves both the patient and the clinician uncertain as to the cause if relapse does occur. Did the symptoms recur from stopping the medication, or from this significant life stress? In general, it is much better to find a relative lull in the patient's life to attempt medication stoppage. Then, if any symptoms do recur, these can be more clearly related to stopping the medication. If the patient is in concomitant psychotherapy while taking medication, it is also preferable not to stop psychotherapy and medication at the same time for similar reasons. Faced with major life stressors, it is preferable to err on

Table 8.1 Issues related to stopping medication

When?
- Usually after 6–12 months of remission
- No simultaneous big life changes
- Include the patient in the decision

How?
- Gradual taper
- Speed of the taper depends on current dose, and the length of administration
- Assess the patient's feelings

the side of continuing a few months "too long" and perhaps finding out that the patient could have done without medication rather than discontinuing medication "too soon" and creating a significant crisis in a patient's life, which is already altered by the current stressor.

In today's society, there are patients for whom a good "smooth spot" in their life cannot be found. Even after several delays, their lives continue to be busy and hectic. Eventually, for these patients, the patient and clinician must decide on an appropriate stopping time even if it is not ideal. On occasion, this can be as long as several years from the initiation of medication.

With depression, there is statistical evidence[1] to help us decide the earliest possible time to stop medication. The rate of relapse curve (i.e. the percentage of patients who relapse when medication is stopped) flattens out 32 weeks (about 8 months) after remission (see Figure 8.1).

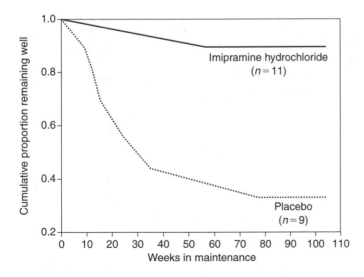

Figure 8.1 Survival analysis for maintenance therapies in the recurrent depression extended study. Difference between the two groups, $p = 0.006$ by the Mantel-Cox test.

As can be seen, the rate of relapse is minimally greater at 10 months or 12 months than it is at 8 months. This suggests that for mild to moderate depression, "the earliest opportunity" when a decision to stop medication could be made is 6 months from the time of remission. If a patient has had a significant major depression or prolonged response time to full recovery, a longer time on medication is desirable. Continuing medication for 9–12 months *from the time of remission* (not the time of starting medication) will allow the patient sufficient opportunity for his or her life to recover from the disruption of a significant depressive episode. These timeframes likewise apply to panic disorder, generalized anxiety disorder, and social anxiety disorder.

Medication for less severe episodes of depression and anxiety can be reasonably stopped 6 months after remission has been achieved. Although the statistical evidence is far less complete, generally medications for a first episode of bipolar disorder and psychosis conditions, which tend to be quite disruptive to the patient's life, should be continued for a minimum of 9–12 months.

Tapering medications

The brain is sensitive to changes in blood levels of psychotropic medications. With a few exceptions (see below), medication should always be gradually tapered rather than discontinued suddenly. The speed of such a taper will depend on the patient's *dose* and *duration* of medication administration (see Table 8.2). When faced with a choice, a slower taper is almost always preferable to (and safer than) a rapid one.

In general, the higher the dose of medication and the longer the patient has been on the medication, the more gradual the taper. For someone who has been on a small dose of medication for a short period of time, a taper may not be necessary.

While this overall regimen is appropriate in the vast majority of patients, it can be modified depending on the special circumstances of each individual patient. These can include their feelings about, and reaction to, the initial taper. A very hesitant patient or one who shows a greater than expected reaction to the initial lowering of doses may benefit from a slower taper.

Table 8.2 **Discontinuing medications**

Low-moderate dose/short administration (less than 6 months)
- Decrease by 25–50% of maintenance dose
- Every 1–2 weeks

High dose/long administration (greater than 6 months)
- Decrease by 10–25% of maintenance dose
- Every 2–4 weeks

Table 8.3 Psychotropics that may cause discontinuation syndromes

■ SSRIs, particularly short half-life compounds such as paroxetine and venlafaxine.
■ TCAs
■ MAOIs

Table 8.4 Psychotropics that do not cause discontinuation syndromes

■ Mood stabilizers, including lithium, valproic acid, and carbamazepine
■ Antipsychotics, both traditional and atypical

"When I stopped, I got worse"

Most psychotropics are not habit-forming, and do not cause "withdrawal" in the traditional sense. Some medications, particularly some antidepressants, do cause a discontinuation syndrome (which is a set of primarily physical symptoms) if the medicine is stopped suddenly. It is important to recognize this syndrome, both to educate and reassure the patient, and to treat it when necessary. Particularly when they occur without warning, the symptoms of discontinuation syndrome can be significantly distressing to patients. The medications that do, and do not, cause a discontinuation syndrome are listed in Tables 8.3 and 8.4, respectively. Clues that a discontinuation syndrome is occurring are listed in Table 8.5.

The following sections will discuss discontinuation syndromes as they occur in specific medication groups.

SSRI discontinuation syndrome

The most common SSRI discontinuation symptoms are dizziness, nausea, lethargy, and headaches[2] (see Table 8.6). The dizziness and lack of equilibrium are often the most bothersome symptoms to patients, and are most noticeable when patients rotate their head quickly. They may feel that they will lose their balance, although they seldom do.

Table 8.5 Tips-offs that a discontinuation syndrome may be occurring

■ A recent stoppage of a medication has preceded the symptoms, especially if it was done suddenly and rapidly. Discontinuation syndrome occasionally happens *during* a taper of medication
■ Patient has been on the medication for at least 5 weeks
■ Onset of symptoms within 1–3 days
■ Symptoms go away, or are substantially improved, in 7–10 days
■ Symptoms remit if the medication is restarted or increased in dose

Table 8.6 Symptoms of an SSRI discontinuation syndrome

- Dizziness, light-headedness, dysequilibrium
- Nausea, vomiting, diarrhea, stomach upset
- Agitation/irritability
- Difficulty sleeping
- Depression/low mood
- Flushing, sweating, tremors
- "Electric shock" sensations in various parts of the body
- "Flu-like" symptoms, muscle aches

*Adapted from Antidepressant discontinuation syndromes: common, under-recognized and not always benign. *Drug Ther Persp* 2001;17(20):12–15.

Table 8.7 Symptoms of a TCA discontinuation syndrome

- Nausea, vomiting, diarrhea, stomach upset
- Agitation/irritability
- Difficulty sleeping
- Depression/low mood
- Flushing, sweating, tremors

TCA discontinuation syndrome

TCA discontinuation syndrome, as shown in Table 8.7, includes the symptoms mentioned above for SSRIs, but the dysequilibrium and the sensory, "electric shock," and "flu-like" symptoms occur far less often.

Benzodiazepine discontinuation

Tapering benzodiazepine anti-anxiety medication may also lead to some confusion on the part of the clinician. When benzodiazepines are stopped suddenly from moderate doses, there can be symptoms of true physiological withdrawal that can include those listed in Table 8.8.

These symptoms can overlap with, and be confused with, relapse of the initial anxiety condition for which the patient was being treated. Therefore, a gradual taper of benzodiazepines is useful and gives the clinician and patient the best chance to distinguish any mild withdrawal symptoms from relapse of the anxiety

Table 8.8 Symptoms of benzodiazepine withdrawal

- Sweating
- Tremor
- Agitation
- Nausea
- Rapid pulse

disorder. Rapid, sudden stoppage of very high doses of benzodiazepines can cause seizures; therefore, patients on large amounts of benzodiazepines should always be tapered slowly.

Antipsychotics and mood stabilizers

Although antipsychotic medications and mood stabilizers do not cause a discontinuation syndrome, they still should be tapered as gradually as possible for other reasons. Because of the intense and potentially life disrupting symptoms of bipolar disorder and psychosis, lengthy tapers are preferred. This gives both the clinician and the patient an opportunity to see any return of symptomatology at a low level, long before full-blown mania or psychosis occurs. The clinician may then quickly raise the dose if psychotic or manic symptoms appear, before a serious episode emerges. Although it would be pharmacologically safe to taper the medication over a several-week period, it is often clinically more helpful to taper over several months, with intermittent visits, appointments and evaluations by the clinician to observe for potential relapse. *Stopping antipsychotic medications and mood stabilizers does not cause a discontinuation syndrome.*

Stimulants

Stopping the chronic use of a stimulant medication, particularly if large doses have been taken for more than several weeks, can result in a withdrawal syndrome that presents a clinical picture quite different from the antidepressant and benzodiazepine withdrawal syndromes described above. Since stimulants promote wakefulness, decreased appetite and increased energy, and are antidepressant, sudden withdrawal of these compounds results in transient reversal of these effects. Stimulant withdrawal is characterized by the symptoms listed in Table 8.9.

With the exception of the depressed mood that, when severe, may be accompanied by significant suicidal ideation (a "crash"), the physical signs of stimulant withdrawal are annoying to the patient but are not intrinsically dangerous. They generally pass in 3–7 days.

Management of discontinuation syndromes

Once mild discontinuation symptoms have been identified and the time-limited nature of their occurrence outlined, most patients can tolerate them satisfactorily

Table 8.9 Symptoms of stimulant withdrawal

- Increased somnolence
- Decreased motivation, lethargy/fatigue
- Increased appetite and eating
- Poor concentration
- Depressed mood

Table 8.10 Management strategies for discontinuation syndromes

- Slow the taper
- Return to a previous comfortable dose to accommodate a more gradual subsequent taper (when an extra or higher dose is prescribed and the symptoms remit, it is a useful indicator that discontinuation syndrome is active and is the likely cause of the symptoms)
- Substitute longer half-life medications for short half-life compounds, and then taper the long half-life medications

without treatment. If reassurance and support are not sufficient to make the situation tolerable, or the symptoms are severe, active management may be necessary as shown in Table 8.10.

Common examples of the last strategy in this table include substituting fluoxetine (a long half-life compound) for paroxetine (a short half-life compound). Fluoxetine plus nortriptyline can substitute for venlafaxine. These longer half-life products, or combinations, can often be tapered more comfortably with fewer symptoms of discontinuation.

Relapse vs discontinuation syndrome

Since symptoms of discontinuation may overlap, in part, with the symptoms of the original condition being treated with the antidepressant, it is important to make the distinction between these two phenomena. *The most important criterion to differentiate relapse (return of original depressed symptoms) from a discontinuation syndrome (caused by stopping the medication) is the time in which symptoms progress or disappear.*

Discontinuation syndrome symptoms almost invariably go away within 10 days. If symptoms have not gone away, or have not substantially improved, by the seventh day, the possibility of relapse is more likely.

Other signs suggestive of relapse are:

- Increasing intensity, rather than decreasing intensity over time
- A repetition of the signs and symptoms of the original illness (rather than new symptoms)
- Gradual occurrence rather than sudden onset (which is more likely with discontinuation syndrome).

If a patient experiences significant symptoms of relapse during a taper, it is usually of little value to continue the taper. Once relapse is definitively diagnosed and distinguished from rebound, "getting over the hump" does not occur. If the taper is continued, the clinician is usually forced to restart the medication later, but with a more severely depressed patient.

Most patients "know" when they are having a relapse of symptomatology, and their report can generally be trusted. It bears repeating that antidepressants are not, in general, habit-forming, and are not abusable. There is, in general, no street market for SSRIs, tricyclics or other new-generation antidepressants. Therefore, when patients say, "I need the medicine again," they are usually right.

When to stop medication more quickly

The exceptions to the "gradual taper" rule are few but important. They include when the patient becomes *pregnant*, develops *an allergy*, or suffers *serious side effects*.

Most patients when they become pregnant will want to discontinue medication as rapidly as possible. If, after a discussion of the risks and/or benefits of stopping medication, it is decided to discontinue medication, do so quickly. While it is possible that this may lead to some discontinuation phenomena with antidepressants or benzodiazepines, it is medicolegally preferable, and often fits with most patient's wishes. Many women would rather take the risk that rebound symptoms may occur than extend the medication period significantly into the first trimester of pregnancy. This is discussed more in depth in Chapter 11.

If the patient develops an allergy to the medication, it is better to stop the medicine, if necessary precipitously, than risk the intensification of allergic symptoms that themselves may be life threatening.

While rare, serious side effects (including seizure, fainting episodes, dramatic decreases in white blood cell count, severe vomiting, documented heart rhythm irregularity, or gastrointestinal bleeding) are other reasons to stop medication at once. While the statistical likelihood of each of these side effects is low (see Chapter 17), when they occur in a particular patient they become a crisis. It is much easier to justify stopping the medication and dealing with any rebound symptomatology than to continue the medication that may perpetuate these intense and life-threatening side effects.

New episode or relapse?

For purposes of documenting whether returning symptoms are part of a new episode of illness or part of a relapse from a current episode of illness, it is arbitrarily assumed that if patients have not experienced any similar symptoms within a 2-month period following stoppage of the medication, they have recovered from this particular episode. If the symptoms do recur within that 2-month period, it is again (rather arbitrarily) assumed that this is a relapse of the initial episode.

Side effects pass quickly

When medications are stopped, *side effects often disappear before therapeutic effects*. If a patient decides prematurely to stop medications, and some objectionable side effects resolve, the patient may believe that he or she is better off not taking the medication. This may be true in terms of the objectionable side effects, and the patient, if initially feeling well emotionally, may be resistant to restart the medication. In this circumstance, both clinician and patient need to observe carefully for signs of relapse over the next 1–6 weeks. If such relapse occurs, a return to medication should be suggested. If the objectionable side effects were sufficiently uncomfortable and the patient is resistant to restarting the original medication, a change of medication may be more favorably received.

Unplanned stoppages of medication

The above sections of this chapter refer to planned stoppages of medication. Patients may, however, stop medication on their own without contacting the clinician. When this occurs, the clinician should not automatically assume that this is a significant problem. The situation can be a useful opportunity to assess the outcome, renegotiate a contract, and form a more workable agreement with the patient. These unplanned stoppages can occur in a number of ways, as shown in Table 8.11.

Commonly, a patient who has made a unilateral decision to stop medication fails to follow through with an appointment. If there is a missed appointment and no contact from the patient, the clinician should always call to discover the reason for the absence. The clinician needs to find out if the patient has just forgotten the appointment, has decided to stop medication, has decided to see another clinician, or has not come for another reason. If the medication has been prematurely stopped, written documentation of the patient's decision should be made in the chart.

At other times, patients will come for their assigned follow-up session, but indicate to the clinician that they have unilaterally decided to stop one or more of the medications they have been taking. This is often cloaked in the notion that they "forgot" a dose of medicine for several days, and decided to use this as an opportunity to see what would happen when they were medication-free. In other cases, patients may have been experiencing a particularly problematic side effect, decided they could not tolerate the medication, and stopped it without contacting the clinician.

Some patients may present for an appointment and insist on stopping the medication, even though they have not yet done so. Despite a recommendation from the clinician that they stay on the medication longer, patients may insist that they cannot, or will not, continue medication.

Table 8.11 **Possible causes of unplanned stoppages**

- The patient fails to show up for an appointment and has no more medication
- The patient makes a unilateral decision to stop medication
- The patient is experiencing side effects
- The patient thinks he or she is well and no longer needs medication
- The patient cannot afford to purchase the medication

In any of these scenarios, patients' decisions may represent an open, overt wish to stop medication because:

- They no longer wish to take it
- They are having trouble tolerating it
- They think they are well.

At other times there will be a hidden agenda in stopping of the medication, such as:

- They are having a *side effect* they have not told you about (e.g. sexual problems)
- They may be receiving resistance from someone important to them. A spouse, parent or child may have been giving them information that counters what you have been telling them, and convinced them that being off medication is the better course of action. Occasionally, this other person may be another medical professional who has told them that the medication may be harmful or that they "don't need it"
- They perceive an unspoken downside to "successful" medication treatment (for example, manic patients may not want to give up the ability to work long hours in a day because it keeps their income high or raises their stature in the eyes of a supervisor).

Regardless of the reason, when patients stop medication prematurely, it does not mean that the clinician must stop contact and involvement with them. It can be a useful opportunity to reassess the status of the current treatment and, if necessary, revise the plan in a mutually agreed fashion. Some patients will wish to continue contact with the clinician even if they are not taking medication. They will continue using the clinician for support, guidance, clarification, and help with their life problems, even though they stopped taking their pills. A clinician can stay in contact with a patient, and continue to be a support, without agreeing that stoppage of the medication was a good thing. It may be quite appropriate to take a "wait and see" approach to medication stoppage, while both clinician and patient watch for any significant change.

When patients stop medication prematurely, the clinician may be surprised to find that they do reasonably well off medication. Even experienced clinicians have had the experience of thinking that a patient needed medication, and was likely to seriously relapse without it, only to find that the patient stopped medicine safely and satisfactorily without relapse. We are far from omniscient in knowing how medication will affect patients.

Ambivalent patients who have stopped medication and then do relapse may become much more cooperative than they were initially in retrying the same or another medication. Many reticent patients need to prove to themselves that they are going to relapse before continuing medication. Only when they do so are they willing to become more engaged in the treatment process, and to take medications on a regular basis.

After stopping medication, some patients experience a partial relapse, but decide that limited symptoms are tolerable. The clinician may have no choice but to go along with this, even if this level of symptomatology leaves the patient partially handicapped in the clinician's eyes. Although some patients will see relatively quickly that they are not doing well and need to be back on medication, others may take months or years to make that decision. Sometimes, only at this later date when a patient returns does the clinician hear about a hidden agenda that was not discussed when the patient initially stopped medication.

References

1   Kupfer D *et al*. Five-year outcome for maintenance therapies in recurrent depression. *Arch Gen Psych* 1992;49:769–773.
2   Haddad P. The SSRI discontinuation syndrome. *J Psychopharmacology* 1998;12(3):305–313.

Chapter 9

The long-term patient

Chapter 8 described the issues involved in stopping medication. Once discontinued, many patients do well off medication without recurrence of symptoms. While it is incorrect to assume initially that all patients will need long-term or life-long medication for their mental health problems, a significant percentage of patients do relapse when they discontinue medication. If relapses are frequent or occur quickly after medication is stopped, the clinician and patient together should consider the possibility of maintenance, longer-term medications to block further relapses or minimize their extent. As with many issues regarding mental health medication, it is important to include the patient in the decision regarding if, and when, a maintenance medication program is begun.

For some patients, the decision to continue on medication "for the foreseeable future" can be relieving and reassuring. When medication serves to prevent or minimize future illness, patients' lives are considerably smoother and more comfortable, and have a consistency that allows them to grow, maximize work potential and have greater satisfaction in relationships. For other patients, the decision to stay on medication is an extraordinarily difficult one that will be resisted, sometimes strongly. For these patients, staying on medication long-term raises many of the same issues they felt when starting medication: "Am I weak?" "Shouldn't I be able to control my symptoms with my mind and will?" "Am I a constitutionally inferior person?" "Why does this keep happening to me?" Concerns about side effects of long-term medication usage, medication interactions, pregnancy or menopause can also arise.

Even some persons who consent to take medication chronically do so with resistance, reluctance and a feeling of having "failed." Internally, such patients may never feel that this is a positive decision, and consent only because of a feeling that there is no other choice. Some patients who resist the clinician's suggestion for a maintenance medication regimen will relapse, sometimes seriously. Despite repeated relapses, some patients remain doggedly resistant to the concept of taking medication over the long term.

Who should receive long-term treatment?

Several factors are important in deciding when to suggest long-term medication treatment to a patient. This decision is seldom made after the initial (index) symptom episode, except in unusual and high-risk situations. More likely, a plan for maintenance will occur after one or several relapses off medication.

Factors that the clinician should consider in recommending maintenance medication include:

1 Relapse characteristics
   - The *speed* with which the onset of relapse occurs
   - The *number of relapse episodes*
   - The *intensity and strength* of each relapse episode
   - The *length of time that it takes to return to health and full functioning* after re-starting medication.
2 The patient's condition while on medication
   - Assessment of *the intensity and interference from medication side effects* that a patient experiences while on medications
   - The *level of symptom control* when taking medication. Is the improvement mild, modest or significant?
3 Personal characteristics and preferences
   - The *patient's level of insight and awareness* regarding his or her own psychological state
   - The patient's *ability to recognize signs of relapse*
   - The *patient's wishes.*
4 Support System
   - The extent and consistency of *family or other support*
   - Sometimes, the *wishes of the patient's family.*

In general, patients with mild to moderate depression, anxiety disease, or symptoms of bipolar disorder will have had a minimum of two relapses after the initial index episode before chronic medication is likely to be considered. For some patients, this principle may be shortened to one relapse following the initial index episode. If the first relapse after the index episode is particularly serious, long lasting or slow to recovery, the clinician may decide to suggest maintenance treatment with medication without waiting for a third episode. A first relapse of psychosis will generally require strong consideration of prophylactic long-term medication.

Other indications that may prompt a clinician to suggest an earlier institution of long-term medication are relapse episodes that include:

- Significant deficits of functioning
- Severe loss of work productivity
- Deep marital discord
- Threats or episodes of self-harm, or harm to others.

Since patients vary greatly in their feelings about taking medication long term, it is important to assess such feelings and take them into account when deciding whether or not to use medication chronically. Patients who have been intensely dysphoric or have had significant lifestyle interruptions because of their illness are often justifiably frightened about further relapses, and these patients may request chronic medication even before the clinician is ready to consider it. When patients raise this issue it becomes an important point of negotiation, and one that should be openly discussed with them and, if indicated, with their family.

At other times, patients may be resistant to maintenance medication even when the clinician feels it would be desirable. Assuming that they are legally competent, patients may need to experience relapses and the consequences of the relapses more often than the clinician feels is helpful. While clinicians may advise and recommend maintenance medication, patients remain masters of their own domain and may choose medication-free intervals, even if the likely result, in the clinician's judgment, is future relapses.

A situation that occurs with some frequency is that of the family wishing to have an identified patient remain on maintenance medication when the patient does not agree. The patient may be overtly opposed to this medication plan, does not see the need for it, or feels that the side effects of the medication are unacceptable. Patients who become angry, disagreeable, less productive, socially isolated, or substance abusers when they relapse can be a significant irritation or worry to their families. Unless the patient has become an acute danger to self or others, however, families may need to accept relapses and persistent symptoms when the patient refuses chronic medication. Except in the case of an incompetent patient with a legal guardian, it is the identified patient, not the family, who will make the final decision. The clinician may see the problem and recommend, or even suggest strongly, that medication could be useful, but the final decision rests with the patient and not with the family.

At times, the family may use incentives or disincentives to induce the patient to take medication. These incentives may include willingness to offer housing, financial support or transportation that are provided only on the agreement that the patient complies with long-term medication treatment. A spouse or partner may only agree to stay in a relationship with the patient if medication is continued. Patients may complain about such arrangements, but ultimately have the choice of whether or not to participate.

A symptomatic crisis in a stable patient – general principles

Long-term patients, who may be doing well on medication maintenance with minimal symptomatology, can present to the clinician describing a new onset of depressive, anxiety, manic or psychotic symptoms. The challenge then facing the clinician is assessing these breakthrough symptoms. The most difficult issue, but also the most important, is determining whether or not the new symptoms represent a true relapse (and hence a medication failure), for which additional medication intervention is likely to help. A relapse indicative of medication failure needs to be differentiated from new or transient symptoms that would respond best to psychotherapy, lifestyle alteration, or other interventions that do not require medication change. Sometimes utilizing both pharmacological and non-pharmacological methods is necessary.

In order to assess this important but sometimes complicated question, issues regarding both medications and lifestyle need to be addressed by the clinician. It is often necessary to revisit areas of evaluation that have been initially assessed during the early stages of evaluation and treatment. A specific guideline for this process is outlined in the next section of this chapter.

When the issues below are evaluated, it may be quite clear to the clinician what is most likely to account for the patient's new symptoms. In some cases, inappropriate dosing, changes in regimen, or other medical causes have altered the physiological blood level of the patient's psychotropic medication. If so, patient education along with a change of psychotropic dosage may re-establish equilibrium fairly rapidly.

In other circumstances, medication issues have little to do with the new symptoms. Major life stressors alone may have precipitated symptom emergence. It is remarkable how often patients do not see or understand the connection between major issues in their life, and the triggering of symptoms or relapse. It is only after the clinician has raised such a possibility that the patient begins to see the connection. When this is the case, making the connection may be sufficient for the patient to understand and endure the symptoms and/or make appropriate changes to improve the situation. At other times, it may be necessary to recommend new or increased psychotherapy sessions, or some other behavioral intervention to deal with the patient's stressors. For occupational stressors, a change of work hours, intervention with a supervisor, or a leave of absence may be necessary to allow the symptoms to remit. On those occasions when behavioral stressors are time-limited and likely to be concluded within a short period, observation and waiting may be all that is necessary. To deal with personal stressors, individual, marital or family treatment may be indicated.

As with the initial decision to start medication, *the most important criterion to determine whether more or different medication is necessary is the amount of functional disruption that is occurring because of the symptoms.* When functional disruption is significant, in spite of a seemingly adequate medication regimen or environmental stressors that may need be amended, a change of medication is often warranted. When possible, a change to another medication within the same classification can be useful. If monotherapy is ineffective, the addition of a second or even a third medication may be necessary. For some conditions, medications within one classification (e.g. antipsychotics or mood stabilizers) may achieve a satisfactory response and renewed equilibrium. Combining different classifications of medications, such as adding an antidepressant to a mood stabilizer, adding an anti-anxiety medication to an antidepressant, or adding an antidepressant or anti-anxiety medicine to an antipsychotic medication, may also yield positive results. Each patient must be individually evaluated to determine the medication formula to be adopted.

"The medicine stopped working" – getting back on TRACCCC

For a patient who has experienced relapse or has breakthrough symptoms after a long period of stability on medication, a useful acronym for the clinician is "getting the patient back on TRACCCC" (see Table 9.1). This acronym guides the clinician to those elements that should be addressed in evaluating significant breakthrough symptoms. The acronym is a useful memory device, although in real world clinical situations the practitioner applies these items in a slightly different order (Re-evaluation, Alcohol, Compliance, then Talking therapy and Changing medication followed by Combination therapy and Consultation).

Talking therapy

Many patients who are managed on medication alone and develop a symptomatic crisis may need the initiation of psychotherapy or *talking therapy*. Patients who have developed new stressors in life may find it considerably useful to have a short course of individual therapy, cognitive therapy, couples treatment or family therapy to deal with new or worsened stressors in their life. Patients who may have been resistant to psychotherapy when medication was first begun can be more amenable to such therapy when a symptomatic crisis emerges. For patients who have been on a "medication only" regimen, the clinician may wish to be more insistent on the necessity of psychotherapy. In doing so, the clinician

Table 9.1 Getting back on TRACCCC

Talking therapy
Re-evaluation
Alcohol and drugs
Compliance
Change medication
Combination therapy
Consultation

reinforces the known benefits of the combination of psychotherapy and medication in the treatment of most emotional illnesses.

Re-evaluation

The clinician should consider a diagnostic and symptomatic *re-evaluation*. A re-evaluation is the cornerstone of assessing relapse and should cover five different areas:

1 Diagnosis
2 Medication
3 Lifestyle
4 Alcohol and drugs
5 Compliance.

If a patient has developed new or returning symptoms, it is sometimes because the clinician's initial assessment was only partially correct, or was incorrect. A depressed patient may in fact have bipolar disorder. A patient diagnosed with panic attacks may develop a depressive episode. A schizophrenic patient may develop a substance abuse problem. A patient with a mood disorder may develop significant anxiety – in the form of either generalized anxiety or panic attacks. Any of these may not have been recognized in the initial assessment. Particularly if it has been a long time since the initial evaluation, it is useful to conduct a fresh assessment of symptoms, even when the patient may have given negative responses in the past to questions about specific symptoms. It is surprising how often new, useful, and previously unrevealed information can be elicited in a re-evaluation done 1 or 2 years after the initial assessment.

There are many reasons why additional or new information may be elicited:

■ Patients may have developed new symptoms that were not present originally
■ Patients have begun to reformulate certain behaviors or feelings as "symptoms" that were not seen as symptoms at the time they were originally seen
■ Patients may have been embarrassed to admit to certain symptoms on an initial visit to a new clinician for fear the clinician would refuse to treat them or look negatively on them because of their symptoms or behavior.

Regarding medication

■ Is the patient getting proper amounts of medication? Exactly how much, how often, and when is the patient taking psychotropic medications? (Sometimes what the clinician is prescribing is *not* what the patient has been taking!)
■ Have any medical conditions arisen that may account for the patient's complaints? Some of these may be related to the medication prescribed, and others may not. For example, has the patient developed an unrelated medical condition that is altering his or her mental health status, such as diabetes mellitus, hypertension, mononucleosis, or hepatitis C?

■ Is the medication prescribed causing a medical complication? For example, if the patient is taking lithium, has he or she developed low thyroid function as a side effect? Have abnormalities of liver function begun as a reaction to the prescription given?

CLINICAL TIP

Appropriate medical screening laboratory tests are indicated for any sudden symptomatic crisis in an otherwise stable patient. This usually includes chemical tests of liver and kidney function, fasting blood sugar, TSH, CBC, and serum psychotropic levels, where appropriate.

■ What *non-psychiatric prescription medications* is the patient taking? Are any of these new?
■ Is the patient taking any new *over-the-counter preparations*? Has the patient begun a new generic preparation or other change in psychotropic preparation recently that could account for the new symptoms?

Symptomatic descriptors and lifestyle issues must also be considered:

■ When did these breakthrough symptoms begin?
■ Was the onset sudden or gradual?
■ Are these symptoms similar to the previous episode, or new?
■ What specific symptoms have occurred?
■ Is the onset of these symptoms associated with any life events?
■ Has the patient had any recent significant life stressors? (At times, significant stressors have occurred, but the patient has not associated these with the symptoms.)

Alcohol and drugs

A re-evaluation of the patient's substance use is necessary even when the patient has claimed limited or no substance use in the past. Alcohol or drug usage is one of the most common behaviors that patients may have minimized or not been willing to admit to when initially seen. At other times, the patient was in fact not using substances at the time of the initial diagnosis but has begun to do so now. If such usage is present, the clinician will need to reaffirm that it may interfere with the medication's ability to control symptoms and may have a substantial negative bearing on the patient's response. If the clinician's suspicion remains high, a blood screen for toxicology, a blood alcohol level, or a serum GGT can be warranted (see Chapter 14).

Compliance

As mentioned at other times in this text, patient compliance with medication is often a significant cause of incomplete response or loss of response. The clinician should evaluate the patient's compliance with the regimen that has been prescribed. It is often best to evaluate this with open-ended questions, such as: "Tell me exactly which medications you are taking and when you are taking them?" This way the clinician is more likely to get an accurate sense of what the patient is actually doing at home. This open-ended question is preferable to the clinician repeating the presumed regimen and then asking if the patient is following that regimen, which makes it far too easy for the patient to say "Yes" whether or not the medicine is actually being taken as prescribed.

Change medication

Changing medication is usually the most common and first remedy that most clinicians consider. It can be helpful in many situations but is not the only option.

Combination therapy

Combination medication therapy has become a common practice in psychopharmacology to treat break-through symptomatology. As has been covered in detail in Chapter 6, addition of another medicine from the same class or medications from different classes may return the patient to symptomatic stability. The synergy generated by two medications taken together can restore symptomatic control.

Consultation

A Consultation is almost always of benefit in a patient who is losing symptomatic response, particularly if a clinician has tried a number of remedies or therapies with minimal or no response. A primary care provider, as well as a mental health specialist, can benefit from consultation with a psychopharmacologist as to possible medication changes or additions. The simple act of having another practitioner evaluate the patient provides a "fresh look" at the patient's problems. Sometimes the current clinician may have fallen into "blind spots" as to the patient's diagnosis or treatment, and these may be relatively easily discovered by a practitioner with another viewpoint. Such consultation can also be of significant benefit to a patient who has been through a number of medications with limited success. Such patients become discouraged and frustrated, and begin doubting whether the primary clinician can help them. By obtaining a consultation, they are often renewed in their willingness to continue efforts toward symptomatic control.

Helping the patient stay well

When psychotropic medications are prescribed, patients often ask, "What else can I do, besides take the medication?" – that is to say, are there any lifestyle changes that may promote recovery and maintain wellness?

While it would be helpful if a specific dietary regimen were beneficial in mental health treatment, numerous studies over several decades have failed to demonstrate that specific *diets*, or specific dietary elements, are curative or have a major role to play in psychiatric wellness. The exceptions to this premise may be the use of omega-3 fatty acids (see p. 338) and folate in the treatment of mood disorders, and caffeine as a factor in producing or worsening anxiety. There is some evidence that less than adequate levels of folate may result in a higher non-response rate to antidepressants,[1,2] and that supplemental folate (500 mg) may[3,4] improve antidepressant response. More information will be necessary, however, before the monitoring and use of folate is routine. Other than these factors, in our current state of knowledge, diet plays a relatively little role in mental health treatment other than in maintaining balanced health and nutrition.

Vitamin supplements have also failed to be shown be as a primary treatment for mental illness. Except for vitamin supplements for the alcoholic patient, the significantly malnourished patient and the pregnant woman, most psychiatric patients do not require additional vitamins. Many of the preparations sold by health-food stores claiming to be helpful for depression, anxiety, or stress have little solid evidence to support their use, and can be quite costly.

Studies of the beneficial effects of *exercise* are numerous and results are generally consistent.[5,6,7] In children,[8] adults,[9] seniors,[10] men,[11] and women,[12] moderate amounts of vigorous exercise can improve mood and anxiety. Physical activity can increase strength and endurance, maintain bone density, improve cardiovascular capacity, lower blood pressure, and heighten the patient's sense of well-being. Clinician attention to the patient's lifestyle, with a focus on physical activity, is therefore clearly warranted.

Contrary to some popular notions, however, it has not been demonstrated that even vigorous physical exercise, alone or in combination with diet, can successfully treat severely mentally ill patients. While there are a multitude of benefits to including exercise as part of an overall regimen for general good health, it should not be assumed that exercise alone can substitute for more specific treatments such as psychotherapy and/or medication. Recommendations for increasing exercise should include doing so gradually, rather than suddenly, to avoid injury in the previously sedentary patient. Suggest that the patient work up to a goal of an exercise regimen of 30 minutes per day three times per week.[6,13]

Helping patients to assess and, when necessary, manage their workload, job expectations, and *work schedule* can also help them stay well. Appropriate diagnosis and targeted medication cannot overcome excessive work hours, failure to take breaks during the work day, postponing or eliminating vacations, or trying to please an overly demanding boss. It may be useful to discuss priorities with patients such that they can realistically meet their financial needs while balancing their work lives.

Missed appointments

Even the most conscientious patient, on occasion, will miss appointments. Emotionally upset and anxious patients are even more likely to do so. While some missed appointments may have psychological significance, not all such absences have deep pathological meaning.

Reasons for patients missing appointments include:

- Simple forgetting (yes, this happens!!)
- Confusion of appointment dates or times
- Unexpected environmental events (traffic, accidents, unexpected business appointments)
- Lack of money to pay for the appointment
- The patient unilaterally deciding to discontinue treatment
- Embarrassment at having to come to a mental health prescriber
- Not feeling it is necessary to monitor medications or keep an appointment
- Resistance to an appointment, because it is a reminder of illness/disability and the need for medication
- Part of a general psychological state of confusion, disorganization, and disorientation.

Patients maintain a wide spectrum of feelings regarding the importance of psychotropic medication management visits. To some, the appointments are crucially important, eagerly anticipated, and the highlight of a week or month. Other patients have little emotional reaction associated with such appointments, and see them as they would any other medical or professional appointments. Lastly, for some patients a medication management visit is an extraordinarily negatively colored chore that they attend only because it is insisted upon. For them such an appointment, like a painful dental appointment, is easily forgotten or attended late. If the clinician provides no incentive to keep an appointment, absences will become increasingly frequent. Repeated missed appointments will usually result in frequent off-hours phone assessments or urgent patient calls for prescription refills. It is important, therefore, for the clinician to have a procedure for dealing with appointments missed by patients to encourage compliance.

The patient should be informed of the clinician's policy regarding missed appointments at the first visit, and this policy reinforced with a written fact sheet. A clinician may not always choose to enforce the policy in every circumstance. If the clinician chooses not to impose the consequence of missing an appointment, it will be perceived as a gift from the clinician to the patient; however, if the clinician does not have a policy and attempts to institute one only after a patient misses an appointment, it will be seen as a punishment.

Financial incentives or disincentives are common in settings where patients pay for their appointments. There is no one system that works for everyone, although a commonly used policy is:

- Cancellation with more than 24 hours notice, no charge
- Cancellation with less than 24 hours notice – half fee or half co-payment
- An unannounced absence – full fee or full co-payment.

Withholding medications when a patient misses an appointment is not a useful first option. Sometimes, however, this becomes the only option if financial disincentives have not been successful, or if the patient has no financial obligation for the appointment. If the clinician must use medication as a lever to ensure timely and appropriate attendance, the following guidelines can be used:

- At the first missed appointment, the clinician will refill the appropriate medications and reschedule a follow-up patient appointment at their mutual convenience. The patient's memory should be refreshed about the missed appointment policy.
- At a second missed appointment, the clinician may refill a small amount of medication and insist on the first possible rescheduling of a follow-up appointment. Identify this as the second and last time that medication will be provided when an appointment is missed.
- For a third missed appointment, provide no medication until an appointment is kept.
- Repeated missed appointments may require the clinician to discuss termination of all therapy, particularly if blood levels and/or patient safety are compromised because of these absences.

Some clinicians will alter and abbreviate the above schedule for certain classes of medications, such as stimulants or benzodiazepines. There is no dangerous withdrawal from low to moderate doses of stimulants, and it is quite appropriate to withhold further stimulant medication until an appointment is kept. Large doses of short-acting benzodiazepines may cause some measure of withdrawal if stopped suddenly; therefore, if medication is to be withheld until the appointment, patients should be advised to taper whatever doses they have left. While they may be uncomfortable without their usual medication, this discomfort usually prompts them to keep future appointments.

When a patient misses an appointment, the clinician or clinic staff should call the patient within 48 hours. This conveys that the clinician has noted the missed appointment and values the visit, and reinforces the importance of the appointment to perform ongoing assessment and monitoring. Placing a call to the patient also possibly prevents a compounding of the problem – if, for example, a patient has genuinely assumed that the appointment was at a later date or time, and then arrives when he or she cannot be seen.

TALKING TO PATIENTS

A friendly way to phrase a contact about a missed appointment is: *"This is Dr Crandall. I missed you for your appointment. Are you okay?"* The patient will usually then discuss the reason for the absence. *"I would like to reschedule to continue your treatment. When are you available?"*

If an answering machine is reached: *"This is Dr Crandall. I missed you for your appointment on Tuesday at 10:30. I hope you are okay. Please call me so that we can discuss the situation and reschedule."*

When the patient asks for more

Clinicians who perform psychotropic medication management can follow patients over many months or years. During this time, requests may be made regarding issues that are related to, but not directly connected with, the psychotropic medication management process. Most often, these requests are totally appropriate and the clinician can be quite helpful in providing advice or directing the patient to appropriate resources. Such areas may include:

- A referral for talking therapy – which may be individual, marital, or family
- Legal services in a divorce or child custody case
- The clinician may be asked to provide a report or testimony to an attorney or court regarding the patient's diagnosis and medication management
- Helping a patient to decide when a family member or relative needs a mental health assessment
- Offering to provide direct assessment and/or treatment of family members who may need medication evaluation.

Often, after a patient has been appropriately diagnosed and medication is successfully used in treatment, the patient will "see," for the first time, the presence of diagnosable and treatable mental health conditions in their parents, spouse, children, or siblings. Except in circumstances where there is significant family strife or potential problematic interactions between the patient and these family members, it can be quite appropriate for the clinician to evaluate and potentially medicate the patient's relatives. It is not uncommon to have several family members, or persons from multiple generations in the same family, being medicated at the same time by the same practitioner. If a patient asks for evaluation services for a spouse, parent, or child with whom they are in significant conflict, however, this can create clinical dilemmas. Confidentiality and practicality may dictate that these new evaluations be performed by other clinicians.

Inappropriate requests

The relationship between the provider of mental health medication and the patient over time may also lead to inappropriate requests for clinician services. When trust is built and judgment respected, patients, often in an unintended way, may ask for additional medical services beyond mental health medication. *Unless the clinician is trained, credentialled and comfortable with providing other medical services, it is generally not appropriate for the psychotropic provider to attempt to be a general medical provider to mental health patients.* It is not uncommon for patients to ask for prescription of non-mental health medications, either as a "one time" prescription or, in some cases, as ongoing medication. Requests for pain medication, headache remedies, cough and cold medications, blood pressure medications, cardiac, respiratory and diabetic medications should, in general, be referred to the patient's family physician, family nurse practitioner, or general health provider. Patients may also ask, "while they are here," to get a refill for ongoing prescriptions usually obtained from their general medical provider, or ask for treatment of conditions that may require further medical assessment. Unless the clinician is trained and routinely provides general medical care, this is an area that may create medicolegal problems and/or be outside the scope of practice for the clinician. When patients request treatment for headaches, backache, respiratory infections, sore throats, or other complaints, they should be referred to their primary care provider. Refills of ongoing non-psychotropic medications should generally be provided by the original prescriber or that person's coverage group.

Another problematic area involves the request for medication refills without appropriate face-to-face contact and follow-up. This practice is often overtly proclaimed or covertly assumed by the patient to be justified under the assumption that: "since you have seen me for so long, you know me. You shouldn't have to continue to see me face-to-face to prescribe my medications." Patients who are doing well, and not having side effects or relapses, may begin to assume that their psychotropic medication can just be renewed without active management, and resist follow-up appointments. The problem of minimal contact patients is covered in more detail in Chapter 20.

Is newer medication better?

Given the pace of change in treating the biological aspects of mental illness, and in medication research and development, new psychotropic medications are continually being introduced. The challenge facing the professional is assessing the value of any new medication in the care of a particular patient. Pharmaceutical companies vigorously promote each new medication, extolling its benefits compared to older medications and competing products. The task for the clinician is to sort out which of these medications offers genuine advantages in therapeutic efficacy, convenience, or possible price.

Of most interest and significance is when a new class of medicine is introduced that may offer a novel or improved biological approach to treatment. New mechanisms of action may offer the patient the opportunity for more targeted and effective treatment, with potentially fewer side effects. Once a class of medications is established, however, it is not uncommon for competitors to produce "sister medications" with similar mechanisms of action and overall efficacy. While these medications are promoted vigorously as superior products, they may in actuality offer minimal therapeutic advantage. There may be some advantages in flexibility of dosing, routes of administration, or cost to the patient, but the new product does not offer fundamental substantive improvements. All parameters of new medications should be carefully evaluated. There may be no substantial reason to alter the patient's medication regimen just because a new medication becomes available.

If a clinician chooses to consider prescribing a new medication based on limited positive response or problematic side effects from the patient's current medication, clear clinical goals need to be established. When a trial of new medication is undertaken, both patient and clinician should evaluate the expected results and agree on a timeframe for such evaluation. A return to the older (often cheaper) regimen may be desirable if substantial clinical improvement is not seen within the allotted time.

What does "atypical" mean?

The term "atypical" has been applied at various times to specific medications or groups of medications. The intent of its use in mental health medications is to identify that the "atypical" medication is different from the currently used medicines or groups. The term often develops if the newer medication is new or different in chemical structure, clinical usefulness, and/or side-effect profile. Unfortunately, it is a term that can be confusing and misleading. Within a short period of time, if an "atypical" medication or group has significant benefits over the existing treatments, it rapidly comes into common acceptance and use. Thus, "atypical" medications may become the norm, and in fact became "typical" in clinical practice. Later, when even newer medications of a third differing type emerge, "atypical atypicals" (or similarly confusing terms) come into use.

In this text, the term "atypical" is solely used for the latest generation of antipsychotic medications, including olanzapine, quetiapine, risperidone, ziprasidone and aripiprazole. Because the term is so widely accepted, it has been used here despite its time-limited usefulness. Thus, members of this group are "atypical" in the sense that they are new and chemically different from traditional antipsychotics (often referred to as traditional antipsychotics, phenothiazines or traditional neuroleptics). With a more benign side effect profile and wider clinical utility (purportedly due to increased serotonergic activity and differing amounts of dopamine receptor blockade), this "atypical" group of antipsychotic medications has become a frequent first choice in treating psychosis.

The heterogenicity of this "atypical antipsychotic" group can be seen from the evolution of the term.[14] It was initially proposed in 1993 by Dr J Lieberman to describe drugs that:

- Showed efficacy in antipsychotic screening paradigms
- Did not induce catalepsy
- Did not up-regulate D_2 receptors
- Did not induce tolerance
- Showed no, or markedly reduced, induction of acute extrapyramidal symptoms and tardive dyskinesia
- Did not elevate prolactin levels (risperidone, although it elevates prolactin, is considered an atypical).

Stahl[15] has suggested further criterion, specifically that atypical antipsychotics:

- Show greater improvement in negative symptoms of psychosis than haloperidol
- Are effective for symptoms that have been refractory to treatment with conventional antipsychotics.

Periodic reassessment

If patients do not fully recover from their initial presenting mental health episode and continue to have moderate or significant functional impairment, restricted work productivity or residual social impairment, periodic reassessment of the diagnosis and treatment plan is indicated.

Long-term medication management patients, particularly those who have not reached optimum response, should have a diagnostic and therapeutic reassessment periodically, even if they do not have a full fledged "relapse" or symptomatic crisis. If the primary clinician's assessment does not reveal significant positive results, consultation with a colleague, supervisor, or psychopharmacologist may yield useful information for possible therapeutic changes.

When reassessment is performed, the following questions highlight the areas to be investigated:

■ Is the original diagnostic assessment correct?
■ Has the patient developed any new medical or psychiatric conditions since the original assessment?
■ If the patient's medical state has changed, how does this affect the overall mental health or medication treatment plan?
■ Are target symptoms being adequately treated?
■ Are there any new treatments or combinations of treatments that might reasonably improve the patient's situation?
■ Have side effects emerged over time?

Concurrence for a change of medication

If the decision to alter a long-standing therapeutic regimen is made, it should not automatically be a unilateral decision on the part of the clinician. Because of the sheer quantity of newer psychiatric products being introduced, there will be many times when a newer medicine might be considered for a patient who has been relatively stable. If the clinician sees no likely therapeutic advantage of the new product, there is no reason even to raise the possibility. When, however, there may be some possible benefit, it is essential to partner with the patient regarding any possible change.

For the patient, changes in a long-standing medication program may have significant psychological consequences or raise anxiety, even if there are potentially gains to be made. A change to a new medication may result in partial response or loss of response before beneficial changes occur. Although this is hopefully mediated by cross-tapering (slowly decreasing the current medication while gradually adding the new preparation), there is the potential for disruption in the patient's functioning. The timing of such a change should be negotiated with the patient and every attempt be made to avoid times of significant stressful events in the patient's life. As with the decision to stop medication altogether (discussed in Chapter 8), it is generally better that medication changes be tried outside of periods of major life stress such as marriage, divorce, job change, buying or selling a house, or a geographical move.

Conflicting advice from others

Every patient, even those who maintain a good therapeutic alliance with the clinician and comply with medication recommendations, may be presented with conflicting advice and differing opinions from other people in their life. Well intended, but possibly misguided, friends or relatives may offer mild, moderate or significant advice and/or pressure about taking psychotropic medication. With the misconceptions, myths, and beliefs listed in Chapter 2, there may be those individuals in the patient's life who do not value (or openly oppose) the use of mental health medication. The patient may experience direct and sometimes strong suggestions to discontinue medications, disregard treatment, or terminate with the mental health provider. These urgings can come from a variety of sources:

- The patient's spouse
- The patient's family, including parents or children
- The patient's friends, neighbors or confidants
- The patient's employer
- Self-help groups
- Internet chat rooms
- The patient's primary care provider
- Other healthcare providers or specialists
- The patient's psychotherapist.

The latter three sources may seem surprising, but even seasoned healthcare providers sometimes have preconceived notions about psychotropics. The medication management provider should always be aware of input from such sources, which may emerge at any time. It is useful for the clinician periodically to assess how the patient is feeling about the medication regimen and overall treatment. It is useful to invite the patient to discuss any input he or she has heard, and any articles or other sources of information read that may call into question the current treatment plan. If uncertainty has arisen, clarification of the plan and reassurance about the wisdom of the treatment is usually sufficient to allay patient anxiety.

If the resistance or conflicting advice is coming from a spouse or close family member, ask the patient about scheduling a three-way meeting involving the clinician, the patient and the relative. This session can allow the relative to ask questions about the patient's diagnosis and treatment, medication prescribed and side effects, the length of treatment, and any other issues about the overall anticipated treatment plan. It will also offer the opportunity for the clinician to get additional feedback about the patient's medication response (or lack thereof) and presentation on a day-to-day basis outside the treatment setting. Concerns or worries that this third person may have about the use of psychotropic medications can be addressed. After receiving solid factual information from the clinician and feeling that they have had input into the patient's care, such resistive family relatives will often feel included in the treatment plan and their resistance usually diminishes. If, by the end of this session, a relative still remains quite opposed to the use of psychotropic medications but medication prescription will continue, the clinician can recognize the relative's right to a personal opinion and request that he or she keeps such opinions to him/herself so as not to make the patient confused, hesitant, or anxious.

Occasionally the clinician must take more active steps if patients indicate that they are getting conflicting advice from other medical or mental health providers. If needed, and with a patient's consent, the medication prescriber should contact such persons and discuss the overall treatment plan. A simple telephone call to a primary care provider, a psychotherapist, a nurse practitioner or other healthcare provider who is involved in the patient's care can often clarify whether, in fact, conflicting information is being given. Even if there has been misinterpretation on the patient's part and there is no active disagreement about the use of psychotropic medications, this presents as an opportunity for the prescriber to strengthen the overall treatment team's position, and ensures that the patient is not caught between prescribers with differing viewpoints.

On rare occasions, the prescriber will need to be forthright and direct with another healthcare provider about the necessity for ongoing psychotropic medications. If the other provider feels that such treatment is unnecessary or inappropriate, he or she must be asked to defer to the prescriber in managing the patient's mental health care. While this is unusual, a direct discussion of the case will usually simplify the situation and allow the patient to continue without confusing input.

References

1   Alpert H et al. Nutrition and depression: focus on folate. Nutrition 2000;16:344–481.

2   Fava M et al. Folate, B$_{12}$, and homocysteine in major depressive disorder. Am J Psychiatry 1997;54:426–428.

3   Alpert JE et al. Folinic acid (leucovorin) as an adjustive treatment for SSRI-refractory depression. Ann Clin Psychiatry 2002;14(1):33–38.

4   Copper A and Bailey J. Enhancement of the antidepressant action of fluoxetine by folic acid: a randomized, placebo controlled trial. J Affect Disord 2001;60:121–130.

5   Salmon P. Effects of physical exercise on anxiety, depression and sensitivity to stress: a unifying theory. Clin Psychol Rev 2001;21(1):33–61.

6   Sexton H et al. How are mood and exercise related? Results from the Finnmark study. Soc Psychiatry Psychiatr Epidemiol 2001;36(7):348–353.

7   Dimeo F et al. Benefits from aerobic exercise in patients with major depression: a pilot study. Br J Sports Med 2001;35(2):114–117.

8   Williamson D et al. Mood change through physical exercise in nine- to ten-year-old children. Percept Mot Skills 2001;93(1):311–316.

9 Toskovic NN. Alterations in selected measure of mood with a single bout of dynamic Taekwondo exercise in college-age students. *Percept Mot Skills* 2001;92(3 Pt 2):1031–1038.

10 George BJ and Goldberg N. The benefits of exercise in geriatric women. *Am J Geriatr Cardiol* 2001;10(5):260–263.

11 Kiernan M *et al*. Men gain additional psychological benefits by adding exercise to a weight-loss program. *Obes Res* 2001;9(12):770–777.

12 Lee RE *et al*. A prospective analysis of the relationship between walking and mood in sedentary ethnic minority women. *Women Health* 2001;32(4):1–15.

13 Hassmen P *et al*. Physical exercise and psychological well-being: a population study in Finland. *Prev Med* 2000;30(1):17–25.

14 Lieberman JA. Understanding the mechanism of action of atypical antipsychotic drugs: a review of compounds in use and development. *Br J Psychiatry* 1993; 163(suppl. 22):7–18.

15 Stahl S. *Psychopharmacology of Antipsychotics*. Martin Dunitz, 1999.

Part III Medicating Special Populations

Chapter 10

Using medication with children and adolescents

In America, between 6 and 9 million pediatric patients have serious mental and emotional illnesses.[1,2] At any given time, approximately 20 percent of children have mental disorders with at least mild functional impairment;[3] 10–13 percent of children and adolescents have symptoms of serious mental illness, and 5–9 percent experience extreme emotional disturbance and functional impairment.[4] Although the use of psychotropic medications in children and adolescents has been less frequent than in adult patients, there has been a dramatic increase in pediatric psychotropic prescriptions over the past several decades.[5-7] This medication practice has been accompanied by relatively limited evidence-based data, however, the need to make prescribing decisions has preceded the information on which we would like to depend. Many of the principles stated elsewhere in this book also apply to pediatric patients, although there are a number of specific facts and techniques that are uniquely useful in child and adolescent psychopharmacological practice. This chapter will highlight those elements.

Outdated views of pediatric mental health prescription

During the latter half of the twentieth century, generalized blanket beliefs by parents, practitioners, and society at large about the use of psychotropics in pediatric patients have unfortunately colored their use and acceptance. Up until the last two decades, a common belief of many practitioners was that psychotropic medications had strong potential for damaging brain function or interfering with developing physiology and growth in children. Within this view, psychotropics would only be used as a last resort. More recently, some practitioners who use psychotropics frequently have taken the opposite (but equally untrue) stance that psychotropic medications should be used liberally and automatically to treat almost every child and adolescent behavioral abnormality. Some parents, families and school authorities still adhere to either of these anachronistic views about using psychotropics. Corollaries of these two opposing extremes describe pediatric behavioral problems as "just a phase" that a child will likely outgrow, or that pills/medications are a "quick fix" for virtually any behaviors found objectionable or undesirable. Neither of these beliefs is categorically true. Each child should be individually assessed, diagnosed and evaluated for the possible role of psychotropic medications in treating specific behavioral or emotional symptoms.

Psychotropic prescription in children is a balance between any real risks of taking psychotropic medication versus "prescribing before it is time." Earlier fears that all psychotropic medications would be damaging to children were not well grounded, nor have they been borne out to be true. In fact, appropriate targeted prescription of psychotropic medications for properly diagnosed psychiatric conditions can often facilitate the achievement of normal development milestones, increase social interaction and appropriate cognitive development, and improve family dynamics. When left untreated, mental illnesses can cause major disruption in any of these areas. The prescriber cannot rationally adhere to a black-or-white, all-or-nothing posture toward prescription in the pediatric population since there are risks to either extreme position.

Risks of premature prescription in children and adolescents include:

- Embarking on a long-term therapy without addressing family dynamics
- Exposing the patient to unnecessary side effects
- Unnecessary labeling of the patient
- Unnecessary damage to the child's self-esteem.

On the other hand, the downsides of excessive waiting for patients to "grow out" of the symptoms of a significant mental illness include:

- Failed or delayed developmental steps
- Poor peer relationships
- Lack of appropriate family interactions
- Poor academic progress
- Shaky self-esteem.

The scope of pediatric psychopharmacology

Pediatric psychopharmacology has gone far beyond the usage of stimulants for attention deficit disorder, which in some countries still dominates the conception of pediatric psychopharmacology. Psychotropic medications are routinely used to treat a wide variety of psychiatric conditions, including psychosis, anxiety disorders, obsessive–compulsive disorders, eating disorders, and personality disorders.

Virtually all of the psychiatric illnesses present in adults are also present in children, although the clinical presentation may vary in the pediatric patient. Some conditions for which medication pharmacotherapy has been used in children and adolescents are summarized in Table 10.1.[8,9] The wide range of uses for psychotropics in children is changing frequently, and this list is not intended to be totally comprehensive.

Principles of psychotropic prescription with children and adolescents

Table 10.2 lists some of the important items to be considered when prescribing for children and adolescents.

Diagnostic and conceptual issues in the prescriptive process

A careful, multi-factorial assessment is crucial to psychotropic prescription to children and adolescents, particularly in clinical circumstances where prescriptions are being written by non-child psychiatrists or non-psychiatric practitioners. There can be a tendency, particularly in primary care settings, to medicate quickly and in an imprecise fashion for perceived behavioral difficulties. The clinician should utilize not only the identified patient, but also the parents and others to gather information about the child's behavior and emotions. Children are often not the most accurate or detailed historians, and they may be poor observers of their own behavior. Although a child's view of the problem is crucially important, interviews with parents, teachers and other caretakers also provide valuable perspective and data.

Use the family history of emotional illness, if any, to assist the diagnostic assessment. For example, hyperactive or overactive children with a strong family history of bipolar disorder are more likely to be bipolar than to have attention deficit disorder (ADD). Likewise, a family history of anxiety disorder may point to a childhood anxiety disorder rather than ADD as the cause of agitation symptoms. Psychotropic prescription can be complicated by lack of family history or developmental history in certain patients who have been maintained in custodial settings. It is often difficult or impossible to obtain previous treatment records from foster care, detention, or jails, which may only arrive after a long delay.

PRIMARY CARE
Primary care providers may or may not have the time and resources to perform a thorough initial evaluation personally. Large pediatric medical settings may benefit from contractual use of a mental health specialist to help with initial assessment and follow-up.

Table 10.1 Some psychiatric disorders in children and adolescents for which pharmacotherapy has been used*

DSM-IV classifications	Medications
Mental retardation	Conventional antipsychotics, lithium, naltrexone, buspirone
Pervasive developmental disorders: autism, autistic disorder	Buspirone, conventional antipsychotics, methylphenidate, atypical antipsychotics, selective serotonin-reuptake inhibitors, fenfluramine, clomipramine
Attention deficit and disruptive behavior disorders	Amphetamine, dexedrine, bupropion, clonidine, methylphenidate, pemoline, tricyclic antidepressants
Tic disorders: Tourette's disorder	Pimozide, clonidine, atypical antipsychotics
Elimination disorders: Enuresis	Imipramine
Other disorders of infancy, childhood or adolescence: separation anxiety disorder	Alprazolam, buspirone, tricyclic antidepressants, SSRIs
Schizophrenia	Conventional antipsychotics, atypical antipsychotics
Mood disorders: Major depressive disorder	Bupropion nefazodone, selective serotonin-reuptake inhibitors, tricyclic antidepressants, venlafaxine
Bipolar disorder	Carbamazepine, divalproex sodium, lithium, atypical antipsychotics
Anxiety disorders: Obsessive–compulsive disorder	Selective serotonin-reuptake inhibitors, clomipramine
Post-traumatic stress disorder (acute)	Benzodiazepines
Eating disorders: Anorexia nervosa	Cyproheptadine
Bulimia nervosa	Selective serotonin-reuptake inhibitors
Primary sleep disorders	Benzodiazepines, imipramine

*Although commonly used by practitioners, efficacy has not been firmly established for many indications, and literature documentation may be sparse.

Table 10.2 Child and adolescent prescriptive issues

■ The clinician must be as precise as possible in assessment, and in use of standardized codification of diagnoses. Accurate diagnosis is essential to targeted prescription.

■ Always evaluate children in their social, family, psychological, developmental, genetic, and biological contexts. There may be many factors besides biological illness that strongly contribute to an individual child's psychiatric disorder.

■ Information should be gathered from sources other than the identified patient.

■ Children are not "little adults." Specific pediatric pharmacokinetic changes may affect blood levels of medications in child and adolescent patients.

■ In general, medications should be used only for serious disruptive behavior or symptoms. Ensure that the prescription is for the benefit of the child, not primarily for the benefit of others.

■ The child is the patient, but alliance with the parent(s) is crucial to effective prescription.

■ Evidence of medication effectiveness in adults does not necessarily predict effectiveness in children, although it has been common psychotropic practice to prescribe medication to young patients without documented evidence of benefit in this population.

■ Maintain informed consent from responsible parties. Attempt to obtain consent from the child at the level of the child's understanding.

■ Address the child's fears and resistances to medication.

■ Medication alone is seldom "the answer."

■ If a clinician does not have child pharmacology training, maintain access to a qualified child consultant.

If the child cannot be referred to a child psychiatrist or another practitioner with pediatric psychopharmacological expertise, there are a number of standardized diagnostic tools that are useful in increasing the precision of diagnosis for the busy primary care practitioner. During a first evaluation, these include:[10,12]

■ the Diagnostic Interview for Children and Adolescents
■ the Child Assessment Schedule
■ the Kiddie SADS.

During follow-up sessions, helpful tools and measurement scales include:[10–12]

■ the Clinical Global Impressions Scale
■ the Symptom Checklist 58
■ the Youth Self-Report and the Behavior Checklist.

During the evaluation process, whenever possible, time should be spent *alone with the child or adolescent* and then *alone with the parent(s)*. Important diagnostic information is often obtained in separate interviews that would not be brought up if the parent and child are only seen together. Examples of this include:

- A parent who might not discuss a family history of mental illness
- A parent who might not discuss his/her own psychiatric or medication history
- A young patient who will not discuss drug/alcohol usage, sexual activity, or possibility of pregnancy.

When possible, use specific diagnostic codes from the *Diagnostic and Statistical Manual* or from the ICD-10 of the World Health Authority. Avoid prescribing for vague or unspecified problems.

When considering medication prescription, evaluate the seriousness, frequency and consequences of the behavior or symptoms, and not just the inconvenience or nuisance factor. Some child patients are thrust into the "need" for medication in order to "control" their behavior, which is reinforced or insisted upon by parents, custodians, or institutional staff. It is particularly important when prescribing to ensure that the medications are also for the benefit of the child, and not solely for the benefit of the parents or staff. A useful criterion that supports the possible need for medication is *when the symptoms or behavior are a problem/worry to the child personally*. While useful, medication may still be indicated even if the child is not keenly aware of the effects of the symptoms.

While many psychotropic medications used in adults are also useful in children, it should not be assumed that studies documenting effectiveness in adults can automatically be used to provide evidence for childhood prescription. While there are some short-term studies of usefulness of medications in child and adolescent populations, there are few long-term studies assessing a medication's effectiveness over time. Since decisions about psychotropics in children may need to be made without the benefit of valid information in the pediatric age group, this issue must be discussed with parents/guardians in the process of obtaining informed consent. This lack of data is usually an issue that younger children may not understand, and is usually omitted from direct discussions with the child patient.

A prime example of this confusion in psychopharmacological prescription for children has been the use of tricyclic antidepressants (TCAs). This group of medications was prescribed for a number of years to children for mood disorders, based on positive outcome research studies with adults. When childhood studies were eventually conducted, the research did not support an antidepressant effect for TCAs in children.[13] On closer study, there was also an increased risk of cardiac arrhythmias with one TCA, desipramine.[14] This lack of effectiveness of TCAs has been speculated to be secondary to the lack of development of the nor-epinephrine system in children – i.e. a child's brain is not physiologically the same as an adult's brain. Major prescription patterns of several decades were ultimately found to have been guided by assumptions that were simply incorrect.

Alliances with both the child patient and the parent(s) are crucial to compliance and safe prescriptive practice. The parents must have a clear picture from the clinician regarding the assessment/diagnosis and the role of medications in the treatment of the diagnosed condition. Many parents, unfortunately, may have either overly optimistic or overly negativistic beliefs about the role of medications in treatment. Some are too concerned about risk and safety, while others are quick to search for a pill to remove any amount of behavioral disruption or distress being experienced.

It is important to manage expectations – on the part of both the parent and the child. Part of the initial prescription is to provide realistic information on what medications can do, and how long it will take for medications to act. At times, it is as important to describe which symptoms medications are *not* likely to change.

TALKING TO PATIENTS

To get at this issue, a useful question to ask the parents is: *"What would you wish that medication will accomplish?"*

TALKING TO PATIENTS

Analogous to the above question, the clinician can ask the child: *"If you could design a medication to do exactly what you would want it to do for you, what would it do?"*

Some parents are prone to see even dramatic signs of significant emotional illness as "just a phase." When significant emotional illness is diagnosed, the clinician must explain possible important sequalae and risks in allowing the illness to remain untreated. Such consequences could include suicidal behavior, accidents, late attainment of developmental milestones, poor self-esteem, and disordered relationships with peers. At times, sharing morbidity and mortality data with parents is useful in emphasizing the seriousness of the condition and the necessity for treatment. An example of this type of data is the suicide rate in childhood depression (2.5 percent) and in adolescents (7.7 percent). Untreated patients with major depression are at twice the risk for suicide as are children and adolescents without diagnosed depression.[15] Children with untreated mental illness also have significantly higher use of alcohol and recreational drugs.[16]

If there is significant parental resistance to the use of medication in their child, it may be useful to try other non-medication remedies first unless there is an urgent or crisis situation. This approach offers time for parents to read about medications or get information from other sources. As the child is treated non-pharmacologically, it is also easier to be more precise in targeting symptoms that may be better treated with medication. Reassurance as to the non-addictive nature of most psychotropics should also be emphasized. With resistive parents, it may be useful to specify a reasonable time period for a medication trial (e.g. 4–8 weeks), after which point a reassessment of the benefits will be done before any further action is taken.

A useful strategy for approaching older children or adolescents who may be ambivalent or resistive to medication is to engage patients in a discussion of *why others (parents, teachers) might want them to take medication.* If patients can identify some appropriate reasons, the clinician can explore if any of the potential effects of medicines would be helpful. Some young patients may be willing to try medication for a set, defined period of time to get their parents "off their back."

Special attention must be paid to informed consent issues before medicating children. Except on an emergency basis, written informed consent must be obtained from parents or legal guardians before medication is instituted. This may be particularly complicated when the parents are separated or divorced. When possible, it is wise to obtain informed consent from both parents. When this is not possible, or when one parent is not involved in parenting duties, informed consent must be obtained from the custodial parent and any efforts made to reach the non-custodial parent, should be documented.

The clinician should be alert to patient resistances that are particularly common in youthful patients. These can include:

- The fear that their mind will be "controlled" by the medication and that they will "lose free will"
- Worries that they will be labeled – either in the family, at school or by their peers – as sick or disabled
- Their own belief that they are "bad" for taking medication or that emotional illness is their "fault"
- Adolescent patients will often stop medications prematurely because they feel they have "outgrown" them
- Adolescents may stop the medication in order to drink alcohol or use recreational drugs.

There are few large-scale, controlled child/adolescent comparisons of medication alone, psychotherapy/family therapy alone, and medication combined with psychotherapy.[17] There is one significant study looking at a comparison of various treatment modalities for ADHD that found that targeted medication treatment plus behavioral treatment was superior to psychosocial treatment or community treatment alone.[18] It is the premise of this book that medication treatment, when indicated, should be combined with psychotherapy (and family therapy, when appropriate) to maximize results. Psychotropic medications need to be part of a comprehensive treatment program involving psychotherapeutic interventions, educational interventions, family intervention, and milieu management. *Medications alone are seldom curative.* However, when appropriately prescribed, medication response can allow for healing and adjustment to occur, with distinctly lessened interference from the symptoms of emotional disease. As with adults, the beneficial symptom reduction from medication may facilitate and increase the effect of psychotherapy or family therapy.

Persons trained in child psychopharmacology are in short supply in most communities, and are particularly scarce in rural areas. Adult psychiatrists with little child training or family physicians/pediatricians/family nurse practitioners who are not mental health specialists will, therefore, make many psychopharmacological decisions for children. Whenever this is the case, the practitioner should seek access to a *child psychopharmacology consultant* or someone trained in child psychiatry to discuss difficult or non-responsive patients. The lack of child-trained practitioners in rural areas can also unfortunately lead to infrequent or almost non-existent follow-up of the psychotropic medications once prescribed. As with adults, children must be seen face-to-face to evaluate medication response.

After appropriate time intervals and stabilization, consideration should be given to a trial of medication discontinuation. Timeframes and practical matters of how/when to do this follow the same principles outlined for adults in Chapter 8. When a trial off mediations is indicated, it is often wise to undertake this during summer vacation or school breaks such that, if there is a relapse, the effects are less likely to disrupt academic performance and school functioning.

A child's goals differ from those of adults

In the same way that a practitioner attempts to find common goals with resistive adult patients, the child prescriber should attempt to find reasons for medication usage that children see to be in their best interest.

Some examples of personal motivations that children can see for taking psychotropic medications are:

- Increased compatibility with peers and schoolmates
- The ability to control their anger, resisting the impulse to throw out their toys or destroy toys that they value
- By being in more emotional control, adolescents may be less likely to upset their friends and better able to maintain their social relationships
- An irritable adolescent can value decreased anger to maintain a specific connection to a boyfriend/girlfriend
- Some adolescents will value the increased self-control and mental focus that will allow their parents to permit them to get a driver's license or have access to a car
- Some young patients will take medication to increase concentration and focus, improve academic performance, and shed the label of "dummy"
- Sad, depressed, or anxious adolescents can value a decrease in symptoms to the point where they can obtain and keep a job to earn spending money.

Parental power struggles over medication

Taking medication can become one part of a larger power struggle between children and parents. In an outpatient setting, if children are fundamentally resistant to and actively refusing medication it is seldom useful for parents to force it, since a child has the ultimate veto power by refusing or "cheeking it" and spitting out medication later. Except in crisis or emergency situations (which are usually in institutional settings), it is preferable to work with children's resistances and obtain at least temporary agreement on the use of medication before it is begun.

The use of medication can also be a cause of disagreement between parents.

They may have legitimate differences of opinion, or medication may become one of a series of contentions between two arguing parents. The clinician should be attuned to sabotage issues between two parents who may not agree on the cause of the symptoms of the mental health condition and the use of medication in its treatment. The parent who opposes medication use can refuse to administer it when the child is with him or her. Disparaging or derogatory messages about the child's need for medication can be subtly or overtly given. When the clinician becomes aware of this interference, a telephone call or meeting with this parent can be helpful.

The medical work-up prior to psychotropics

The necessary medical evaluation of a pediatric patient for whom a clinician is going to be prescribing a psychotropic will depend on the child's medical history, the length of time since their last physical exam, the presence of somatic complaints, and the medication to be prescribed. In general, a physical exam is recommended if:

- It has been more than 6 months since the child's last physical exam
- The child has any somatic complaints
- Toxins, alcohol or street drugs are being used or use is suspected
- High-dose medication is anticipated
- The child has a co-morbid medical condition.

Laboratory screening would include:

- A comprehensive metabolic panel, including blood sugar, electrolytes, kidney functions and liver functions
- A CBC
- Thyroid stimulating hormone level
- Urinalysis.

If a high-dose stimulant or desipramine is to be prescribed, or if there is any history of long Q-T interval in the family, an EKG should also be obtained.

Practical issues in child/adolescent prescription

Physiological differences between children and adults include increased liver mass compared to body weight, a relatively high proportion of body fat, and a high volume of extracellular water. In children, these differences can result in a significantly changed ability to distribute and metabolize medication. Typically, metabolic pathways for drugs function at a low level during the perinatal period, become mature by 6–12 months of age, and peak between 1 and 5 years. Children's ability to more rapidly metabolize medication persists in childhood, and gradually declines to adult patterns by 15 years of age.[19,20] The net effect of these pharmacokinetic changes is that, in general, *children and adolescents require larger doses on a milligram per kilogram basis of weight than adults*, to achieve comparable blood levels and therapeutic effects.[21] There is also a specific study with lithium and children showing that, compared to adults, children and adolescents need a higher maintenance serum lithium concentration to ensure that therapeutic levels are achieved.

While these physiological changes are greater or lesser in an individual child, they may be overridden by changes in pharmacodynamics (i.e. receptor-site responsivity, or lack of responsivity to various medications). These individual response variations can be quite dramatic, and totally overshadow any pharmacokinetic issues. Presumably, as with adults, these individual pharmacodynamic variations are based on genetic differences.

Because of the pharmacokinetic issues mentioned above, which lead to more rapid breakdown and excretion, children may also require split dosing (twice, or even three times daily) in order to maintain consistent blood levels and adequate medication effects around the clock. This is particularly true for short half-life compounds such as paroxetine, venlafaxine, and gabapentin.

SSRI/TCA discontinuation syndromes (see Chapter 8) can occur in young patients as well as in adults. Because of the rapid elimination of these medications in children and adolescents, they may be more prone to such syndromes *between* doses, or if short half-life drugs are given once daily. Likewise, during the stopping of a course of antidepressants a slow, gradual tapering of dose is necessary to minimize the likelihood of discontinuation syndrome symptoms.

CLINICAL TIP

Whenever possible, avoid having child patients take medication at school since this increases their fear that they will be labeled as ill or "different" by needing to go to the nurse's office to take the medication. The most common scenario when midday dosing is an issue is with the use of stimulants for ADD/ADHD. To circumvent this issue, consider using long-acting stimulant preparations such as Ritalin LA, Adderall XR, Concerta and Metadate CD, which maintain therapeutic effect throughout the school day. Most antidepressants, mood stabilizers, and antipsychotics can be given once daily or, at most, twice daily, in the morning and at bedtime. The only exception to this general principle is a child enmeshed in a very chaotic family in which the clinician may suspect that medication may be given at home erratically or not at all. In this case, dosing the medication at school may be more predictable and dependable even at the risk of labeling.

The medication regimen should be kept simple. Whenever possible, doses should be given once daily. When multiple daily doses are required, doses can be tied to events easily recognizable for the child, such as meals or bedtime, rather than specific clock times.

The tendency to polypharmacy in order to meet parental expectations for a "quick" cure must be avoided. Dysfunctional families may often see medication as a cure-all to multiple ills. There can be resistance to looking at family dynamics and at mental after-effects of loss, neglect, abuse, or trauma, even though these may be significant causes of the child's symptomatology. In such families, pressure can be brought to bear on the clinician for rapid improvement and the addition of multiple medications to achieve response quickly. Underlying this pressure is the wish to deny or avoid other dysfunctional elements in the family.

PRIMARY CARE

Particularly when psychotropic medication is prescribed in a general medical/pediatric office, dispel the "aspirin" expectation. In this framework, many parents (and some children) expect psychotropics to work like an aspirin, with relief and effect within minutes to hours of taking the pill. The clinician should describe regular consistent dosing, the need for gradual build-up of dose, and the likelihood of response over several weeks to several months.

PRIMARY CARE

P-450 interactions between medications, as in adults, are more common when children take multiple medications or have multiple medical problems. Increased side effects or lack of therapeutic response in these children, especially when other non-psychotropics are present, can be indicators of altered psychotropic serum blood levels.

It is important to discuss both the *physical* side effects to medication and the *behavioral* side effects of medications that can indicate excessive dosage or toxicity. Most families are aware of physical side effects such as:

- Excessive napping or sleepiness in school
- Nausea, changes in bowel habits
- Changes in vital signs (increased or decreased pulse rate, lightheadedness from decreased blood pressure, headaches from high blood pressure).

Youthful patients and their parents may, however, not anticipate behavioral side effects in the same way as they do physiological side effects. When appropriate, any behavioral side effects to the medication prescribed should be described. These can include:

- Agitation, nervousness, and restlessness, which may occur with SSRIs and benzodiazepines
- Akathisia (internal restlessness), which may occur with antipsychotics
- Disinhibition, which may occur with benzodiazepines
- Mental confusion or "spaciness," which may occur with almost any psychotropic.

Some children may have difficulty in swallowing medications or be fearful of swallowing large pills, so it is useful to ask about this issue prior to writing a prescription. If concern is expressed, it is helpful to show a picture of the pill in the PDR or other drug reference to see if the child feels it is of a size that can be swallowed. It is better to discover this in the office than to find out later that evening when the child balks at the first dose. When a child is unable to swallow the recommended pill, the parent can crush or break the pills into smaller components that can be given in applesauce or ice cream. Even if there is loss of the "timed release" element of a pill that is crushed or opened, this may be less of a problem than a symptomatic child who will not take the pill at all. Liquid preparations, when available, are also a useful alternative. As a last resort, consider prescribing an alternative medication with a smaller pill size.

When prescribing in an outpatient setting, the clinician should start at small doses and go slow with any dosage increase. The response to dosage increases can be evaluated, and pressure to escalate dosage rapidly to quick "fix" the problem resisted.

The clinician should give information about medications to children in age-appropriate phrases, and then ask for questions. Simple phrases, such as "this will help your brain work better," are useful for young children. It is often useful to give the actual paper prescription for the medication to the child to carry out of the office so that he or she "owns it."

The clinician should assess the child or adolescent's ability to manage his/her own medications. Children aged 4 and under will usually accept medication dispensed by parents without difficulty. If older than 4, the child's compliance is strongly desirable, but the pills should still be controlled and dispensed by the parents. In adolescents who are assessed to be dependable, there is value in allowing them to control their own medications. If they are undependable, erratic, likely to be non-compliant, or adversely disposed to the medications, however, parents should be involved in observing them take the medication.

Adolescents are notorious for giving away, selling or trading their medication with peers. When medicating adolescents, the clinician should be particularly attuned to the possibility that patients may be underdosing themselves because they have given or sold their medication to others. Adolescent patients may also be taking medication prescribed for other people.

When prescribing mental health medications, the clinician must maintain contact with the patient's general physician or pediatrician. If the pediatrician is providing follow-up of psychotropic medication, specific improvements expected, potential complications or side effects, or other issues that would constitute a reason for re-evaluation by the mental health prescriber, should be discussed by the mental health prescriber.

Details of uses, doses, side effects, and other specific medication issues for pediatric patients can be found in textbooks specifically devoted to child and adolescent psychopharmacology.[22–25]

References

1 Hodges K. Structured interviews for assessing children. *J Child Psychol Psychiatry* 1993;34:49–69.

2 Kutcher S. *Child and Adolescent Psychopharmacology*. WB Saunders, 1997.

3 Rosenbaum JF and Pollock RA. *Update on Children's Mental Health*. American Psychiatric Association Meeting May 2002. Available on the Internet at www.medscape.com/viewarticle/436402

4 Friedman RM *et al. Prevalence of Serious Emotional Disturbance in Children and Adolescents*. RW Manderscheid and MA Sonnnschein eds. Center for Mental Health Services, 1996, pp. 71–88.

5 DeVane CL and Sallee FR. Serotonin selective reuptake inhibitors in child and adolescent psychopharmacology: a review of published experience. *J Clin Psychiatry* 1996;57:55–56.

6 Findling RL *et al.* Antipsychotic medications in children and adolescents. *J Clin Psychiatry* 1996;45(suppl. 9):19–23.

7 Alessi N *et al.* Update on lithium carbonate therapy in children and adolescents. *J Am Acad Child Adolesc Psychiatry* 1994;33:291–304.

8 Devane CL. Psychoactive drug–drug interactions in children, adolescents and adults. *Essential Psychopharmacology* 1997;2(1):33.

9 Theodore Levin, MD, personal communication.

10 Wilens TE *et al.* Combined pharmacotherapy: an emerging trend in pediatric psychopharmacology. *J Am Acad Child Adolesc Psychiatry* 1995;34:110–112.

11 Aarons L. Kinetics of drug–drug interactions. *Pharmacol Ther* 1981;14:321–344.

12 Guengerich FP. Human cytochrome P450 enzymes. *Life Sci* 1992;50:1471–1478.

13 Birmaher B *et al.* Childhood and adolescent depression: a review of the past ten years. Part II. *J Am Acad Child Adolesc Psychiatry* 1996;35:1575–1583.

14 Varley CK and McClellan J. Case study: two additional sudden deaths with tricyclic antidepressants. *J Am Acad Child Adolesc Psychiatry*. 1997;36:390–394.

15 Isacsson G *et al.* Epidemiological data suggest antidepressants reduce suicide risk among depressives. *J Affective Dis* 1996;41:1–8.

16 Weissman MM *et al.* Depressed adolescents grown up. *JAMA* 1999;281:701–713.

17 Klein RG. Major depression in children and adolescents. *Am Soc Clin Pharm Progress Notes* 2002;11(1):2–4.

18 MTA Cooperative Group. A 14-month randomized clinical trial of treatment strategies for attention-deficit/hyperactivity disorder. *Arch Gen Psychiatry* 1999;56:1073–1096.

19 Perel JM. Inhibition of imipramine metabolism by methylphenidate. *Fed Proc* 1969;28:418.

20 Kraus DM *et al.* Alterations in theophylline metabolism during the first year of life. *Clin Pharmacol Ther* 1993;54:351–359.

21 Hunt RD *et al.* Clonidine benefits children with attention deficit disorder: report of a double-blind, placebo-crossover therapeutic trial. *J Am Acad Child Adolesc Psychiatry* 1985;24:617–629.

22 Jacobson FM. *Psychoactive Medications in the Treatment of Adults and Adolescents*. John Wiley & Sons, 2002.

23 Martin A (ed.). *Pediatric Psychopharmacology: Principles and Practice*. American Psychological Association, 2002.

24 Green WH (ed.). *Child and Adolescent Clinical Psychopharmacology*, 3rd edn. Lippincott, Williams and Wilkins, 2001.

25 Werry JS (ed.) *Practitioners Guide to Psychoactive Drugs for Children and Adolescents*, 2nd edn. Plenum Press, 1999.

Chapter 11

Pregnancy and psychotropics – rewards and risks

Prescribing medication during pregnancy is an area that raises anxiety for some practitioners, but it is a crucially important time that can also provide great reward to the clinician. Although we are gradually obtaining increased amounts of clinical information that will help us provide evidence-based recommendations to patients, there is still much that we do not know.

This chapter focuses on the general approaches to medication and pregnancy as well as the specific recommendations for the various reproductive phases in a woman's life, including:

- Issues for the fertile woman, pre-pregnancy
- When a woman wishes to become pregnant
- While a woman is attempting to become pregnant
- When the patient becomes pregnant
- Medication during pregnancy
- Medication during the postpartum and breastfeeding periods.

Each of these timeframes creates different medication considerations for the clinician in dealing with patients, and thus will be considered separately.

Clinician principles for prescribing to the pregnant woman

As has been outlined in other chapters in this book, almost all treatment decisions with psychotropic medications are collaborative. Nowhere is this more important than in making decisions about the use of mental health medications during a pregnancy. Ultimately, the mentally competent pregnant woman herself, in concert with her partner, makes the decision as to the use or non-use of the medication. These decisions, however, carry a great emotional charge. When a woman takes medication during a pregnancy and then delivers a normal, healthy baby, the patient and her partner are relieved, but may be vigilant for years looking for signs that having taken medication may have caused problems. In the event of a baby with a problem or disability, clinicians may be legally vulnerable if they acted in a way to coerce or strongly influence the patient toward one decision or the other. Therefore, unless the patient is incapacitated or incompetent, *the clinician cannot make decisions about medication during pregnancy unilaterally or for the patient*. In the vast majority of situations, it is the role of the clinician to:

■ Provide up-to-date, balanced information to the patient and her partner about possible risks of medication and/or the possible complications of untreated illness
■ Help the woman or couple choose the best decision for themselves, always being cognizant that the final decision rests with them
■ Once a decision is reached, verbally support their final choice.

Regardless of the classes of medications used and the patient's life circumstances, there are risks and benefits to virtually every medication decision during pregnancy. Clinicians should be open and direct as to what, as professionals, they do and do not know. They should be informative and non-judgmental, but avoid making the decision for the patient, and share a balanced picture of the potential upsides and downsides to various choices (as best they are known) both in general and in the specific light of the patient's history, current status and previous response to medication. The clinician's role is that of information provider, clarifier and objective observer of the patient's history and current state, not of arbiter or decision-maker. Initially the clinician should be familiar with the current literature and present a summary of the data and research known, in understandable terms familiar to the patient. This *verbal presentation is more helpful than simply referring the patient to journal articles or books*, which are often written in technical jargon and easily misinterpreted. If the patient does request further detailed information beyond the clinician's digest of the current literature, she can be directed to specific patient-centered websites devoted to issues of reproduction and psychotropics, such as:

■ Massachusetts General Hospital Center for Women's Health Perinatal Information Resource Center at www.womensmentalhealth.org/index.html

- The Motherisk Program in Toronto Canada at www.motherisk.org or 416-813-6780
- Pregnancy and depression at www.pregnancyanddepression.com/

Although the clinician does not need to shield the patient from specific professional references and articles, these should be a third line source of information. If information is requested beyond this Internet information, the patient can be referred to reputable summary articles on issues of pregnancy, breastfeeding and psychotropics, such as the references at the end of this chapter. (Since this is a rapidly evolving data set, there may have been useful articles and/or book chapters published since this text went to press.) Regardless of which professional material the patient reads, the clinician should always ask that she comes to the office to discuss her understanding of the facts she read and the applicability to her specific clinical situation before decisions are made. It is often helpful to suggest that the patient brings a copy of any material she has read with her to the office for discussion.

Even when the clinician has doubts about a patient's choice, in general, *once she reaches a decision about the use or non-use of medication*, it is most helpful if the clinician finds a way to *support the positive elements of her decision*. The patient needs to know that the clinician is 'with her' throughout this process. If the patient's decision is not the one the clinician would have made, it is important to keep this belief in the background once the choice has been selected. The clinician should focus on the benefits and positive reasons for which the patient has made her choice, rather than highlight the risks of the patient's decision.

TALKING TO PATIENTS

For example, when a patient chooses to stop medication even though there may be a significant risk of relapse, focus on her wish *to give the best possible, medication-free environment to her child even when it means a potential discomfort to herself.*

Similarly, when a patient chooses to continue medication or start medication during a pregnancy, focus on how the mother is *trying to provide the most stable emotional environment for her future baby*. In this situation, the clinician can also recollect with the patient the intensity of the symptoms that she experienced off medication, and how medication has significantly improved her condition.

In either case, empathize with the patient's difficulty in making this decision. Regardless of what she has chosen, underscore how she has given it much thought and consideration. Once the woman has chosen a course of action, there is virtually no benefit in highlighting risk when she has already made what she believes to be the best decision for herself and her baby.

When a patient has attempted to go through a pregnancy medication-free, but then finds she must start medication because her symptoms have become too significant or overwhelming, this decision too will be a difficult one. The patient will need to go through a grieving process for being unable to provide a medication-free environment for her child. She may have significant mixed feelings about this choice, even as she knows the medication will help her. The clinician must be attuned to this possibility and help the patient with appropriate grief work, mourning her ability to carry on without medication.

Working with the fertile woman, pre-pregnancy

If the clinician has followed the suggested initial evaluation guidelines listed in Chapter 3, including questions about pregnancy, last menstrual period, and any pregnancy plans, these issues will already have been documented in the patient record.

If a woman presents for an initial evaluation and is planning to become pregnant in the near future, this may influence the choice of medication or class of medications toward those with a longer track record of safety during pregnancy. For such women, groups of medications with known teratogenic risk may be less desirable choices than those with minimal known risks. For example, with a depressed patient who is planning to become pregnant shortly, a clinician might choose to use fluoxetine, sertraline, nortriptyline, or desipramine (for which there are more documented cases of safe use during pregnancy) and avoid medications with few evidence-based pregnancy data. Similarly, for a bipolar patient, carbamazepine or valproic acid, each of which has known teratogenic effects, would be less desirable choices for a woman who is planning to become pregnant in the near future.

The clinician should reinforce the concept that a planned pregnancy is more desirable than an unexpected one, and that planning will simplify decisions about medication. In an initial medication evaluation, issues of family planning and/or birth control should be discussed with all female patients of childbearing age, even if they are not imminently planning on becoming pregnant, and this discussion documented in their notes. *For any woman of childbearing age where there are any symptoms suggestive of pregnancy, or the possibility of pregnancy cannot be ruled out with certainty, a pregnancy test must be obtained before the patient begins medication.*

When a patient presents for an initial evaluation in the midst of a full-blown mood, anxiety, or psychotic episode and yet is actively trying to get pregnant, the clinician should advise the patient to put off such attempts until her mental health episode is treated. Unfortunately, not all patients will follow this advice. To bolster this advice, it is helpful to provide a timeframe for which the patient is expected to be on medication. Knowing the length of time they are expected to take medication, some women will decide to delay their attempt to become pregnant immediately. Because of severe symptoms or chronicity, the clinician may have to revise this initial estimate at a later date. Hopefully, at that time, the patient will be more focused, stable and able to make the most appropriate decision about medication. Even if the clinician suspects that long-term medication treatment will be necessary, a new patient in an agitated state seldom accepts the recommendation for chronic medication early on in a patient–clinician relationship. Discussion of long-term medication should therefore be put off until the patient is more stable.

Discussion of pregnancy and possible medication complications are particularly important in patients who show impulsive, grandiose, psychotic, or confused symptomatology, since these individuals are more likely to become pregnant in an unplanned way.

When the patient wishes to get pregnant

The mildly/moderately symptomatic cooperative patient

During medication prescription, when a woman states a specific wish to become pregnant it allows the clinician, together with the patient, to gather information that will help the decision-making process when she ultimately does become pregnant. If it has not already been gathered, obtain information about the amount and severity of symptomatology during previous pregnancies. Was any treatment used in previous pregnancies? Was it successful? How long did it take for the patient to become pregnant?

When the patient brings up the desire to become pregnant, *it may possibly be an appropriate time to stop medication in order to assess her response or relapse.* The patient's reaction to a trial off medication prior to attempting to get pregnant may give valuable information to both clinician and patient about whether stopping medication during pregnancy is likely to be feasible. If a patient is firmly committed to attempting to become pregnant soon, the clinician may choose to taper and stop medication early, even if a full course of therapy has not been completed.

A woman thinking about becoming pregnant may raise several other issues for discussion. Women who are particularly sophisticated about medicine and chemistry may inquire about the desirability of switching to a very short half-life medication in the hope that the chemical would be entirely excreted in a matter of hours if she became pregnant. Although some patients believe in the intrinsic logic of this action, there is no evidence to date that shows that use of a short half-life compound provides any defined safety benefit. Although a clinician could agree to change medication for this reason, any small advantage is usually outweighed by the uncertainty of response to a new medication. The vast majority of psychotropics are excreted substantially in 2 to 4 days, and are virtually fully excreted by 1 week. The notable exception is fluoxetine, whose metabolite, norfluoxetine, may be present in small quantities for up to four weeks.

When some patients look forward to pregnancy, they will be interested in switching medications to one that has a longer track record of safety during pregnancy. Although the clinician may accede to the patient's wishes if she feels strongly about this issue, in general, unless patients are taking a known high-risk medication, most of them should be continued on medication to which they have responded rather than switching to a medication that may give an uncertain response.

It is important to ensure that any discussion of the pros and cons of using medication during pregnancy is balanced. In addition to the possible complications of medication usage, which may for some medications include teratogenicity at delivery, neonatal withdrawal, behavioral teratogenicity, and increased risk of miscarriage, the *clinician should discuss the possible effects of untreated depression, psychosis, and anxiety*. Studies have shown that mothers who are significantly depressed during pregnancy have a higher risk of pre-term delivery, low birth-weight babies and small gestational-age babies.[1] Additional information has shown that these children have poor orientation skills, decreased motor tone, lower activity levels, and reduced reflex tone.[1–4]

Prior to attempting to conceive, it is also reasonable at this time to discuss with the patient decreasing or stopping other behaviors that may have additive deleterious effects on pregnancy, such as cigarette smoking, alcohol overuse, or recreational drug usage.

The severely symptomatic, mentally compromised patient

If it is the clinician's assessment that the woman wishing to become pregnant is not thinking clearly and/or may be prone to making impaired judgments, it is useful to involve the spouse/partner before making decisions about medication use. A more stable partner may be able to influence the opinion of an unstable, impulsive, or disorganized patient who is requesting to stay on medication. Before becoming pregnant, if the patient (with or without her partner's agreement) makes a clear choice to refuse or stop medication when she becomes pregnant, this decision must be documented along with details of the discussion regarding any risks anticipated.

If a patient has a psychotic or bipolar illness that has resulted in serious psychotic behavior and life-disruptive symptoms, it is generally better to maintain her on antipsychotic and/or mood stabilizing medication for as long as possible prior to attempting pregnancy. If the patient is mentally competent and is insistent on stopping medication despite her history, it may be preferable to wait until the patient becomes pregnant and stop medication quickly, rather than discontinue medication while she is trying to become pregnant. It may take the patient months or years to become pregnant, during which time a psychotic episode could be devastating.

While the patient is actively trying to become pregnant

By this time in the process with an ongoing patient, if the woman is taking medication, a plan should be documented and agreed upon as to how medications will be handled once she does become pregnant. If the decision is that the patient will be taken off medications as soon as she becomes pregnant, she should be advised to notify the clinician as soon as any signs or symptoms of pregnancy occur, or a positive pregnancy test is obtained. If the patient's medications are discontinued before attempting to get pregnant, the clinician should monitor the patient's condition closely to observe for any clinical worsening. This is particularly important if it takes a long period for the patient to conceive. Some patients who have decided to stop medications while they are trying to get pregnant may find that their symptoms worsen to the point that restarting medications becomes a clinical necessity prior to conception.

If the patient is taking carbamazepine, valproic acid, or other anticonvulsant mood stabilizers while trying to conceive, she should be started on folate (minimum of 4 mg a day) to reduce the likelihood of neural tube defects,[5] – a known complication of these medications when used during pregnancy.

When pregnancy occurs

Once the patient becomes pregnant, the clinician should document when he or she was informed of the possibility of pregnancy, when pregnancy was confirmed by test, and the estimated date of delivery. Medicolegally, it is also useful to document any other medications taken at the time of conception beyond the psychotropic being prescribed. Any history of alcohol or drug abuse that is ongoing should also be included. If necessary, the mental health clinician can order a serum pregnancy test to confirm the possibility of pregnancy, and assist the patient in finding an obstetrical provider or other care provider for prenatal care.

Once the woman is pregnant, the previously agreed plan for stopping or continuing medication should be implemented. The clinician should be aware that some patients who may have made a plan to continue medications may have second thoughts, and decide to stop them once they actually do become pregnant. If medications are to be stopped, this should occur as quickly as possible once pregnancy is suspected or confirmed. In general, the patient's wish to be medication-free will be stronger than her experience of any discontinuation phenomena. It is better to stop medications quickly rather than maintain a prolonged taper, even if this might be the preferred schedule during other, non-pregnant circumstances.

If medication is to be continued during the pregnancy, it should be decreased to the lowest possible dose that provides reasonable symptom control. In some cases, it may be possible to give medications every second or third day rather than every day. It is particularly important to decrease the medication load during the first trimester, when organ development occurs. In general, the time of maximum teratogenic potential is approximately 17–60 days after conception; therefore, medication dosage should be minimal during that period whenever possible.[6]

If the patient has been maintained on a combination of medications, monotherapy can be considered – even if it results in only partial symptom control.

Particularly with an unplanned pregnancy, the prescribing clinician may also raise the issue of the patient's feelings about having become pregnant. Some patients will use the clinician as an objective sounding board to verbalize the positive and negative options for them, given that they have become pregnant in an unplanned way. It is crucial that the clinician help the patient with a balanced point of view toward keeping or terminating the pregnancy, and help the patient make her own choice, rather than imposing the clinician's values on her situation.

During pregnancy

Although an initial plan of action regarding medication has been established, it is important for the clinician to remain flexible during the pregnancy as clinical circumstances may change. Patients who have decided to remain off medications may worsen to the point that reinstitution of medications may be necessary. Within the second or third trimester, when the risk of teratogenicity is less, some patients may decide to reinstitute medications that they have avoided during the first trimester. Regardless of whether the patient is on medication or not, her mental health condition should be monitored frequently for changes. This can be done directly, face-to-face, or through a psychotherapist, who may be seeing the patient more frequently.

Each patient and each pregnancy is unique. Any decisions about medication should be made *ad hoc*, with careful consideration of risks of using medications versus the risk of untreated illness *for this patient, at this time*. Open discussion with the patient (and her partner) about these changing issues should be documented in the patient's chart. Most obstetricians are quite willing to have the mental health prescriber monitor any psychotropics used during pregnancy. Be sure to include any obstetrical provider in the treatment process from the beginning, and at times of clinical worsening.

Medication prescription for symptoms occurring during pregnancy

The clinician should follow these basic guidelines when symptoms worsen or emerge during a pregnancy:

- First consider non-pharmacological interventions. These can include cognitive behavioral therapy, individual or group therapy, or light therapy for depression.[7] For the mildly to moderately symptomatic patient, evaluate life stressors, including job, family, and relationship issues, to see if lifestyle interventions may be helpful in decreasing symptomatology.
- If medication is used, maintain the lowest possible dose that treats the symptoms. Use intermittent dosing, when possible. However, when symptoms are not adequately controlled, increase medication doses to pre-pregnancy doses if necessary.
- Once a decision is made to return to medication, be positive, encouraging and supportive, even if there are known risks.
- For severe symptoms of psychosis, depression or bipolar disorder, make a strong case for starting or continuing medication. In general, the medication risk to mother and fetus is small in comparison to the sequelae of a major mental breakdown. Consider hospitalization and/or the use of ECT for treatment and safety.
- For the woman who is not thinking clearly, is psychotic, exceptionally anxious, or depressed, be sure to include the partner or caretakers to help discern the extent of symptomatology and the behavioral risk of the illness, if

any. For legally incompetent patients, involve the guardian in any decision about restarting medication.

■ Avoid polypharmacy whenever possible.

■ In general during pregnancy, unless the medication previously used by the patient is significantly higher in risk than other choices, it is best to return to a medication that was therapeutically effective and tolerated. Pregnancy is not a time to be experimenting with a new regimen.

■ Avoid complicated or risky medications such as monoamine oxidase inhibitors.

■ Monitor the patient's weight, since increased weight and the presence of gestational diabetes are increased risk factors for fetal neural tube defects.[5] Assist in diet and exercise counseling to maintain reasonable gradual weight gain during the pregnancy.

■ During pregnancy, serum concentrations of medications may change with time because of increase in total body water, decreased protein binding, decreased absorption of drug, and increased renal excretion rate. Serum tricyclic levels as well as serum lithium levels can decrease over the course of a pregnancy. When these medications are used, check serum blood concentrations at frequent intervals to maintain consistent, clinically adequate, nontoxic blood levels.

■ As the pregnancy progresses, if a patient remains medication-free, discuss with her any plans for reinstituting medication postpartum. Document the discussion and assessment of the risk for intensification of symptoms after delivery. In some cases, medication doses that have been decreased during the pregnancy will need to be brought back to full dosage shortly after delivery.

■ Before delivery, discuss with the patient her plans for breastfeeding and the issues regarding psychotropic medication and lactation (see below).

Specific conditions and medication groups

Although our evidence-based information about specific medications is far from thorough, it is better for some medications than for others. This section describes recommendations for clinicians regarding specific medications and classes, based on the limited information available to date at the time of publication.

Of necessity in this text these recommendations are not exhaustive, and the reader is referred to excellent summary articles.[12,19,20]

Depression and antidepressants

When medication is used for mild/moderate depression, consider medications with the most evidence-based information about their use in pregnancy. In general, almost all commonly used antidepressants appear relatively safe when used during pregnancy. These include the SSRIs and TCAs. Fluoxetine, paroxetine, sertraline, and citalopram have a relatively benign track record when used during pregnancy.[8–11]

Tricyclic antidepressants, particularly nortriptyline and desipramine, also have been evaluated in many studies and have generally been shown to pose few side effects or risks of teratogenicity.[12]

Expectant patients may also find reassuring the gradually emerging data about children born to mothers who took fluoxetine or tricyclics during their pregnancy. These studies have shown that such exposure has not affected global IQ, language development or behavioral development in these children to date.[13,14]

For severe, incapacitating or psychotic depressions, consider hospitalization and/or the use of electroconvulsive therapy (ECT).[15]

Bipolar disorder and mood stabilizers

In contrast to the use of antidepressants described above, which appears (within the scope of our data) to be relatively safe, the use of mood stabilizers and the treatment of bipolar disorder in pregnancy is considerably more complicated. No mood-stabilizing medication is clearly risk-free. If the patient's course has been relatively mild and severe episodes have not emerged, it may be reasonable gradually to decrease and stop mood-stabilizing medication so that the patient will be medication-free for 4 weeks prior to conception. Whenever possible, the fetus should not be exposed to mood stabilizers during the first trimester. Of particular concern would be the use of carbamazepine, valproic acid or benzodiazepines, all of which have had documented teratogenic effects.[16,17] Since each of the major mood stabilizers has a somewhat different risk profile during pregnancy, they will be discussed separately.

Lithium carbonate

Exposure to lithium during the first trimester has long been known to be related to an increased incidence of the cardiovascular malformation, Ebstein's anomaly (a malformation and downward displacement of the tricuspid valve into the right ventricle, causing backward leakage and weakening of the ventricular outflow to the lungs). Although the risk is known, the incidence of this anomaly is relatively small (estimates of 0.05–0.1 percent).[17] Recent studies[18,19] also suggest that the incidence may be less than originally thought, although it is still 10–20 times more common in babies exposed to lithium during the first trimester than in the general population. Cardiac fetal ultrasound evaluation performed at 16–19 weeks of pregnancy can reveal the presence of Ebstein's anomaly, and may be a useful diagnostic tool in patients who have had first-trimester lithium exposure.

For a number of reasons, serum lithium levels from constant oral dosage may drop over the course of a pregnancy. Therefore frequent monitoring of serum blood levels is important and gradually increasing doses may be necessary for the first $8\frac{1}{2}$ months.[16,20] In the *several weeks prior to delivery, the dosage of lithium should be dramatically decreased* since increased serum levels and toxicity may result from the drastically decreased blood and fluid volumes immediately following childbirth. This dosage can then be quickly reinstated after delivery, when the risk of postpartum mood episodes is high (see below).

Carbamazepine and valproic acid

Both of these anticonvulsants, frequently used for mood stabilization, have known risks of minor and major malformations, especially neural tube defects and spina bifida. Each should be avoided during the first trimester. When the risk/benefit ratio is sufficient to prescribe them, there may be some lessened risk of use during the second and third trimesters.[19]

When taking anticonvulsants, women should begin folate supplementation (4 mg/day) as soon as they attempt to get pregnant, since supplemental folate has been shown to reduce the risk of neural tube defects.[21]

For those women who do use anticonvulsants after the first trimester, there is a risk of neonatal hemorrhage after delivery. This risk can be reduced by giving vitamin K 20 mg daily during the 1–2 months prior to delivery, with 1 mg of vitamin K given intramuscularly to the newborn at birth.[22]

The weight gain that the woman experiences during pregnancy should be monitored, since exceptionally high weight gains have been associated with increased risk for neural tube defects.[23,24] If such weight gain occurs, the clinician should assist the patient in dietary consultation or refer her to a dietician.

Other mood-stabilizing medications

Lamotrigine has had an ongoing naturalistic study of first-trimester exposure with known outcomes collected by the manufacturer. Although data are limited, the rate of major congenital defects is below the baseline rate in the general population.[25] There are very limited data on other anticonvulsant mood stabilizers (including gabapentin and topiramate). These agents should only be used when there is a clear, positive benefit/risk ratio.[20] Atypical antipsychotics (which may be used for mood stabilization) can be useful and are covered in the section below. Other mood stabilization considerations for a severely bipolar woman include hospitalization, electroconvulsive therapy, or a calcium channel blocker. There is no causal link between haloperidol, chlorpromazine, fluphenazine and teratogenicity. These typical antipsychotics are generally thought safe during gestation in smaller doses.[19,20] Verapamil appears safe in pregnancy, but data are limited.[26]

Bipolar and depressed individuals are at serious risk for recurrence of their illness in the immediate postpartum period.[27] This risk may be as high as 50 percent. Therefore, any mood stabilization medication that has been discontinued either before or during pregnancy should be restarted immediately after delivery, and adequate serum therapeutic levels reached quickly.

Psychosis and antipsychotic medications

Typical antipsychotic medications have been studied much more thoroughly than atypical antipsychotics. In general, if medication is required for psychosis, the clinician might consider well-studied, high potency agents such as haloperidol and trifluoperizine, and avoid, if possible, low potency phenothiazines such as chlorpromazine.[26] Of the atypical antipsychotics, only olanzapine has had any significant amounts of data collected. With use during pregnancy, its rate of major congenital malformation is less than one half of baseline rates in the general population. Rates of other perinatal complications are within normal historical control rates.[25] Risperidone, quetiapine and ziprasidone all have minimal human exposure data. Use of clozapine in pregnancy shows no association with congenital abnormalities, but there have been two cases of new-onset or worsening of gestational diabetes with shoulder dystocia.

Routine prophylaxis against extraparamidal symptoms is generally not advised during pregnancy. If extraparamidal symptoms (EPS) do emerge, anticholinergic medications should be avoided. When some medication treatment is necessary for EPS, consider diphenhydramine in small doses.

Anxiety and anti-anxiety medications

In general, anxiety, stress, and tension during pregnancy should be treated with non-pharmacological methods, including cognitive behavioral techniques, hypnosis, relaxation exercises and decreasing stressful events in the patient's life.

If medication is necessary, benzodiazepines have been the most studied group. However, because there is a clear association between benzodiazepine exposure in the first trimester and increased risk of specific anomalies of the oral cleft, use of these medications should be avoided during that period.[19]

If benzodiazepines are necessary during the second and third trimester, consider using agents such as lorazepam, which are less likely to accumulate in fetal tissue than longer acting agents such as diazepam.[20]

Clonazepam is also a reasonable choice in that cord blood levels have been undetectable in most cases if the maternal daily dosage is less than 1 mg a day. Although no maternal or neonatal toxicity have been seen in doses up to 3.5 mg per day, there is increased risk of neonatal toxicity at higher doses (greater than 5 mg a day[17]).

When benzodiazepines are used in the period approaching delivery, discontinuation should be attempted gradually at a rate no greater than 10 percent per day. Such gradual discontinuation is recommended prior to delivery, since women taking benzodiazepines at the time of delivery have shown an increased duration of labor and possible withdrawal symptoms in the neonate.[28]

The use of buspirone has not been systematically investigated, and there is little information to guide its use during the pregnant period.

Postpartum and lactation

In a pregnancy where the clinician has been actively involved throughout the process, a plan for medication use or non-use in the postpartum period will have been discussed and documented. In women with histories of bipolar disorder and depression, the clinician should be particularly vigilant for serious postpartum depression or the infrequent, but potentially catastrophic, postpartum psychosis. Those patients with a bipolar history are at significant risk for postpartum worsening of their mood disorder. In the patient who will not breastfeed, a rapid institution of full mood-stabilizing and/or antipsychotic medications in the several days postpartum is indicated.

Systematized, evidence-based data on the usage of psychotropics in breastfeeding mothers are virtually absent. The evidence on which recommendations are made consists primarily of isolated case examples, and retrospective reviews of data from these isolated case examples over time. Such data are further complicated by the fact that not all case examples are documented through physician examination, but may be based solely on maternal report.

One final complication is that older medications used over a longer time often have many more case reports than more recently introduced medications. It is not clear whether an increased frequency of side-effect reports represents a true increased risk for that particular medication, or whether it is only a statistical artifact of the larger number of cases observed over time. It is possible that newer medications may appear safe based on small amounts of data, but would perhaps show equal or greater complications if more case reports were available.

To gather information on which to make recommendations, research has relied on several "objective" data sources. The most easily collectible data are measurements of the concentration of psychotropic in breast milk. By estimating the consumption of breast milk by the infant during the day, an extrapolation is made as to how much medication the infant is exposed to. Other "objective" measures include comparing the plasma psychotropic concentration in the mother's serum to the concentration in breast milk, resulting in a fraction. If this fraction is less than one for a particular medication, it is assumed to be safer than if it is greater than one (which could indicate active accumulation of drug in breast milk or higher rates of passive diffusion into breast milk). Relatively few reported cases involve checking the serum concentration of psychotropic in the infant, and most of those reports are measures of parent compound only without measurement of any metabolites. Furthermore, none of these "objective" measures take into account factors of infant physiology (namely immature liver function, decreased liver gomular filtration rate, immature blood/brain barrier and other infant pharmacokinetic issues).

These data sources are quite inconclusive, and there is little (if any) proof that any of these measures relate directly to infant/child behavioral or emotional outcome. There are virtually no long-term studies of the effects of neonatal exposure to psychotropics. Because of this dearth of information, women and their partners must be advised that recommendations given have little documented supporting evidence. Having said this, from the information we do have, it appears that psychotropic medications, in general, do not *seem* to have long-term effects. Those adverse effects from psychotropics seen in infants are generally reversible side effects rather than brain toxicity.[29]

As with decisions about medication during pregnancy, decisions about prescribing psychotropic medications during breastfeeding should be made on an individual basis for each patient and each pregnancy. It is important to take into account what information is known about the medication, as well as the past psychiatric history of the patient, the seriousness of any symptoms during previous episodes, and the wishes of the patient and her partner.

If the patient does wish to breastfeed her infant and medication use is being considered, the clinician should explain that virtually all psychotropic medications taken by the mother do seep into breast milk in varying concentrations. In general these concentrations are small, and the effect of these small medication amounts is uncertain over the long term. If the patient is going to be using medications while breastfeeding, several principles to minimize risk are useful:

■ Mothers may have a strong predisposition to breastfeed, in spite of any medication risk, in that there is clear evidence that breastfed infants may have lower rates of gastrointestinal and respiratory ailments, anemia, and otitis media.[30,31] The breastfeeding experience also provides an opportunity for mother/child bonding.

■ Although the exact incidence is not known, in general, currently measured risks to infants from psychotropic medication exposure during breastfeeding are low. Risks of harm or neglect to the infant from a mother who is profoundly depressed, anxious, manic, or psychotic can be significant and, at times, catastrophic. In patients with serious symptoms, the treatment should favor the maintenance of the mother's mental health, which may include psychotropic medication.

■ Maintain the least possible dose that controls the patient's symptoms.

■ Consider discarding breast milk product in the 7–10 hours following a dose of medication (the so called "pump-and-dump" technique). Use formula for feeding during this time period, when concentrations of medication may be high. Utilize only breast milk secreted after the 10-hour window, which is likely to have a lower concentration of psychotropic contained therein.

■ Another timing strategy is to breastfeed the child just before his or her longest period of anticipated sleep and then have the mother take the psychotropic just after feeding, which will allow for a lesser concentration of drug in breast milk when the infant awakes and needs to be fed again.

■ Premature infants have less well-developed hepatic and kidney function, and therefore may be more at risk to medication exposure effects than full-term infants.

■ Have the mother consider weaning the infant sooner than might otherwise be desired, to limit exposure to the medication.

■ Monitor the condition of the baby through maternal report and examination by a pediatrician. If symptoms of irritability, somnolence, psychomotor slowing or inappropriate delay in achieving developmental milestones occur, measure the amount of psychotropic medication present in the baby's serum. If the concentration is high, decrease the dosage of psychotropic or discontinue it. If the concentration is low but infant symptoms persist, stop the medication or stop breastfeeding, and obtain a pediatric consultation.

■ As with pregnancy itself, the breastfeeding period is not a time to try a new medication previously not used and shown to be effective and tolerable. The only time to consider using a new medication is if the patient has had no previous medication trials, or if all previous medications tried have been unsuccessful or poorly tolerated.

Specific medicines and medication groups in breastfeeding

The following recommendations are taken from excellent review articles and these sources should be seen for further details on individual medications.[20,26,29,32] Further information, including additional case reports (or lack thereof) will inevitably emerge in print.

Antidepressants

SSRI antidepressants, which as a group are in common usage, have shown minimal problems during breastfeeding. Sertraline and paroxetine, with no reports of adverse side effects and relatively short to medium half-lives, are desirable alternatives. Fluoxetine, with its long half-life and possible reports of complications, is less desirable during breastfeeding. There is minimal information regarding the use of citalopram and fluvoxamine.

Other new generation antidepressants, such as bupoprion, venlafaxine, mianserin and trazodone, have minimal data on their use during breastfeeding, and should only be considered as alternatives if other medications are ineffective and/or the risk/benefit ratio is favorable.

Collected reports of tricyclic usage during breastfeeding have shown no adverse reports of those infants whose mothers took imipramine, amitriptyline, nortriptyline, desipramine, and clomipramine. Doxepin, which has had at least one potential possible adverse effect, is not recommended.

Two medications that are available only in the UK, dothiepin and meclobomide, have not been shown to have adverse effects, but are generally less likely to be recommended, given their potential toxicities.[32]

Mood stabilizers

Each of the most common mood stabilizers has potential complications. Lithium has been associated with possible accumulation and excessive blood levels in the infant; carbamazepine use has shown transient hepatic dysfunction; and valproic acid has had one case of reported thrombocytopenia and anemia. Since the risk of postpartum exacerbation of bipolar disorder is significant, the use of medication may be highly indicated or mandatory. The clinician may wish to take a stronger-than-usual stance with a patient regarding the use of medications, without breastfeeding for these highly at-risk patients.

There are a few case reports of lamotrigine or gabapentin being used without obvious complications. Similar early and small numbers of case reports of the use of risperidone and olanzapine have likewise not shown problematic reactions. Although data are limited, these may be considered as alternatives to the above mentioned mood stabilizers if the patient insists on breastfeeding during the immediate postpartum period, and has symptoms necessitating medication.

Chlorpromazine, fluphenazine, and thiothixine are excreted in breast milk, but have not been associated with definitive problematic outcomes. Usage is based on a risk/benefit analysis.[20] Haloperidol and clozapine have had case reports of possible drowsiness and toxicity with their use during breastfeeding, and are generally not recommended alternatives for psychotic patients in the postpartum period. Olanzapine and risperidone are excreted in animal breast milk, but human case reports of infant exposure are scant. Olanzapine has not been associated with any adverse effects in these infants. It is unclear whether risperidone is excreted in human milk, and caution should be advised.[20]

Anti-anxiety medications

There are case reports of adverse neonatal effects with diazepam, clonazepam and alprazolam, which make them less desirable alternatives to lorazepam, oxazepam and temazepam, for which there are none. These latter three medications also have relatively short half-lives, and may be desirable in terms of rapid excretion from the mother's body. If anti-anxiety medication is used, it should be used intermittently. Timing of doses is best when the medication is given to the mother just *after* breastfeeding, to allow for maximum excretion prior to the next feeding. Based on the current lack of reported adverse effects, the infant may incur less risk if SSRI antidepressants are utilized as the primary medication for panic disorder, generalized anxiety disorder, OCD and other anxiety disorders.

Data will change; the decision process will not

Two facts about prescribing medication during pregnancy and lactation are almost inevitable:

1 Data on individual medications and classes of medications will change continuously
2 As clinicians, we will unfortunately likely always be using the same limited data for our prescribing decisions.

Significant differences in prescribing patterns may emerge year-to-year, based on increasing amounts of safety or risk data that are collected on an on-going basis. Medications that enjoy wide prescription and maintain high therapeutic effectiveness will gradually, over time, develop increasing pools of data reflecting a medication's safety or risk during pregnancy and/or breastfeeding. Within the first 3–5 years after the introduction of a medication that is prescribed frequently, a few medication case reports documenting uneventful usage or possible potential problems emerge. Based on these isolated reports, the medication usually moves relatively quickly into a group of medication that *appears* to be relatively safe (and becomes a first- or second-line choice), or shows one or more significant adverse effects (and becomes contraindicated or a less desirable fourth- or fifth-line alternative).

Ten or twenty years from now, we will certainly have significantly more data on some of the medications we currently prescribe, assuming they continue to be used with frequency. By definition, however, newer medications within the first several years of their introduction will still have very little data on which to base prescribing decisions about their usage in pregnancy and lactation.

Due to the ethical considerations and the practical obstacles of recruiting research subjects for systematized prospective research with pregnant or breast-feeding women, there is a distinct possibility that we will *never* see a well-designed study of a medication's safety in pregnancy or during lactation. Therefore, in all likelihood 20 years from now we will still be using the same *types* of data that we have now – isolated case reports and, eventually, pooled data summaries of these case reports. Because of the rapid evolution of psychopharmacology, the rapid rise in the number of medications we prescribe and the emergence of new classes of medications, we may, in fact, actually have smaller amounts of data on any one particular medication. Unless a new medication is overwhelmingly superior to its prescribing alternatives, and vast numbers of women are prescribed this medication, we will continue to have only small numbers of isolated case reports with any one particular product.

The ongoing and increasing frequency of diagnosable emotional illness and the obstacles to prospective, controlled studies will virtually certainly require us to be making prescribing decisions with less information than we or our patients are totally comfortable with. During our prescribing lifetimes, therefore, we will continue to:

- Present the evidence-based information, limited as it may be
- Include the pregnant woman and her partner in the decision-making process
- Help balance the risks of untreated illness versus possible medication effect for each individual woman and each individual pregnancy.

Studies evaluating the emotional, physical and behavioral effects on children born to women taking any particular psychotropic may take 7–10 years from the time a medication is introduced. Long-term studies of the behavioral, emotional and physical effects on a child when a mother takes psychotropic medication are logistically very difficult, may never be done, or will often become available long after a medication is out of common usage.

The principles discussed in Chapter 27 regarding keeping current in the prescribing process are nowhere more important than regarding the issue of medication use during pregnancy and lactation. Each new case report of a particular medication used during pregnancy or lactation will bolster our level of confidence when no problems occur, or will increase our concern if potential problems ensue. Whenever a woman presents to us seeking to become pregnant, having become pregnant or desiring to breastfeed, yet is at risk for emotional illness, we must re-evaluate the current literature so that we can present the most up-to-date information to aid her decision. There is little doubt, however, that our role in the prescribing process will change little. We must become comfortable with helping a patient to make a difficult decision, with less-than-adequate, evidence-based data.

References

1 Newport DJ. The neuroendocrinology of maternal depression and stress during pregnancy. *J Gender Spec Med* 2001;(Suppl. 8):6–7.

2 Abrams SM *et al.* Newborns of depressed mothers. *Infant Mental Health J* 1995;16:233.

3 Jones NA *et al.* Newborns of mothers with depressive symptoms are physiologically less developed. *Infant Behav Devel* 1998;21:537.

4 Lundy BL *et al.* Prenatal depression: effects on neonates. *Infant Behav Devel* 1999;22:119.

5 Koren G. Use of atypical antipsychotics during pregnancy and the risk of neural tube defects in infants. *Am J Psychiatry* 2002;159:136–137.

6 *The Maudsley Prescribing Guidelines*. Martin Dunitz, 2001, p. 107.

7 Oren D *et al.* An open trial of morning light therapy for treatment of antepartum depression. *Am J Psychiatry* 2002;159:666–669.

8 Pastuszak A *et al.* Pregnancy outcome following first-trimester exposure to fluoxetine (Prozac). *JAMA* 1993;269:2246–2248.

9 Chambers CD *et al.* Birth outcomes in pregnant women taking fluoxetine. *N Engl J Med* 1997;336:258–262.

10 Kulin NA *et al.* Pregnancy outcome following maternal use of the new selective serotonin reuptake inhibitors: a prospective, controlled, multicenter study. *JAMA* 1998;279:609–610.

11 Ericson A *et al.* Delivery outcome after the use of antidepressants in early pregnancy. *Eur J Clin Pharmacol* 1999;55:503–508.

12 Miller L. Pharmacotherapy during the perinatal period. *Essent Psychopharmacol* 1998;2(3):263.

13 Nulman I *et al.* Neurodevelopment of children exposed *in utero* to antidepressant drugs. *N Eng J Med* 1997;336:258–262.

14 Mattson SN *et al.* Neurobehavioral follow-up of children prenatally exposed to fluoxetine. *Teratology* 1999;59(3):376.

15 Kahn DA *et al.* Major depression during conception and pregnancy: a guide for patients and families. www.womensmentalhealth.org

16 Erlick Robinson G. Women and psychopharmacology. *Medscape Women's Health* 2002;7(1).

17 Altshuler LL. The use of medication in bipolar women during pregnancy and postpartum. Presented at the Third International Conference on Bipolar Disorder, June 1999.

18 Jacobsen SJ *et al.* Prospective multicentre study of pregnancy outcome after lithium exposure during first trimester. *Lancet* 1992;339:530–533.

19 Altshuler LL *et al.* Pharmacologic management of psychiatric illness during pregnancy: dilemmas and guidelines. *Am J Psychiatry* 1996;153:592–606.

20 Masud Iqbal M *et al.* Effects of antimanic mood-stabilizing drugs on fetuses, neonates, and nursing infants. *Southern Med J* 2001;94(3):305–322.

21 Dansky LV *et al.* Mechanisms of teratogenis: folic acid and antiepileptic therapy. *Neurology* 1992;42(suppl. 5):32–42.

22 Delgado-Escueta AV. Consensus guidelines: preconception counseling,

management and care of the pregnant woman with epilepsy. *Neurology* 1992:42(suppl. 5):149–160.

23 Goldstein DJ *et al.* Olanzapine-exposed pregnancies and lactation: early experience. *J Clin Psychopharmacol* 2000;20:399–403.

24 Stones SC *et al.* Clozapine use in two full-term pregnancies. *J Clin Psychiatry* 1997;58:364–365.

25 Ernst CL *et al.* The reproductive safety profile of mood stabilizers, atypical antipsychotics and broad spectrum psychotropics. *J Clin Psychiatry* 2002; 63(suppl 4):42–55.

26 Miller L. Pharmacotherapy during the perinatal period. *Essent Psychopharmacol* 1998;2(3):274.

27 Cohen LS *et al.* Postpartum prophylaxis for women with bipolar disorder. *Am J Psychiatry* 1995;152(11):1641–1644.

28 Stowe ZN and Nemeroff CB. Psychopharmacology during pregnancy and lactation. In: CG Schatzberg and CG Nemeroff (eds), *American Psychiatric Press Textbook of Psychopharmacology.* American Psychiatric Press Inc., 1995, p. 823.

29 Buist A. Treating mental illness in lactating women. *Medscape Women's Health* 2001;6(2).

30 Wilson IT. Determinents and consequences of drug excretion in breast milk. *Drug Metab Review* 1983;14:619–652.

31 Chen Y *et al.* Artificial feeding and hospitalization in the first 18 months of life. *Pediatrics* 1988;81:58–62.

32 Burt VK *et al.* The use of psychotropic medications during breastfeeding. *Am J Psychiatry* 2001;158:1001–1009.

Chapter 12

Prescribing psychotropics for older patients

Statistics regarding medication use in older adults are impressive. Although they make up only 13 percent of the American population, patients over 65 years account for 30 percent of the use of prescription medications.[1] The average individual over the age of 65 fills 13 prescriptions each year, which is almost twice the national average.[1] In the geriatric population, prescription medication is complicated by frequent use of over-the-counter and herbal preparations (often seen as a way to save money on a limited budget). As many as 10 percent of the elderly use medications prescribed for other people, and 20 percent take medications not currently prescribed by a clinician.[2]

The reasons for increased medication usage in this population are several:

- Compared to a younger person, geriatric patients have more illnesses (both medical and psychiatric) for which medication is used
- Many elderly patients believe that every problem should have a remedy ("a pill for every ill") and seek medication for relief
- Particularly in nursing homes, institutional or care settings, patients may not have had a thorough re-evaluation of their medication regimen and can accumulate a long list of medications over the course of their lifetime.

Prescribing psychotropic medications to older individuals presents specific challenges to the clinician. The prescriber must specifically attend to issues regarding the patient's understanding of why the medication is being prescribed, and the ability to cooperate and comply with the treatment regimen.

Seniors at risk

Geriatric patients are physiologically at increased risk for medication problems with the use of psychotropics for several reasons. These include:

- Pharmacokinetic changes
- Pharmacodynamic changes
- Increased frequency of medication interactions
- Side effects with lack of compensating physiological mechanisms.

Pharmacokinetic changes

As the body ages, there is a decrease in lean body mass and total body water with a consequent increase in body fat. These changes lead to changes in distribution, half-life and elimination of many psychotropics that are lipophilic and are stored in the body fat. Metabolic breakdown of these lipophilic drugs is into water-soluble forms that can be more readily eliminated, and occurs primarily in the liver. Effects of aging include decreased blood flow to the liver, and decreased liver size and mass.[3,4] Therefore, the drugs that are metabolized from the systemic circulation via first-pass hepatic metabolism are excreted more slowly, have a reduced clearance, and are at risk for accumulation and prolonged half-life. Elimination and excretion, usually through the kidneys, are also affected by aging. As a person ages, there is a decline in the glomerular filtration rate, decreased kidney size, decreased renal blood flow, and a decrease in the number of nephrons.[5,6]

Clinically, the end result of these pharmacokinetic changes is that *older patients may have larger concentrations of medication in their bloodstream when given a "standard" or typical adult dosage*. Medications with a long half-life, that are slow to be eliminated, may accumulate, resulting in exaggerated side effects. Lipophilic medications with long half-lives, such as diazepam, flurazepam, and amitriptyline, are particularly poor choices in the geriatric population because their distribution and elimination are altered by several of these mechanisms.[7,8]

Pharmacodynamics

In addition to measurable changes in the blood serum concentration of various psychotropics, elderly patients may have unexpected or unusual pharmacodynamic responses to medications.[10] Within the elderly brain, receptor response can be more sensitive to the action of psychotropic drugs. Therefore, as a patient ages the therapeutic response and/or excessive response can begin to occur at lower than "normal" therapeutic levels.

Medication interactions

It is well known that the larger the number of medications a patient takes, the more likely it is that the patient will have medication interactions. A patient taking four prescriptions is twice as likely to experience an adverse medication interaction than a patient taking just one medication. If a patient takes seven medications simultaneously, the risk of an adverse reaction increases fourteen-fold![1] We also know that the greater the number of diagnoses, the greater the number of medications likely to be prescribed. Because seniors have a greater number of diagnosed illnesses and take a significantly increased number of medications (often of several classes), they are statistically much more likely to have drug interactions and their sequalae than their younger counterparts.

Particularly troublesome side effects for the elderly include sedation, confusion, dizziness, and decreased sleep – all of which can be common with psychotropics. Also problematic are anticholinergic effects, including decreased urination, blurred vision, and dry mouth.

Elderly persons are less able to compensate for the side effects of many medications.[10] Especially problematic is decreased sensitivity of baroreceptors, which can predispose the senior to postural hypotension, dizziness, and the likelihood of falls.

Side effects alone can be severe enough to require hospitalization. One study documented that 16.8 percent of general hospital admissions for the elderly were due to side effects of medication.[11]

Non-compliance – a major problem

Although estimates of non-compliant medication usage in the elderly vary, almost all estimates are high – ranging from 40 to 75 percent.[12] Non-compliant usage may lead to overusage, underusage, sporadic, or changing usage of medications. The causes of non-compliance are multiple, but include:

- Not understanding the reasons for medications being used, and therefore using them incorrectly
- Unintentional non-compliance due to confusion about dosing schedules
- Forgetfulness
- Intentional non-compliance because of inability to afford the medication and/or omitting doses to "make them last"
- Intentional non-compliance because of increased sensitivity to bothersome side effects/toxic reactions to medications.

The geriatric population's tendency toward increasing cognitive changes with advancing age leads to significant forgetfulness and unintentional underdosing, overdosing, or missed dosing (see Chapter 15). Not remembering that they have taken the dose, patients may take a second or third dose unknowingly and unintentionally. Particularly when anticholinergics or sedative hypnotics are included in the regimen, memory interference is common. With impaired memory, patients may also forget to take prescribed doses altogether.

Deliberate overuse of non-prescription drugs (which are usually less costly than prescription medication) is a common occurrence.[13] Patients may use their experience with rapid-acting non-psychotropic medications (e.g. pain pills) as a guide to how they believe psychotropics may act. They will take too much prescribed psychotropic medication in the hope that by taking a larger dose they will get well more rapidly. By being able to improve sooner they believe they can stop the medication sooner and ultimately save money.

Underusage of medications is a more significant problem in the elderly than in other age groups. Besides the memory problems mentioned above, seniors may take less than prescribed amounts of medication for various other reasons as well. Owing to the high cost of prescription drugs, consistent use of medication may be a major concern for many pensioners who live on a fixed income. Patients will attempt to make their supply of medication last longer by taking doses intermittently to spread them out. Likewise, they may be even more prone than other mental health patients to stopping medications at the earliest opportunity, often as soon as they begin feeling well, believing that they no longer need the psychotropic. Misunderstanding the mechanism of action and the need for continuing doses of psychotropics contributes to a failure to take adequate medication for an adequate period of time. Elderly patients may also stop a prescription medication prematurely and begin an over-the-counter remedy in the hope that it will sustain the effect, be just as useful, and be less expensive.

Frequently, side effects common to the use of psychotropics can cause elderly patients to underdose themselves. Anticholinergic, sedative and hypotensive side effects of psychotropics, which are especially bothersome to seniors, can lead geriatric patients to underdose themselves or stop medication early.[14]

Principles of psychotropic medication prescription in the elderly

Two statements can guide the clinician in the prescribing of psychotropic medications to the elderly:

1 *Less is more* with regard to:
   ■ Dosage of medication prescribed
   ■ Number of medications prescribed
   ■ Length of time medications are prescribed.
2 *More is better* with regard to:
   ■ Giving instructions
   ■ Vigilance for side effects
   ■ Frequency of follow up evaluations.

Although many of the principles described in this section are important for all age groups, they are particularly crucial when prescribing psychotropic medications to the geriatric population:

■ Minimize the number of medications used
■ Start low and go slow with dosage increase

■ Remember that the ultimate therapeutic dose of drug may be lower than that used in younger adults

■ For the patient taking chronic psychotropics, the amount of drug necessary for therapeutic response can change with advancing age (and usually decreases)

■ Lengthen the time period between dose changes to allow the patient to adjust to any new or increased side effects, and to observe for response (positive or negative)

■ Avoid psychotropic medications for minor or non-specific diagnoses

■ Use medication for agitation and behavioral control only when necessary, and then in minimal doses (see Chapter 15).

Because of the increased sensitivity to side effects and the decreased ability to compensate for them, clinicians should always consider whether non-pharmacological means are useful in treating a mental health condition in the elderly (see Chapter 15 for a discussion of these non-pharmacological alternatives). If medication is used, monotherapy is always preferable to polypharmacy. However, despite the downside of using multiple medications, some geriatric patients may require intentional polypharmacy by the clinician to obtain an adequate therapeutic response.

In general, when starting a medication in a geriatric individual, the clinician should use half the dose typically used for an adult patient. Further dosage increases should be done more gradually and at greater intervals than those timeframes used in younger adults. This will allow elderly individuals to adapt to both the therapeutic effect and any side effects from the medication. Because lower starting doses are used and dosage increases leading to a final therapeutic dose are spread out, it may take a longer period of time to assess the therapeutic response to a particular medication. A trial of medication may take several months to be done safely and yet allow for assessment of adequacy of response.

Regular re-evaluation

Particularly in elderly patients who are followed over time, or patients maintained in an institutional care setting, the clinician must regularly re-evaluate the patient's medication regimen. During such an assessment, it is important for a clinician to consider eliminating any unnecessary medications and minimizing the overall medication prescription burden.

Questions to be asked by the prescriber during re-evaluation should include:

■ Is each of these psychotropics still necessary to this patient?

■ Has the patient had an interval without medication to observe for ongoing clinical necessity?

■ Could any medications be discontinued that were added during a crisis that has now passed?

■ Would a lowering of dosage accomplish a continuing satisfactory therapeutic result?

■ Is the patient experiencing any new or added side effects from the psychotropics?

■ Is the patient cognitively and physically still able to manage his or her own medications safely?

■ Has the patient's mental, physical, or financial circumstances changed such that the medication prescription regimen should be altered?

■ Has the patient been compliant with his or her regimen? (Are refills being filled on time, early or late? Are there more pills left over from a previous prescription than there should be if the patient were taking the medication as directed?)

■ If non-compliance is suspected, is further education or reinforcement necessary to emphasize why, how and when the medication should be taken?

Senior medication problems – general strategies

During evaluation and initial prescription

At the initial evaluation of any geriatric patient, the clinician should perform a comprehensive review of all prescription, non-prescription, and herbal medications that the patient takes. Prior to the actual patient visit, it is often useful to ask the patient or caregivers to prepare a list of medication names, doses, frequency of administration, and length of time taken. This gives patients and/or their caregivers the opportunity to formulate such a list at their leisure in a more organized and complete way, rather than attempting to produce the information on the spur of the moment in the office.

In addition to other considerations of effectiveness and therapeutic benefit for a geriatric patient, the clinician should consider the following information in recommending medication.[2]

■ How many prescription medications does the patient take?
■ How many non-prescription medications does the patient take?
■ How many clinicians does the patient consult?
■ Can the patient tolerate the addition of another medication?
■ What side effects are likely to occur?
■ Does the initial starting dosage need to be modified?
■ What medication interactions are likely?
■ Is the patient mentally, physically or financially impaired in a way that will affect the choice of medication or its administration?
■ Does the patient have sensory or literacy problems that may affect the patient's understanding of instructions or ability to carry them out?
■ Does the patient live alone?
■ Can the patient self-administer the medication prescribed?
■ Is special packaging required?
■ What frequency of re-evaluation is necessary to determine if the medication is safely tolerated and effective?
■ If the medication is effective, what target date is appropriate to evaluate when it may be stopped?

Communication between the clinician and patient is crucial in obtaining medication compliance. It is vitally important that geriatric patients understand the nature of their mental health condition, the role of medications in treatment, and the limitations of the medications' effect. Patients must know what the medications can do and will not do, and the timeframe in which a therapeutic response is expected. The clinician must explain possible drug interactions and side effects. Once explained, it is important to obtain at least a verbal response from patients that they understand the regimen and will comply with it. For this medicine, is taking extra doses helpful or, in fact, harmful? Whenever possible, PRN (as needed) dosing should be minimized and the patient given a schedule that is consistent day to day. If extra doses are permitted or recommended, at each patient's discretion, how much medication can be taken and how often?

In prescribing a dosage regimen, the clinician should attempt to match the regimen to the particular patient's daily schedule. When possible, dosages should be attached to predictable elements of daily routine such as meals or bedtime, rather than middle of the day dosing. It may be necessary to ask about the timing of these daily events in *this* patient's life. Some persons who live alone may have idiosyncratic eating and sleeping times. The drug regimen should be kept simple, using once-daily dosing whenever possible.

Visual or mechanical aids are very helpful to the prescriptive process with the geriatric population. Written instructions as well as charts are useful ways to explain medication dosing. The patient can be advised to obtain a partitioned "pill minder" at the pharmacy to organize dosages for a day or a week, which will minimize unintentional repeat dosing. Color-coded bottles may be helpful in distinguishing one medication from another. Large lettering on any instructions or on pill bottles is also useful. Patients with arthritis or hand pain should have medication bottles without safety caps, which may be difficult to open. The pharmacist should be alerted on the written prescription of the necessity to utilize these aids for a patient. The patient should be encouraged to use one pharmacy for all medications – both psychotropic and non-psychotropic. Computerized pharmacy medication profiles at a single pharmacy can alert the pharmacist to potentially problematic drug interactions of medications prescribed by multiple clinicians.

It is important to avoid referring to pills solely by color ("the little white pill"), as patients with multiple medications often have several pills of the same color.

When discussing medications with geriatric patients, clinicians should realize that they have a decreased attention span and may need repetition in order to understand the nature of their medication regimen. When a patient will self-administer medication, a caregiver or family member can be included at the time of giving prescription and dosing instructions so that that the caregiver may repeat and reinforce the instructions at a later time.

Senior patients may need specific direction on what to do if a medication supply runs out and any consequences that can occur (e.g. discontinuation syndrome) if the medication is stopped suddenly. If there is risk involved in allowing the supply to run out, the patient needs specific directions to contact the clinician before using the last dose. Patients must be aware that it is not routinely good practice to decrease the dose to try to make the current amount last longer or, worse yet, stop the medication without notifying the clinician.

During follow-up visits

Patients should bring a list of all medications they are currently taking to each follow-up visit, and update the list with any new medications from other pre-scribers. At the first follow-up visit, the clinician should ask the patient to explain how many pills of each psychotropic medication he or she is taking and at what time of day. It is surprising how often the patient is not taking the medication in the amount or frequency that the clinician has prescribed!

Once a year, patients should bring in all pill bottles of medications they are currently taking so the clinician can review with the patient each of the psy-chotropics, how they are taken, for what condition they are being taken, and any side effects that may have occurred. For long-term patients, the patient's advanc-ing age may justify a dosage decrease, or it may be possible to discontinue one or more medications.

Specific psychotropic medication considerations in the elderly

No psychotropic medication choices are ideal or risk-free in geriatric patients, given the inherent potential fragility of the aging body and mind. Certain psy-chotropic medications, however, carry added risk for elderly patients, and should be avoided whenever possible. These medications are listed in Table 12.1.[1,7,12]

In general, drugs with a narrow therapeutic index such as lithium carbonate and tricyclic antidepressants are medications where changes in blood level can lead to serious side effects or toxicity in the elderly. More frequent monitoring of

Table 12.1 Psychotropic medications to be used with caution in elderly patients

Class of medication	Medications	Effect
Tricyclic antidepressants	Amitriptyline, doxepin	Strong anticholinergic and sedating properties; may induce arrythmias
	Desipramine	Sleep interference
Long-acting benzodiazepines	Chlordiazepoxide, diazepam, flurazepam	Long half-life, oversedation, high fall risk
Antihistamines	Diphenhydramine, cyproheptadine	Strong anticholinergic activity and effects
Beta blockers	Propranolol	May worsen respiratory function
Traditional antipsychotics	High doses of any antipsychotic medications	Hypotension, sedation, falls

serum blood levels is necessary, with vigilance for the addition of any agent that could alter blood levels, in order to minimize risk.

Antidepressants

Virtually all SSRI and other new generation antidepressants offer advantages over TCAs in the elderly population.[15] Another useful class of medication to treat depression for this group is stimulants that have been shown on multiple occasions to have rapid antidepressant activity with minimal drug interactions and side effects.[16–18] Issues of habituation and abuse are lessened in the geriatric age group, and stimulants can be especially useful in the medically ill, depressed elderly because of their rapid onset of action and minimal medication interactions.

Anti-anxiety agents, sedative hypnotics

If benzodiazepines are necessary, shorter acting medications, such as alprazolam, lorazepam, oxazepam, triazolam, and temazepam, are preferable to longer acting agents. Benzodiazepines should be used judiciously in small doses, since no benzodiazepine is without some increased sedation/fall risk in the elderly. Anxiety disorders may be better treated with antidepressants if longer-term medication is necessary.

Any sedative medication from any classification, whether of short or long half-life, can cause excess sedation and increase the risk of falls and subsequent hip fractures.[19] Patients can awaken confused or ataxic in the middle of the night as they arise to use the bathroom. The clinician should carefully assess the risk/benefit ratio before prescribing anything as a sedative/hypnotic.

Antipsychotics

With the exception of clozapine, which has major potential side-effect concerns for the elderly, new atypical antipsychotics (risperidone, olazapine, quetiapine, aripiprazole, and ziprasidone) have safety and tolerability advantages over traditional antipsychotics.[20] Markedly lower incidence of movement and neurological complications (see Chapter 17) make these agents preferable choices to earlier agents for seniors.[21] Clozapine, with a side-effect profile that includes lowered seizure threshold, blood dyscrasia, strong anticholinergic properties, and significant orthostatic hypotension, is generally a fourth or fifth choice after the other atypical antipsychotics for elderly patients.

Mood stabilizers

There are no controlled data studies of mood stabilizer effectiveness specifically in the geriatric population. Safety and side-effect profiles have been more thoroughly collected for the anticonvulsant mood stabilizers in the epileptic population rather than the mental health population. None of the commonly used

Table 12.2 Possible adverse effects of medications*	
Drug	Possible adverse effects
Carbamazepine	Ataxia, dizziness, hyponatremia, cardiac conduction disturbance
Valproic acid	Ataxia, dizziness, weight gain, tremor
Gabapentin	Somnolence, dizziness, ataxia
Lamotrigine	Somnolence, dizziness, ataxia, diplopia, rash
Topiramate	Dizziness, ataxia, difficulty concentrating, tremor, word-finding difficulty

*Adapted from Bourdet SV *et al*. Pharmacologic management of epilepsy in the elderly. *J Am Pharm Assoc* 2001;41(3):434.

mood stabilizers is without at least one potential side effect that could be troublesome or hazardous to an elderly patient (see Table 12.2). Therefore, mood stabilizer decisions should be made on a case-by-case basis using a risk/benefit assessment for each patient.

Atypical antipsychotics, such as olanzapine, risperidone, quetiapine, aripiprazole, and ziprasidone, may have usefulness as mood stabilizers in this population.[22] Further safety and risk issues for these compounds may emerge from a large multicenter trial currently in process under the auspices of the National Institute of Mental Health.[23]

Other considerations

Of particular concern in the elderly is the risk of hypotension, dizziness, and falls. Seniors who use psychotropic drugs, particularly benzodiazepines and antidepressants, are at almost twice the risk of hip fracture secondary to a fall than are patients not taking these medications.[8]

Medication-induced cognitive changes are also a major concern in the elderly. Since the incidence of delirium and dementia increase with age, before factoring in any effect of medication (see Chapter 15), the addition of medication can further complicate cognitive ability. Even mild cognitive impairment may negatively impact patients' day-to-day functioning and their ability adequately to comply with their overall medication regimen. This is a particular issue if the patient lives alone.

References

1 Beers MH *et al*. Drugs and the elderly, part 1: the problems facing managed care. *Am J Manag Care* 2000;6(12):1313–1320.

2 Lamy PP *et al*. Drug prescribing patterns, risks, and compliance guidelines. In: C Salzman (ed.), *Clinical Geriatric Psychopharmacology*, 2nd edn. Williams & Wilkins, 1992, pp. 15–37.

3 Wynne HA *et al*. The association of age and frailty with the pharmacokinetics and pharmacodynamics of metoclopramide. *Age Ageing* 1993;22:354.

4   Wynne HA *et al*. The effect of age upon liver volume and apparent liver blood flow in healthy man. *Hepatology* 1989;9:297.

5   Rowe JW *et al*. The effect of age on creatinine clearance in men: a cross-sectional and longitudinal study. *J Gerontol* 1976;31:155.

6   Lindeman RD *et al*. Longitudinal studies on the rate of decline in renal function with age. *J Am Geriatr Soc* 1985;33:278.

7   Gareri P *et al*. Conventional and new antidepressant drugs in the elderly. *Prog Neurobiol* 2000; 61:353–396.

8   Turnheim K. Drug dosage in the elderly: is it rational? *Drugs Aging*, 1998; 13(5):357–379.

9   Hammerlein A *et al*. Pharmacokinetic and pharmacodynamic changes in the elderly: clinical implications. *Clin Pharmacokinet*. 1998;35(1):49–64.

10 Offerhaus L (ed.) *Drugs for the Elderly*, 2nd edn. WHO Regional Publications, European Series, 1997.

11 Col N *et al*. The role of medication noncompliance and adverse drug reactions in hospitalizations of the elderly. *Arch Intern Med* 1990;150:841–845.

12 Zubenko GS and Sunderland T. Geriatric psychopharmacology: why does age matter? *Harv Rev Psychiatry* 2000;7(6):311–333.

13 Kiernan PJ and Isaacs JB. Use of drugs by the elderly. *J R Soc Med* 1981; 74:196–200.

14 Gryfe CI and Gryfe BM. Drug therapy of the aged: the problem of compliance and the roles of physicians and pharmacists. *J Am Geriatr Soc* 1984;32:301–307.

15 Preshorn SH and Catterson M. Antidepressants and the elderly: focus on newer agents. *Int J Geriatr Psychopharm* 1998;1:66–77.

16 Massand PS and Tesar GE. Use of stimulants in the medically ill. *Psychiatr Clin North Am* 1996;19(3):515–547.

17 Emptage RE and Semla TP. Depression in the medically ill elderly: a focus on methylphenidate. *Ann Pharmacother* 1996;30(2):151–157.

18 Pickett P *et al*. Psychostimulant treatment of geriatric depressive disorders secondary to medical illness. *J Geriatr Psychiatry Neurol* 1990;3(3):146–151.

19 Wang PS *et al*. Zolpidem use and hip fractures in older people. *J Am Geriatr Soc* 2001;49:1685–1690.

20 Blake L *et al*. Optimal management of psychosis and agitation in the elderly. On the Internet at www.medscape.com, March 2002.

21 Borson S. Side effects of atypical antipsychotics: issues for geriatric psychiatry. Presented at the American Association for Geriatric Psychiatry Conference, 2001. Available at www.medscape.com/viewarticle/430714

22 Keck PE. Clinical management of bipolar disorder. CME June 2001, on the Internet at www.medscape.com

23 Schneider LS *et al*. National Institute of Mental Health Clinican Antipsychotic Trials of Intervention Effectiveness (CATIE). *Am J Geriatr Psychiatry* 2001;9:346–360.

Chapter 13

Medication of sleep problems

Sleep disorders affect 60 million adults per year worldwide.[1] Fifty percent of adults at some point in their lives are affected by insomnia.[2] Many of these people with a sleep problem will approach their medical practitioner for help and request medication.[3]

Difficulty in sleeping is one of the most common presenting requests to a medication clinician. Based on accurate diagnostic assessment, the prescription of medication to aid sleep is generally safe, can be extraordinarily helpful for patients, and can help to speed recovery from a primary mental health disorder. On the other hand, poor prescribing habits and/or overprescription of sleeping medication can cause daytime sleepiness, accidents, falls, exacerbation of medical illness, and possible habituation. Some clinicians, unfortunately, withhold the prescription of sleeping medication unnecessarily, while others prescribe prematurely, lacking sufficient evaluation and follow-up. The prescription of sleeping medication is neither an area to be feared and avoided, nor should it be the immediate, automatic response to a patient who is having difficulty sleeping. This chapter will discuss the principles of assessment of sleep problems and the informed prescription of sedative/hypnotic medication.

Facts and definitions

Several key definitions are important in order to discuss the issue of sleep. These include:

- *Insomnia* – difficulty in initiating or maintaining sleep or having sleep, that is non-restorative.[4]
- *Psychophysiological insomnia* – a condition in which a patient who begins having difficulty sleeping becomes increasingly anxious and worried that he or she will not sleep, which then makes it more difficult to fall asleep, perpetuating a problematic cycle leading to further insomnia.
- *Rebound insomnia* – increased difficulty sleeping after a patient who has been taking a sleep medication on a chronic basis stops the medication suddenly.
- *Sleep latency* – the interval of time between when patients lie down to sleep and the time they actually fall asleep.
- *Sleep efficiency* – the amount of time that a patient actually sleeps divided by the amount of time a patient spends in bed trying to sleep, expressed as a fraction or percentage (e.g. a patient who is actually asleep for 5 hours while in bed for 8 hours has a sleep efficiency of 5/8, or 62.5 percent).
- *Phase-shifted sleep* – when persons get adequate hours of sleep, but do so at unusual times or at times that interfere with usual day and evening functioning (e.g. they sleep from 6 pm to 3 am – phase advanced sleep – or 4 am until noon – phase delayed sleep).
- *Sleep apnea* – transient periods of breathing cessation during sleep. *Central* sleep apnea results from failure of the respiratory centers in the medulla; *obstructive* sleep apnea (OSA) is caused by collapse or obstruction of the airway during REM sleep.[5] Both types of apnea result in disrupted sleep, unrefreshing sleep, and daytime fatigue.
- *Restless leg syndrome (RLS)* – a common central nervous system disorder characterized by uncomfortable "creepy, crawly, bubbly, or tingling" sensations in the legs, which usually appear at rest, are relieved temporarily by movement, worsen during the evening or night, and can interrupt the ability to fall asleep.[6]
- *Periodic limb movements of sleep (PLM)* – stereotypical flexing motions of the legs that occur in clusters of 20–40 seconds during sleep, which can cause arousal and daytime sleepiness.[6] PLMs occur frequently in persons with restless leg syndrome.
- *Insufficient sleep syndrome* – a condition that results from persons who recurrently consciously attempt to "get by" with less than usual amounts of sleep in order to accommodate shift work, exams, multiple jobs, social or family expectations, and leads to fatigue and irregular sleep patterns.[7]
- *Narcolepsy* – recurrent, irresistible, brief episodes of sleep during the day accompanied by spells of muscle weakness when emotionally upset (cataplexy), and visions or vivid dreamlike states in the drowsy state just before sleep (hypnogenic hallucinations) or just prior to awakening (hypnopompic hallucinations).[7]

Stages of sleep

Sleep is not a consistent, uniform activity. There are distinctly demarcated stages of sleep that can be easily differentiated on an EEG. Broadly, sleep is divided into non-rapid eye movement (non-REM) sleep and rapid eye movement (REM) sleep, which is the stage in which we dream. Non-REM sleep is divided into stages one, two, three, and four, with stage one being the lightest stage and stage four the deepest. The vast majority of our sleep is taken up in the non-REM stages, and routinely occurs in a cycle. The cycle begins with stage one, progressing in depth to stages two, three, and four. The cycle then reverses itself back to stages three, two, and one, followed by a REM period. This cycle repeats itself three to four times per night, and can be seen most clearly in the top graph in Figure 13.1, which shows the typical stages in a child's sleep. The subsequent graphs show sleep patterns for young adults and elderly individuals. The most important element of these comparison graphs is that as we age, we have significantly less

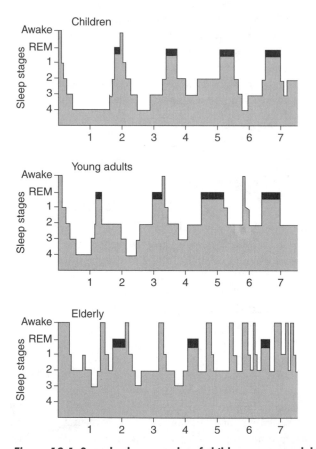

Figure 13.1 **Sample sleep graphs of children, young adults, and seniors**
*Source: Kales A and Kales JD. Sleep disorders: recent findings in the diagnosis and treatment of disturbed sleep. *N Engl J Med* 1974;290:487.

stage-four deep sleep and more of the lighter stages of sleep, with many more frequent awakenings. This becomes particularly important when discussing sleep with elderly individuals, since it is a normal, expectable, physiological phenomenon that their sleep is lighter and more disrupted than it was when they were younger.

Evaluating a sleep problem

The important factors to be addressed in an evaluation of a sleep problem are listed in Table 13.1 and elaborated on in the subsequent text.

When a patient first presents describing difficulty with sleep, the clinician should find out how long this sleep problem has been occurring. Sleep problems are divided into *transient insomnia* (limited to a few nights), *short-term insomnia* (less than 3 weeks) and *long-term insomnia* (of more than 3 weeks' duration).[8] Generally, transient and short-term insomnia have a different set of causes to chronic (or long-term) insomnia.

Transient and short-term insomnia can often occur owing to:

- Periods of emotional distress or bereavement
- Initiation or discontinuation of pharmaceuticals
- Use/abuse/withdrawal of streets drugs or alcohol
- Recent onset of a physical or painful illness, such as musculoskelatal injury or peptic ulcer disease,
- work-shift changes
- jet lag.

Table 13.1 Factors in a sleep evaluation

1   Duration of the sleeping problem (How long has the patient had difficulties with sleep?)
2   When during the night does the problem occur? For example, does the patient have:
- Difficulty falling asleep
- Awaken in the middle of the night (sleep continuity disturbance)
- Early morning awakening
3   Are there recent events that may have precipitated the sleep problem?
4   Evaluation for the various causes of sleep disorders including:
- Medical diseases
- Psychiatric disorders
- Substance abuse and withdrawal
- Prescription medications
- Non-medication substances
- Primary sleep disorders
- Sleep apnea
- Restless leg syndrome
- Periodic limb movements of sleep

When evaluating short-term insomnia, it is important to ask about *recent stressors and lifestyle changes*. Patients are not always cognizant of the effect that certain lifestyle changes, such as jet lag, changes in work shift, personal crisis, or the initiation of a chemical or pharmaceutical, can have on their sleep, even if it may be obvious to the clinician. At times the patient may be aware of the event(s), but not have made the connection to their insomnia.

A clinician must know *when* during the night patients are having trouble. Are they having difficulty falling asleep, but once asleep stay asleep? Are they having minimal difficulty falling asleep, but awaken in the middle of the night (sleep continuity disturbance)? Or are they having trouble awakening before they have completed a full night's sleep (early morning awakening)? If medication is to be prescribed, these timing factors will strongly affect the choice of medication to be recommended. Is the amount of sleep normal in duration but occurs at the "wrong time" (phase-shifted sleep)? In this case sleep medication is unlikely to be the best treatment or may not be prescribed at all (see below).

In general, insomnia that has lasted for more than 3 weeks (and may have persisted for months or years) has other causes than those listed above for short-term insomnia. Long-term insomnia is much more likely to have at its root significant medical disease, major psychiatric conditions or substance abuse. For some of these patients a psychophysiological cycle of insomnia has been established, where worrying about continued inability to sleep produces even more difficulty in falling or staying asleep.

The prescriber should screen for *medical diseases* associated with insomnia, including hypertension, hyperthyroidism, respiratory insufficiency, cardiovascular insufficiency, and chronic pain. *Prescription medications* that can be associated with difficulty sleeping include antihypertensives, diuretics, steroids, stimulants, bronchodilators, decongestants, histamine antagonists, and xanthines such as theophylline.[9-12]

Many *psychiatric disorders*, including depression, bipolar disorder, a variety of psychotic conditions and anxiety disorders such as PTSD, panic attacks and generalized anxiety disorder can present with difficulty sleeping either as a primary or a secondary complaint.

Onset of insomnia temporarily associated with the recent initiation of any psychotropic medications should be noted, since many antidepressants, stimulants, and atypical antipsychotics have been linked with sleep disturbance. In some cases, a recent dosage increase in one of these medications may also lead to disordered sleep.

Approximately 10–15 percent of patients with insomnia have substance abuse problems.[12] Many patients do not understand that alcohol, although it may help initiate sleep for some individuals, will generally lead to middle of the night awakening and the perception of insomnia. Although alcohol is often referred to as a central nervous system "depressant," in this context it means that it decreases overall neuron firing and may have a calming or sedative effect. (It does not mean that it causes depression or is "depressogenic.") Particularly when the alcohol consumption is heavy, it may initially induce sleep. When the alcohol levels drop owing to metabolism and excretion, however, the CNS rebounds in activity and neuron firing becomes more active, leading to awakening or disrupted, non-restful sleep.

Patients should also be questioned about their daily intake of caffeine and particularly whether caffeine is taken after 3 pm.

Other useful screening questions of a patient with long-term insomnia that may elicit symptoms suggestive of a *primary sleep disturbance* include:

■ In the evening or night, has the patient had any unusual, restless, painful, or "creepy, crawling" feelings in their legs that are temporarily relieved by movement? (restless leg syndrome)
■ Has anyone told the patient that he or she snores heavily, coughs/chokes repeatedly, or has irregular breathing at night? (sleep apnea)
■ Is there any history of spells of muscle weakness triggered by emotional upset? (narcolepsy)
■ Is there any history of "burning the candle at both ends" and trying to "make yourself get by with less sleep than you need"? (insufficient sleep syndrome).

For those with chronic sleep problems, information from the patient's sleep partner is helpful. Ask the partner specifically about any periods of difficulty in breathing, choking, coughing, or apneic spells. It is also helpful to evaluate the *patient's daily routine*. How much exercise does the patient get? How much, and when, does he or she eat? What is the evening routine, particularly in the several hours before bedtime?

For chronic insomnia, a *physical exam* should be performed with specific focus on the presence of nasal obstruction, a low-hanging palate, an unusually small mandible size, or an enlarged thyroid, any of which could lead to obstructive sleep apnea. The patient's weight and blood pressure should be recorded. Hypertension and/or obesity are positively correlated with obstructive sleep apnea.

The patient should be referred for polysomnography in a sleep lab if:

■ Any of the above questions for primary sleep disorder are answered positively
■ Appropriate therapy for a short-term sleep disorder is unsuccessful and the condition persists
■ A patient is exhibiting daytime sleepiness to the point of having difficulty staying alert while driving, or if the patient is experiencing academic/occupational problems secondary to tiredness and fatigue
■ A sleeping partner notices distinct apneic periods.

Principles of treating sleep disorders

How much sleep is normal? The old adage that everyone needs 8 hours of sleep is commonly believed, but is not true for many people. A range of $6\frac{1}{2}$–9 hours of sleep is common, and sleep within these parameters does not generally indicate sleep pathology or psychopathology. More or less sleep than this on a regular basis can be indicative of a sleep disorder.

It is crucial to have a diagnosis for the type of sleep disorder being treated or at least to have performed a thorough evaluation to attempt diagnosis, even if a firm diagnosis cannot be made. To prescribe sleeping pills routinely after a minimal or negligible assessment of what kind of sleep problem the patient is having will often mean that underlying medical or psychiatric causes of a sleep disturbance are missed, and will likely result in overprescription of sleeping medication.

The underlying condition must be treated. If there is an underlying medical condition (e.g. hypertension, pulmonary problems, cardiovascular disease with cardiac insufficiency, thyroid disease), this must be appropriately evaluated and treated to have reasonable success with improving a patient's sleep. Likewise, if a patient is suffering from depression, bipolar disorder, an anxiety disorder or psychosis, these too must be appropriately evaluated and treated in order for the sleep to improve. If there is any evidence of a primary sleep disorder, including restless leg syndrome/periodic limb movement disorder, sleep apnea or narcolepsy, these must be adequately evaluated rather than simply prescribing sleeping medications that may actually worsen the condition.

Before sleeping medication can be prescribed, the patient's personal history of alcohol and drug use should be assessed and any family history of alcohol or drug abuse noted. Persons with a family history of substance abuse are at more risk for abusing sleep medications than those without. If sleeping medication is prescribed for a patient with substance abuse, or a family history of substance abuse, extra vigilance should be maintained for misuse of medication (see Chapter 19).

Treatment of sleep problems

When sleeping medications are prescribed, the least amount of medication that permits restorative sleep should be used for the shortest period of time until the patient's normal sleep pattern re-emerges.

For the responsible patient who is having transient or short-term sleep problems secondary to a clear personal stressor and who does not have a substance abuse problem, or underlying medical or psychiatric illness, sleeping medications can generally be prescribed safely. In these patients there is minimal risk and the clinician can generally feel comfortable prescribing sleeping medications for several days to several weeks. Appropriate patient warnings about the possibility of excess sedation during the day, potential interactions with other sedative medications and increased sensitivity to alcohol are warranted. The clinician can reassure the patient about the lack of habituation, if the medication is taken in the dose prescribed for a several-week period. Over this timeframe, there is minimal risk of rebound insomnia.

If a short-term trial of medications is insufficient to resolve the patient's problem, or if the patient has had a history of sleep difficulties for longer than 3 weeks, a more in-depth evaluation is necessary. This intensity of the sleep problem is often a sign of a more serious underlying medical illness, psychiatric disorder or primary sleep disorder. Asking the patient to record bedtimes, hours of sleep and times of arising in a sleep diary for 2 weeks may also elicit further useful information. It is essential, in patients with long-term sleep problems, to get historical information from the patient's sleep partner.

Non-pharmacological treatment

The following suggestions should be made to patients routinely, whether or not sleeping medication is ultimately prescribed. These issues are especially crucial in dealing with patients who experience chronic insomnia:

- Advise a regular schedule with approximately the same bedtime and morning arising time each day. Counsel against "sleeping in" on weekend days, and marked variations in bedtime.
- Avoid naps during the day.
- Although a light snack may be useful at bedtime (particularly for geriatric patients with insomnia), heavy meals should be avoided prior to sleep.
- Suggest regular exercise three to four times per week, although it is best not done after dinner since adrenaline stimulation may exacerbate sleep difficulties. Inform the patient that any exercise regime that aids sleep will take up to 6 weeks to have a beneficial sleep effect.
- Control the bedroom temperature and surroundings. Patients generally do not sleep well in rooms that are excessively hot or cold, noisy or brightly lit. If necessary, advise the use of earplugs, sleep masks, white-noise machines or fans to maintain comfortable, consistent bedroom conditions.
- Encourage relaxing activities and a "ritual wind down" in the hour or two prior to going to bed. This can involve reading, television, relaxation exercises, or yoga. At times, progressive relaxation training is useful.
- Avoid stimulating or emotionally charged issues (e.g. preparing taxes, reading an excessively arousing book, or discussing emotionally-loaded issues) before going to bed.
- Avoid caffeine-containing substances after the noontime meal.
- Avoid alcohol after dinner.
- Advise that the bed be used only for sleeping or sexual activity, and not as a place for watching television, eating, or other activities.
- If the patient has not fallen asleep within 30 minutes of going to bed, advise him or her to get up and do a pleasant, relaxing activity, such as reading, listening to music, or watching television, until drowsy. Only then return to bed. Advise against staying in bed, tossing, turning, and looking at the clock.
- Similarly, if the patient awakens in the middle of the night and has not fallen back to sleep within 30 minutes, advise him or her to get up and do a relaxing, pleasant activity until drowsy.

In patients with a phase-shift sleep problem, a sufficient number of sleep hours are experienced but patients sleep and awaken at inconvenient or unusual times. They may fall asleep very early in the evening and wake up very early in the morning (advanced-phase sleep, which is common in seniors), or stay up until the middle of the night and then sleep until noon (delayed-phase sleep, which is common in younger people). These patients may benefit from the use of high-intensity artificial light therapy, which can gradually readjust the timing of their abnormal phase. For advanced-phase sleep (e.g. 7 pm to 3 am), use 10 000 Lux of light in the early evening beginning with a 30-minute exposure and gradually increasing to 90 minutes. For delayed-phase sleep (e.g. 4 am to noon), instruct the patient to arise 30 minutes earlier every 3 days and begin using a 10 000 Lux light for 30 minutes each day at that time. Medication is seldom a satisfactory treatment for phase-shifted sleep patterns.

Pharmacological treatment

Once it has been determined that medication would be beneficial and is indicated for a patient's sleep problems, the clinician can choose from one of the following categories:

■ Over-the-counter (OTC)/herbal sleep aids
■ Sedative hypnotics (benzodiazepines, non-benzodiazepines)
■ Psychotropic medications that may be used for sedation in addition to its mental health effect
■ Non-psychotropic prescription medications used for their sedative properties.

For a patient who does not have a primary psychiatric disorder, and for whom a "pure" sleeping medication is desired, over-the-counter alternatives may first be considered for mild sleep disorders. These can include antihistamines (including diphenhydramine and hydroxyzine), melatonin, l-trytophan (not available in the USA), or valerian root. If the patient fails a trial with an OTC preparation or has severe sleep problems, a prescription medication is needed.

If a patient has a primary psychiatric disorder with a sleep problem as one of its symptoms, consider "killing two birds with one stone" by using a sedative medicine that has activity in treating the primary psychiatric illness as well. For example, a psychotic patient might benefit from a relatively sedative antipsychotic such as quetiapine or risperidone, which would treat psychosis as well as aid sleep, if given at bedtime. For depression, an antidepressant with sedative properties (such as mirtazapine, nefazodone, or paroxetine) may, for some patients, help the sleep disorder when given as a once-daily dosage at bedtime.

Other medications used for sleep, even though this is not their primary indication, are sedative antidepressants (particularly trazodone, doxepin or trimipramine), gabapentin (used for seizures and pain), and clonidine (an antihypertensive). With appropriate monitoring, these medications may be used effectively as sleep aids. When used in this context, these medicines are used solely for their sedative and non-habituating properties. Although using these medications as sedatives is an off-label usage, it can be a useful, safe, rational prescription for some patients with intermittent sleep problems, even if no other medical or psychiatric diagnosis is present.

Medications specifically designed for sleep are generally divided into benzodiazepine compounds and non-benzodiazepine compounds. These compounds are listed in Tables 13.2 and 13.3, respectively.

Table 13.2 Benzodiazepine hypnotics with the recommended adult dosage for treatment of insomnia*

Compound (proprietary name)	Usual adult dosage (mg/day)	Half-life
Alprazolam (Xanax)	0.50–1.00	Intermediate
Clonazepam (Klonopin)	0.5–1.00	Long
Estazolam (ProSom)	1	Intermediate
Diazepam (Valium)	5–10	Long
Flurazepam (Dalmane)	15–30	Long
Lorazepam (Ativan)	2–4	Long
Temazepam (Restoril)	15–30	Intermediate
Triazolam (Halcion)	0.25	Short

* From Karakan I *et al*. Pharmacotherapy of insomnia. *Essent Psychopharmacol* 1996;1:2.

Table 13.3 Non-benzodiazepine sedative hypnotics

- Zolpidem
- Zaleplon
- Zolpiclone

Benzodiazepines as a class have been in common use as sedative/hypnotics for several decades. They are among the most commonly prescribed medications for sleep and anxiety in primary care and mental health patients alike. As many as 11.5 percent of Americans report using a benzodiazepine at least once in a one-year period and 1.5 percent used a benzodiazepine on a nightly or regular basis.[13] This high degree of usage reflects their predictable anti-anxiety effect at low doses and sleep-inducing effects at moderate doses with relatively few serious side effects.[14] Although abuse, dependence, discontinuation syndrome, and oversedation are well-known possible complications, these compounds are remarkably useful and safe when prescribed intelligently and used in moderation. Despite their common prescription by many practitioners, there are those who will unnecessarily avoid their prescription and virtually refuse to do so, fearing that the patient will become addicted, or that the clinician's willingness to prescribe tranquilizers will be abused.

It is of crucial importance in the choice of a benzodiazepine or other sedative hypnotic to match the half-life of the compound chosen with the type of difficulty the patient is having. A patient who is having difficulty in falling asleep, but stays asleep once asleep, would benefit from a short-acting hypnotic that would induce sleep but would likely be metabolized and excreted prior to awakening, leaving minimal morning medication hangover. Such a short-acting compound would not be used in a patient with sleep continuity disturbance, since the patient needs help in the middle of the night, not shortly after taking the medication. A short-acting compound would be metabolized and excreted, and be of minimal help when the patient needs it most.

A patient with sleep continuity disturbance would benefit from an intermediate acting compound, which would still be present when the patient needs to remain asleep. Similarly, patients with early morning awakening would be better treated with an intermediate-acting compound, which would hopefully be present in sufficient amounts to keep them asleep longer, until their normal awakening time. In general, long-acting sedative hypnotics such as flurazepam (with a half-life of 2–5 days) or quazepam (with a half-life of 2–3 days) are problematic for many patients since they give significant sedative effect during the day, and make it difficult for the patient to rise without a morning medication hangover. Older patients in particular are at risk for drug accumulation and drug hangover, leading to increased risk of falls or accidents.

Some patients will lose the hypnotic effect of benzodiazepines over time with repeated usage, although others can comfortably utilize the medication safely over the long term, particularly if taken less than every night. Those who take benzodiazepines nightly for several months can experience some rebound insomnia, lasting 1–7 days, when the medication is stopped. With very high doses of benzodiazepines taken over extended periods of time, frank physical withdrawal and seizures may result from sudden discontinuation. This is seldom a problem if the clinician actively monitors the patient's condition and progress, and limits the quantities of medication prescribed.

Geography and politics have altered the availability of high potency benzodiazepines in different countries. Triazolam has been withdrawn from the UK market because of its ability to cause retrograde amnesia (loss of memory for events that occurred in the several hours before the medication was taken). Triazolam remains fully available in the USA, with recommendations to use smaller doses (0.25 mg) to avoid this complication. Rohypnol, in contrast, is fully available in the UK and Europe, but has never been available in the USA, having gained the label of a "date rape" drug, and thus being too dangerous to use. The commonality to these two seemingly opposite situations is that both compounds are high potency benzodiazepines that may cause increased side effects at higher doses in sensitive individuals, or when combined with alcohol. Used in smaller doses, under appropriate medical oversight, neither drug is likely the dangerous compound portrayed, but they are both medications that should be prescribed with caution in modest doses.

Non-benzodiazepine hypnotics are listed in Table 13.3, and are currently limited to three compounds: zolpidem (Ambien), zaleplon (Sonata), and zolpiclone (Zimovane and generic, available in the UK only). These medications are presumed to exert their mechanism of action at the benzodiazepine receptor site in the brain, but have some advantages over benzodiazepines themselves. Compared to benzodiazepines, the habit-forming potential is less and is relatively small, although some measure of physical dependence has been reported with long-term use of very high doses. Disruption of normal sleep architecture, medication interactions and rebound insomnia are minimal compared to benzodiazepines.[5,15–19] Their primary downside is cost, as they are considerably more expensive than generic benzodiazepines. Zaleplon's very short half-life makes medication hangover very unlikely. This same property may render it mostly excreted by the middle of the night, when it might be needed for patients with middle of the night sleep continuity disturbance. It can, however, be taken as a repeat dose in the middle of the night. Although the incidence of side effects and dependence is less than with benzodiazepines, these medications may cause confusion or memory impairment when used in large doses or in sensitive individuals (e.g. seniors or brain injured individuals).

Old-line sleep medications, particularly phenobarbital or other barbiturates, are poor choices of sleep medications due to their high risk of habituation and the availability of multiple safer alternative medications.

Necessity of follow-up

Follow-up assessment of response and/or side effects is important whenever a sleep medication is prescribed. The patient must be evaluated for daytime sleepiness, lack of attention or coordination, or other side effects of overdosage/drug accumulation. Also, a patient should virtually never be prescribed chronic sleep medications without several trials off medication at varying intervals to assess continued need. Unfortunately, patients in institutional care settings or nursing homes have often been prescribed sleep medication with minimal follow-up, and can remain on such medication for months, years or indefinitely, without appropriate follow-up and attempts to discontinue the medication. When a trial off medication is attempted, it should continue for a long enough period of time to allow any rebound insomnia to resolve, since this is temporary and should not be confused with ongoing therapeutic necessity.

Although every effort should be made to stop sleeping medication, for some responsible patients (particularly those with documented psychiatric and/or medical comorbidity that exacerbate their sleep problems) long-term, chronic prescription of sleep medication may not be poor medication practice.[20] This is especially true when trials off the medication have consistently resulted in clinical deterioration.

Special populations

Patients with substance abuse

Those patients who have a history of substance abuse or have otherwise abused medications are, in general, poor candidates for benzodiazepine and other sedative hypnotics. When these individuals are sleep disordered and non-pharmacological methods have been unsuccessful, some appropriate medication considerations would be:

- Over-the-counter preparations such as antihistamines, melatonin, l-tryptophan, or valerian root
- Gabapentin
- Trazodone, doxepin, or trimipramine.

Patients undergoing withdrawal from alcohol can expect to have disrupted sleep for several days to several weeks. In general, it is not helpful routinely to prescribe sedative hypnotics to such patients except as part of a detoxification profile. If a patient has elevated vital signs, including rapid pulse and raised blood pressure, benzodiazepines are often used to manage withdrawal (see Chapter 14). When used this way, these medications may simultaneously have a beneficial effect on sleep.

There is a select small number of patients who have had a history of substance abuse, but have been substance-free for extended periods of time, and who are dependable and reliable. If the above measures have been tried and are unsuccessful, these patients could be carefully tried on sedative hypnotics, including benzodiazepines. When this is the case, it should only be done with careful assessment, follow-up and patient education about the potential risk of habituation. Patients with a history of substance abuse should be encouraged to use sleeping medications intermittently rather than on a regular basis, even if they do not sleep well on the nights they do not take medication. The clinician should be acutely aware of any signs of medication misuse, "lost" prescriptions, or requests for increasing dosage of sleeping medications in this patient group.

Liver-impaired patients

Patients who have significant liver impairment from hepatic disease have limited medication options for sleep, as most of these medications are hepatically metabolized. Gabapentin is one good choice for such patients, since the majority of its excretion is through the kidneys. A hepatically impaired patient with bipolar disorder might also be tried on lithium or lamotrigine as a mood stabilizer, which might also assist with sleep. Other hepatically metabolized medications are not totally contraindicated for liver-impaired patients, but should be prescribed in small doses with frequent follow-up evaluation when other measures have failed (see Chapter 5).

Older patients

As seen in the previous chapter, geriatric patients are at increased risk for insomnia and are often at greater risk for side effects from medications.[21,22] In choosing sleeping medications for elderly patients, shorter-acting medications and intermittent dosing are always preferable to longer-acting preparations and nightly dosing, which may lead to drug accumulation. Shorter-acting preparations such as zaleplon or triazolam in small doses may be helpful.

In addition to medication, clinicians should consider the following non-pharmacological issues with elderly patients:

■ Increase the patients exercise, decreasing a sedentary lifestyle
■ Evaluate the patient's daily routine. Particularly if the patient lives alone, he or she may have developed an excessively unusual routine that contributes to sleep difficulty (e.g. staying up very late, performing routine activities in the middle of the night, eating at unusual times)

- Advise the patient to avoid daytime naps
- Suggest removing a clock from the patient's room so he or she is not constantly looking at the clock and worrying about sleep
- Suggest a light snack before bed, but avoiding a heavy meal
- Control patient's pain and medical illnesses, such as cardiovascular disease
- Eliminate any unnecessary medications that may be complicating sleep
- Avoid late-day diuretics, which increase the need for night-time urination
- Evaluate for substance abuse that can disrupt sleep (most clinicians do not wish to believe that anyone their grandmother's age abuses alcohol or drugs, even though the prevalence in this age group is significant!)
- Evaluate closely for medication-induced drug hangover, poor balance or coordination, which can lead to falls
- Re-evaluate the patient frequently to attempt discontinuation of any sleep medication started.

References

1 Karacam I *et al*. Pharmacotherapy of insomnia. *Essent Psychopharmacol* 1996;1(2):167–181.

2 The Gallup Organization. *Sleep in America: A National Survey of US Adults*. National Sleep Foundation, 1995.

3 Radecki SE and Brunton SA. Management of insomnia in office-based practice: national prevalence and therapeutic patterns. *Arch Fam Med* 1993;2:1129–1134.

4 Gillin JC. Relief from situational insomnia: pharmacologic and other options. *Postgrad Med* 1992;92:157–160.

5 Lippman S *et al*. Insomnia: therapeutic approach. *South Med J* 2001;94(9): 870–872.

6 Clark MM. Restless leg syndrome. *J Am Board Fam Pract* 2001;14(5):368–374.

7 Yoshihawa N *et al*. A case of insufficient sleep syndrome. *Psychiatry Clin Neuro* 1998;52(2):200–201.

8 Meyer TJ. Evaluation and management of insomnia. Hospital Practice 1998. www.hosppract.com/issues/1998/12/Meyer.htm

9 Hartmann PM. Drug treatment of insomnia: indications and newer agents. *Am Fam Physician* 1995;51:191–194.

10 Becker PM, Jamieson AO and Brown WD. Insomnia: use of a "decision tree" to assess and treat. *Postgrad Med* 1993;93:66–85.

11 Ancoli-Israel S. All I want is a Good Night's Sleep. Mosby Year Book Inc., 1996, p. 116.

12 Brunton SA. When your patient can't sleep. *Fam Prac Recertif* 1992;14:149–170.

13 Salzman C. Benefits versus risks of benzodiazepine. *Psychiatric Ann* 1998;28:139.

14 McGee M and Pres R. Benzodiazepines in primary practice: risks and benefits. *Resident Staff Physician* 2002;48(4):42–49.

15 Stimmed GL. Future directions in drug treatment of insomnia. *Psych Times* 1999, May, suppl. 1–8.

16 Darcourt G. Safety and tolerability of zolpidem – an update. *J Psychopharmacol* 1999;13(1):81–93.

17 Bowes M. Sedative hypnotic medications for insomnia. *Psych Times* 1999, May, suppl. pp. 9–16.

18 Doghranji K. Treatment of insomnia in aging patients. *Sleep Disorders* 1999; July: 5–6.

19 Richardson GS *et al*. Management of insomnia – the role of Zaleplon. On the Internet at www.medscape.com, *General Medicine* 2002; 4(1).

20 Schenck C and Mahowald MW. Long-term benzodiazepine treatment of injurious parasomnias and other disorders of disrupted nocturnal sleep in 170 adults. *Am J Med* 1996;100:333.

21 Mosier WA, Nelson AS and Walgren KD. Wanted: a good night's sleep. *Adv Nurse Pract* 1998;6:30–35.

22 Nakra BRS, Grossberg GT and Peck B. Insomnia in the elderly. *Am Fam Physician* 1991;43:477–483.

Alcohol and mental health medications

Alcohol abuse and alcohol dependence is extraordinarily common. Depending on the study and the definitions used, the prevalence of alcohol abuse and dependence ranges from 10 to 16 percent of the American population (28 percent in men and 8 percent in women).[1-4] There is also a strong overlap of persons with an alcohol use disorder and a comorbid mental disorder, this being as high as 53 percent in one study.[4] Individuals with both a mental disorder and a substance abuse disorder (commonly called dual diagnosis patients) present a clinical challenge to all healthcare professionals, and particularly to a clinician prescribing psychotropic medication. This chapter will focus on interactions between psychotropic medications and alcohol, and the ways that psychotropics are used in alcohol abuse. Specifically, the following areas are covered:

- Routine warnings regarding alcohol use and psychotropics in the non-substance abusing patient
- Warning signs to the clinician of possible alcohol abuse
- Comorbid alcohol abuse and mental health prescription
- Evaluation issues with the intoxicated patient
- Psychotropics and the treatment of alcohol abuse.

Routine warnings in the non-substance abusing patient

When prescribing psychotropic medications to patients without a personal or family history of alcohol abuse, a recommendation regarding possible interactions with alcohol should still be routinely given. This should cover the specifics of permitted alcohol usage and the risks of overutilization of alcohol, even if the patient denies that this is likely to be a problem. In general, *patients should be advised to refrain from alcohol for the first several weeks of medication prescription while they are becoming accommodated to the medication and its effect is being evaluated.* Once stable on the medication, the general rule of thumb for non-substance abusing patients is that they may *have no more than one drink in an evening and no more than four drinks in a week* without seriously compromising the effect of their mental health medication or creating a serious health hazard for themselves. This is discussed in the following dialogue.

TALKING TO PATIENTS

"For the first several weeks, while you are adjusting to the medication, I would prefer that you do not drink any alcohol. If and when you do choose to drink alcohol, I would recommend that it be in moderation. I am defining moderation as no more than one drink in an evening and no more than four in a week. If you stay within this framework while you are taking medication, you are unlikely to have problems from use of alcohol. Do be aware that approximately 20 percent of patients notice increased intoxication if they drink while taking medication.

If you are in that 20 percent, your ability to drive or perform coordinated activities could be affected when you drink. The majority of patients, however, will experience no significant increased intoxication. Remember that the medication I am prescribing is still in your system and may be affected by alcohol regardless of when you took your dose." (The latter fact is important, since some patients think that if medication is taken in the morning it is no longer in their system at night, and they can therefore drink freely with abandon.)

"There are two significant effects of heavier alcohol intake that you need to be aware of when taking medications.

First, heavy drinking may work against the effect of the medication. More than just feeling hung over, you may feel the medication is 'not working' for several days after heavy alcohol intake.

Secondly, if you drink heavily, you may unpredictably *experience an alcoholic blackout in which memory is lost for activities surrounding the drinking episode. You can wake up the next morning and not realize how you got home or what you did. You may not have 'passed out,' and may have continued to do potentially dangerous activities such as drinking and driving.*

If your intake of alcohol remains moderate, as I have defined, you are not likely to have either of these two problems."

Signs of alcohol abuse

When prescribing psychotropics, it is important that the clinician be vigilant for indications of excessive alcohol use. People's drinking behavior does not always match what they describe in the office. Patients' alcohol intake may also change over time with their emotional state. Many signs of alcohol overutilization are well known and easy to discern in a clinical setting. These can include:

1 Alcohol on the patient's breath
2 Staggering gait
3 Slurred speech
4 Reddened eyes
5 Signs of mild to moderate alcohol withdrawal, including
   ■ Hand and body tremors
   ■ Sweating
   ■ Rapid pulse
   ■ Elevated blood pressure
   ■ Dilated pupils
   ■ Elevated temperature
   ■ Behavioral restlessness or overactivity
   ■ Clouding of consciousness.

Some more subtle signs that may alert the clinician to possible covert alcohol abuse can include the following:

1 Abnormal laboratory findings suggestive of alcohol abuse, including:
   ■ Elevated serum gammaglutamyl transferase (GGT), which is raised in 80 percent of those who overutilize alcohol. If there is a GGT greater than 30 units, 70 percent of these individuals will have been involved in persistent heavy drinking (greater than eight drinks per day).
   ■ Carbohydrate deficient transferase (CDT) greater than 20 units also indicates persistent heavy drinking. Both of these latter tests revert to normal within several days to 1 week of the cessation of heavy alcohol intake.[5,6]
   ■ High normal or elevated mean corpuscular volume (MCV) of erythrocytes. Elevated MCV is a direct toxic effect of alcohol on the formation of red blood cells.
   ■ Increased liver function tests will gradually occur with long-term and persistent alcohol usage.
   ■ Increased triglyceride and lipoprotein levels may also be present.
2 The clinician should also be alert to evidence of cross-tolerance with other addictive medications. Patients who show an elevated need for narcotic pain medications, sedative/hypnotics and benzodiazepine anti-anxiety medications may also have developed a measure of cross-tolerance because of abuse of alcohol.
3 Lack of intoxication when it would be expected can also signal high regular usage. If a person has a blood alcohol level of greater than 100 milligrams of

ethanol per deciliter and does not show some sign of intoxication, this indicates a degree of alcohol tolerance. At a blood alcohol of greater than 200 milligrams per deciliter, most non-tolerant individuals will be severely intoxicated. While blood alcohol levels are not regularly drawn in an outpatient practice, a clinician may get reports from an emergency room or hospital that document a blood alcohol level and lack of signs of intoxication, which can alert the clinician to the possibility of alcohol abuse.

While not all of these signs or symptoms are pathognomonic or automatically valid indicators of alcohol abuse in isolation, several of the signs present together should alert the clinician to the suspicion that alcohol abuse is occurring.

The remaining sections of this chapter will deal with issues regarding psychotropic medications in individuals who have acutely and/or chronically abused alcohol, and in whom their problems with alcohol are known and recognized by the clinician.

Evaluation of the intoxicated and withdrawing patient

The presence of acute alcohol (or drug) intoxication or withdrawal will confound the diagnostic acumen of even the best clinicians. The physiological state of intoxication and withdrawal generally lasts no more than several hours to several days. During the states of acute intoxication and withdrawal, assessment for psychotropic medications is difficult, if not impossible. Given the short length of time it takes for these states to resolve, evaluation for psychotropic medication should be delayed until the patient is sober and free from the acute signs and symptoms of withdrawal, except in unusual circumstances.

There has been an ongoing belief by some clinicians, which persists currently, that persons with substance abuse problems must be totally substance-free for an extended period of time in order to assess accurately and treat any emotional problems with psychotropic medication. While not totally untrue, the fact is that it depends on the clinical situation. The willingness of practitioners to medicate with psychotropics in patients abusing alcohol will vary markedly from practitioner to practitioner. There are practitioners who insist on patients being substance-free before they will medicate at all, whereas other practitioners (including the author) are willing to prescribe for clearly diagnosed mental health conditions despite the presence of mild to moderate alcohol usage. The hope, in the latter situation, is that when the patients are appropriately medicated they will be better able to decrease or eliminate their alcohol usage. The premise of reduced substance usage once psychotropics are prescribed requires constant re-evaluation, and is certainly not universally true for all patients. For those patients who, despite adequate medication, continue to abuse alcohol, ongoing medication prescription may not be in their best interest and may indeed present some medical hazard.

Months or years of sobriety are not necessary prior to a mental health evaluation and the possible prescription of targeted psychotropic medications. While some risk of blurred diagnosis or interaction between alcohol and medication may occur, these risks are relatively small compared to the much larger risk of untreated emotional illness (including suicidal and homicidal behavior, lost jobs and disrupted families). It is reasonable to undertake an evaluation for medication within several days of an episode of acute intoxication, and within a week after a period of significant alcohol withdrawal.

To expect that patients who have been using substances for a long time, particularly as "self-medication" (see below), will cease their habit for a lengthy period prior to being medicated is, in most cases, unlikely and unreasonable. Often such a prerequisite with an alcohol-dependent person, if strictly and uniformly enforced, will drive a patient from treatment before medication can offer improvement. If, however, the clinician has a patient history suggesting that a person has abused the combination of medication and alcohol before, it is reasonable to insist that he or she be detoxified before medication is prescribed.

Psychotropic medications and dual diagnosis patients

Patients who have both diagnosable mental health conditions and a diagnosable alcohol use disorder are common. As many as 53 percent of individuals with an alcohol disorder have a comorbid mental disorder.[6] Individuals with alcohol abuse suffer from mood disorders at significantly higher rates than in the general population.[3,7]

Dual diagnosis – the comorbidity of mental health and substance abuse diagnoses – can overlap in several ways:

■ A psychiatric disease with increased alcohol usage as "self-medication" for emotional symptoms. The alcohol use may be episodic or continuous.
■ A psychiatric disorder with a separate alcohol abuse disorder, which occurs sporadically or continuously, regardless of the presence of mental health symptoms.
■ A continuous alcohol use disorder with episodic psychiatric symptomatology.

Although clinicians have attempted in the past to sort out which illness came first – the alcohol abuse or the mental illness – this differentiation is really less important than ensuring that both conditions are adequately treated.[8] What is unequivocally clear is that the presence of dual diagnoses has a negative impact on medication compliance, lengthens the time to recovery, and increases the rate of relapse for both conditions. Conversely, adequate treatment of both the mental health problem and of the alcohol abuse improves the outcome of the other.[9]

Biases of philosophy, training and experience have unfortunately complicated the principles of treatment for dual diagnosis patients. There is a common tendency of purely "mental health" clinicians to miss the seriousness of and necessity of treatment for alcohol abuse. Primary "substance abuse" clinicians often inadequately assess and undertreat emotional illnesses, focusing solely on the abuse. These biases have led to two opposite and equally untrue conclusions:

1 Mental health medications will treat alcoholism
2 Appropriate alcohol treatment will solve most mental health symptoms.

Since there is significant overlap between many emotional illnesses and sub-stance abuse, there is much 'self-medication' with alcohol. Certain mental health patients, once they begin feeling better as a result of psychotropic medication treatment, no longer feel the need for increased alcohol use. *It is not reasonable, however, to assume that all persons with substance abuse problems will necessarily decrease their substance abuse when they are appropriately medicated for their emotional illness.* Some may continue to abuse alcohol despite their mental health improvement. These individuals will need separate, independent substance abuse treatment. Similarly, patients engaged actively in alcohol abuse treatment (whether within the 12-step Alcoholics Anonymous model or some other treatment program) will not *automatically* resolve any underlying mental illness by stopping their alcohol use. In fact, some patients become even more acutely aware of their mental health symptoms when they are sober.

After medicating those patients assessed to have a primary psychiatric diagnosis who also abuse alcohol, it is reasonable to allow several weeks to several months for adequate symptom control to occur before determining that separate substance abuse treatment is necessary. If ongoing substance usage is occurring at that time, specific alcohol abuse treatment should be recommended and undertaken. Even with considerable symptom relief from emotional symptoms, however, some patient's alcohol abuse will take on a life of its own and persist indefinitely without treatment. Alcohol abuse is a chronic relapsing illness with frequent relapses and remissions. Therefore, waiting many months or years for the psychotropic medications to "do their job" while expecting alcohol use to stop is not reasonable.

Additional evaluation issues in dual diagnosis patients

In addition to performing a thorough evaluation of mental health symptoms as well as alcohol and other substance abuse, the clinician should be alert to the high prevalence of other medical illnesses in patients who abuse alcohol. These include:

- HIV
- Tuberculosis
- Hepatitis
- Sexually transmitted diseases.

Falls, motor vehicle accidents, homicides, and suicides are also more common in patients with alcohol abuse disorders.

Another issue of relevance to medication prescription for an alcohol abusing patient is the presence of family history of mood or psychiatric disorder. A positive family history should alert the clinician to the possibility of a genetic predisposition toward an underlying mood disorder, and thus the clinician should be even more vigilant than usual regarding a possible underlying anxiety or mood disorder that could be treated with medication.

Some clinicians with a strong background in substance abuse treatment, particularly of the 12-step model, believe that using medications in patients with a history of substance abuse is simply "trading one chemical dependency for another." This is not generally true. If mental health symptoms persist and if a diagnosis can be made, particularly (but not exclusively) in light of a positive family history of emotional disorder, the clinician should not hesitate to utilize appropriate psychotropics in the treatment of the dual diagnosis patient. Antidepressants, mood stabilizers, and antipsychotics are, in general, not abused, and may be of significant benefit to an appropriately diagnosed patient.

Habituating medicines, particularly benzodiazepines for anxiety and stimulants, should *not* be used liberally with dual diagnosis patients. Non-pharmacological means and non-habituating medicines should be tried first. If, however, these fail, and the patient is firmly engaged in treatment and shown to be responsible in the use of medication, it may be reasonable to use small amounts of these medication groups judiciously with close monitoring.

Some patients, when given psychotropics, will correlate side effects from the medication with uncomfortable feelings they have experienced with intoxication or withdrawal from their alcohol usage. Sedation can mimic a hangover, and nervousness can mimic withdrawal. To minimize this problem in dual diagnosis patients, start with low doses of medications and titrate very gradually with an aim toward a modest final therapeutic dosage and minimal side effects.[10]

Psychotropics used in the treatment of alcohol use disorders

The above sections have focused on the interaction between alcohol and psychotropic medications, issues of comorbidity, and the place of medications in the treatment of comorbid conditions. This last section will discuss the direct usage of psychotropics in the treatment of alcohol abuse and withdrawal. It is necessary to focus on these issues since the specific medications used – disulfiram, naltrexone, and acamprosate (UK only) – are used in relatively unique ways compared to the psychotropics otherwise discussed in this book.

Disulfiram

Disulfiram (antabuse) is unique in psychopharmacology in that its purpose is to discourage a particular behavior (alcohol intake) by causing intense negative physiological symptoms when alcohol is ingested. Disulfiram has neither a direct effect on psychiatric symptoms, nor a direct effect on the patient's craving for alcohol. Its sole purpose is as a negative deterrent to drinking alcohol, such that the patient knows that drinking while taking antabuse will lead to severely unpleasant sensations. Disulfiram is usually dosed between 250 mg and 500 mg a day on a daily basis, or three to four times a week for some patients sensitive to its effect.

Disulfiram disrupts alcohol metabolism and inhibits the action of aldehyde dehydrogenase, thus blocking the conversion of acetaldehyde to acetate. Alcohol, when ingested by a person who is taking disulfiram, will have an accumulation of acetaldehyde, leading to distinct unpleasant physical sensations including:

- Sweating
- Flushing

- Difficulty breathing
- Nausea and vomiting
- Throbbing headache
- Weakness and hypotension.

After alcohol ingestion, several of the above symptoms will occur rapidly within 15 to 60 minutes, and persist for 30 minutes to 2 hours.

An important part of the prescription of disulfiram is educating the patient about "hidden" sources of alcohol that, in particularly sensitive individuals, can cause an alcohol–antabuse reaction. Common but unexpected sources of alcohol include tonics, liquid potions, aftershave lotion, mouthwash, colognes and perfumes. The patient must also be advised to be assertive regarding food preparation, particularly when foods are being prepared by another source (at a restaurant or at another person's home). Such inquiry is necessary to ensure that alcohol is not included in the food ingredients, which could precipitate a reaction.

Naltrexone and acamprosate

These two medicines, naltrexone (Revia) and acamprosate (Campral EC – currently widely available in Europe, but under investigational status in the USA) are discussed together. While they are distinctly different drugs with presumed different mechanisms of action, their purpose is similar – to decrease craving for alcohol in patients who abuse alcohol.

Naltrexone (Revia), an opiate antagonist, was originally approved for treatment of opioid dependence under the theory that the endogenous opioid system may have been involved in the development of alcohol dependence.[11] When the compound was tested in alcoholics, several large-scale studies showed naltrexone to be useful in decreasing alcohol craving, lowering the number of drinking days, and reducing the rate of full-blown relapse.[12,13]

Alcoholics who have stopped alcohol consumption show hyperexcitability in the glutamate system. Structurally resembling the naturally occurring amino acid mediator γ aminobutryic acid (GABA), *acamprosate* restores normal receptor tone in the glutamate system. Numerous studies involving over 4500 patients have shown acamprosate to decrease alcohol craving, prolong abstinence, and reduce the rate of relapse.[14–17]

Psychotropics in treatment of alcohol withdrawal

Acute alcohol withdrawal syndrome is a serious medical condition. In its milder forms it is characterized by sweating, tremor, elevated blood pressure, tachycardia, insomnia, elevated body temperature, and irritability. In its more severe form, it can be accompanied by delirium tremens, hallucinations, *grand mal* seizures progressing to status epilepticus, and, rarely, death. Various psychotropics have been used over the past 50 years to modulate the progress of alcohol withdrawal. For much of the past 15 years, benzodiazepines have been the mainstay of treatment for alcohol withdrawal. In the past, other psychotropics (e.g.

barbiturates) have been used to manage withdrawal, however use of these agents has fallen out of favor.

Various institutions and academic bodies have developed many benzodiazepine protocols by using diazepam, lorazepam, and chlordiazepoxide to treat withdrawal. Some of the protocols have fixed decreasing doses of the benzodiazepine as the patient's withdrawal symptoms improve; others have flexible dose regimens depending on the presence or absence of certain measurable criteria, such as elevated pulse, elevated blood pressure and elevated body temperature. Examples of such protocols are shown in Table 14.1.

Table 14.1 Alcohol detoxification with diazepam or lorazepam*

Mild withdrawal	Moderate withdrawal	Severe withdrawal
Diazepam 5–10 mg p.o.	Diazepam *Day 1:* 15–20 mg p.o. q.i.d. *Day 2:* 10–20 mg p.o. q.i.d. *Day 3:* 5–15 mg p.o. q.i.d. *Day 4:* 10 mg p.o. q.i.d. *Day 5:* 5 mg p.o. q.i.d.	Diazepam 10–25 mg p.o. every hour while awake PRN
Lorazepam 1–2 mg p.o. every 4–6 hours PRN for 1–3 days	Lorazepam *Days 1 & 2:* 2–4 mg p.o. q.i.d. *Days 3 & 4:* 2 mg p.o. q.i.d. *Day 5:* 1 mg p.o. b.i.d. (May need to adjust, based on signs and symptoms of alcohol withdrawal)	Lorazepam 1–2 mg i.v. every hour while awake PRN for 3–5 days (to sedate)
Systolic blood pressure >150 mmHg	Systolic blood pressure 150–200 mmHg	Systolic blood pressure >200 mmHg
Diastolic blood pressure >90 mmHg	Diastolic blood pressure 100–140 mmHg	Diastolic blood pressure >140 mmHg
Pulse >100 bpm	Pulse 110–140 bpm	Pulse >140 bpm
Temperature >100°F	Temperature 100–101°F	Temperature >101°F
Tremulousness	Tremulousness	Tremulousness
Insomnia	Insomnia	Insomnia
Agitation	Agitation	Agitation

*Monitoring in intensive care is recommended for cardiac and respiratory function, fluid and nutrition replacement, vital signs, and mental status. Restraints are indicated in the confused and agitated state to protect the patient from self and others. (Delirium tremens can be a terrifying and life-threatening state.)
From Miller NS. Pharmacological detoxification from alcohol and other drugs. *Essent Psychopharmacol* 1997;1(3):273–290.

References

1 Heizer JE and Pryzbeck TR. The co-occurrence of alcoholism with other psychiatric disorders in the general population and its impact on treatment. *J Stud Alcohol* 1991;49:219–224.

2 Myers JK *et al*. Six month prevalence of psychiatric disorders in three communities, 1980–1982. *Arch Gen Psychiatry* 1984;41:959–967.

3 Regier DA *et al*. Comorbidity of mental disorders with alcohol and other drug abuse. Results from the Epidemiologic Catchment Area study. *JAMA* 1990;264:2511–2518.

4 American Psychiatric Association, *Diagnostic and Statistical Manual of Mental Disorders*, 4th edn. American Psychiatric Association, 2000.

5 Anton RF *et al*. Carbohydrate-deficient transferring as an indicator of drinking status during treatment outcome studies. *Alc Clin Exper Res* 1996;20:841–846.

6 Arndt T. Carbohydrate-deficient transferrin as a marker of chronic alcohol abuse: a cricital review of preanalysis, analysis and interpretation. *Clin Chem* 2001;47:13–27.

7 Kessler RC *et al*. Lifetime co-occurrence of DSM-III-R alcohol abuse and dependence with other psychiatric disorders in the National Comorbidity Survey. *Arch Gen Psychiatry* 1997;54(4):313–321.

8 Stratowski SM *et al*. Twelve-month outcome after a first hospitalization for affective psychosis. *Arch Gen Psychiatry* 1998;55(1):49–55.

9 Tohen M *et al*. The effect of comorbid substance use disorders on the course of bipolar disorder: a review. *Harv Rev Psychiatry* 1998;6(3):133–141.

10 Albanese MJ. Assessing and treating comorbid mood and substance use disorders. *Psychiatric Times* 2001;18(4).

11 Cohen G and Collins M. Alkaloids from catecholemines in adrenal tissue: possible role in alcoholism. *Science* 1970;167:1749–1751.

12 Volpicelli JR *et al*. Naltrexone in the treatment of alcohol dependence. *Arch Gen Psychiatry* 1992;49(11):876–880.

13 O'Malley SS *et al*. Naltrexone and coping skills therapy for alcohol dependence. A controlled study. *Arch Gen Psychiatry* 1997;49(11):861–887.

14 Alquatari M and Littleton J. The anticraving drug acamprosate inhibits calcium channel antagonist binding to membranes from the rat cerebral cortex [extract]. *Alcohol Alcohol* 1995;30:551.

15 Naasila M *et al*. Mechanism of action of acamprosate. Part 1. Characterization of spermidine-sensitive acamprosate binding site in rat brain. *Alcohol Clin Exp Res* 1998;22:1–8.

16 Pelc I *et al*. Efficacy and safety of acamprosate in the treatment of detoxified alcohol-dependence patients: a 90-day placebo-controlled dose-finding study. *Br J Psychiatry* 1997;171:73–77.

17 Mason BJ *et al*. Methodology of the US multicenter study of acamprosate in alcohol dependence. Presented at the American College of Neuropsychopharmacology (ACNP) Annual Meeting, Kameula, Hawaii. 1997.

Chapter 15

The confused and cognitively impaired patient – medication pitfalls

While not a specific diagnosis, mental confusion may be caused by any of a variety of conditions, both medical and psychiatric. Either self-referred or brought by their families, patients with mental confusion, poor memory and cognitive disorganization will frequently present to clinicians for mental health evaluation, in the hope that medication will help their cognitive difficulties. At other times, patients present for an evaluation of physical or mental health symptoms and the clinician perceives a confused state during the evaluation process. When aware of their deficiencies, patients may use phrases such as "I'm spacey," "I just can't focus," "My memory is going," or "I'm losing my mind." Other profoundly confused and forgetful patients are almost oblivious to their mental state, despite ample evidence to those around them. Behavioral historical information from family or caregivers may alert the clinician to possible cognitive problems. The family may identify that the patient is having difficulty with finances, transportation, taking medication, grooming, organization, planning, or performing tasks of daily living.

Clinical tip-offs that may alert the clinician to the presence of mental confusion that is not a primary complaint are listed in Table 15.1.

Primary care and non-mental health providers, when confronted with a patient who is disorganized, forgetful, confused, or inattentive, can often quickly jump to the diagnostic assumption that this is a "psych" case with need of a treatment referral to

---

Table 15.1 Signs and symptoms that can alert the clinician to patient confusion

- Perplexed, confused facial appearance
- Disorganized thinking
- Disorientation to person, place, or time
- Poor memory for details
- Rambling, disjointed speech
- Seeming inability to understand or respond appropriately to questions
- Easy distractibility
- Perceptual distortions (e.g. seeing things out of the corner of the eye), darting glances
- Easy startle response

---

a mental health specialist. If consultation is unavailable, reaching for the prescription pad to treat the symptoms can also be a common, but unhelpful, solution.

The role of medications in the treatment of disorders of cognitive impairment is quite variable and, in general, different to the direct, target symptom approach described in most other portions of this text. Although psychotropic medications may help for specific diagnoses and indirectly decrease confusion, in general, psychotropic medications are at best neutral, and may actually cloud the initial assessment process of the confused patient. As will be seen, medication prescription is often *not* one of the appropriate first steps in dealing with a confused patient unless that person is acutely, behaviorally out of control.

This chapter will discuss the stepwise assessment of confusion, and recognization of the limited number of situations when medication may be appropriate.

General principles of dealing with the confused patient

Mental confusion has many causes (see Table 15.2). While some are traditionally thought of as "psychiatric," many confused people have a medical problem that results in delirium, which has mental confusion as one of its symptoms. Assessment and evaluation to discover the cause of the mental confusion is essential to appropriate management.

Recent onset confusion, particularly when severe, is cause for an urgent medical evaluation. This is especially true in an adult without a past history of a definitive psychiatric disorder. *Unless urgent behavioral control is necessary for the patient, evaluation of the cause of confusion is the primary task and the use of psychotropic medications should be minimized.*

Cognitive disorders – delirium and dementia

Cognitive disorders (disorders that affect thinking, learning, and memory) are one of the most common causes of mental confusion, forgetfulness, and inattention. Cognitive disorders are broadly divided into *delirium* and *dementia*, which are described here.

Table 15.2 Causes of confusion

1. Cognitive disorders
   - Delirium
   - Dementia
2. Substance use
   - Alcohol intoxication or withdrawal
   - Drug intoxication or withdrawal
3. Psychiatric causes
   - Psychosis
   - Mania
   - Depression
4. Anxiety
5. Attention deficit disorder

Delirium and dementia are symptom complexes of an underlying medical condition, and are not illnesses in and of themselves. There is a vast array of systemic medical conditions, as well as direct illnesses of brain tissue, that affect normal brain functioning and cause delirium or dementia. In the past, cognitive disorders have often been referred to as "organic" brain disorders or "organic brain syndromes." This classification is not particularly helpful, since it implies that these conditions are due to "organic" causes and that other "functional" conditions (such as psychosis, bipolar disorder, and depression) are a separate, clearly differentiated group without medical cause. As our understanding of these latter so-called "functional" illnesses has progressed, it has become clear that they too have clear biological underpinnings, and therefore are also "organic."

PRIMARY CARE

In the mentally confused patient, especially when there is no history of previous psychiatric illness (and at times even if there is), think of delirium and dementia first and psychiatric disease second.

During an evaluation, when a clinician detects that a patient being evaluated has mild or moderate confusion, a formal assessment of mental status should be promptly performed (see Chapter 3 and Appendix 1) to document the level of confusion and disorganization. If the patient is significantly confused, further history taking from the patient will be at best inaccurate, and may be an inefficient use of the clinician's time. Rather than gathering information from a significantly confused patient, initial history should be obtained from other sources, including patient records, family members, friends, caretakers, and other individuals familiar with the patient's day-to-day life. If the confused patient shows signs of intoxication, regardless of the source, it is usually of little use to attempt to elicit extensive historical information. Beyond simple basics such as medications taken, recent ingestions, substance use, and medical illnesses, detailed history taking should be postponed to a later time when the patient is not intoxicated.

Because psychotropic medications take an entirely different role with delirium and dementia than in other conditions, further detail about the evaluation of delirium and dementia is necessary at this time. In almost all situations discussed in this text, medications are used to treat specific symptoms or a diagnosis in a positive, symptom-specific way. However, when treating problematic behavior associated with delirium and dementia, most psychotropic medications do not treat the diagnosis or the underlying cause. Any excess medication may complicate the assessment process and potentially worsen the patient's clinical state. The sole exceptions to this are the cholinesterase inhibitors that target one possible underlying mechanism of Alzheimer's dementia (see below).

After a clinical description, the appropriate evaluation process and treatment for delirium will be outlined.

Delirium

Delirium is defined as an acute mental syndrome primarily involving changes in cognition, disturbance of consciousness, and impaired attention. It is divided into two groups, depending on the cause:

1   Delirium secondary to a medical condition
2   Delirium secondary to drug intoxication or withdrawal.

Delirium is considered a sign of acute dysfunction of the brain and should be considered a medical emergency requiring urgent diagnostic evaluation and treatment. Delirium is quite common in emergency room settings and intensive care units, and on medical/surgical wards. The common symptoms of delirium are listed in Table 15.3.

In general, a delirium develops quickly and progresses rapidly. It may be highly reversible once the medical cause is discovered and corrected. Although there are intracranial causes of delirium, as can be seen in Table 15.4, *the majority of causes of delirium exist outside the central nervous system.*

Delirium may precede the symptoms of its medical cause. If the cause is not immediately identified in a first-round of diagnostic tests, but delirium continues to be present, it is incumbent on the clinician periodically to re-evaluate the patient's medical condition to attempt specifically to identify the cause.

Dementia

Dementia is a cognitive disorder that involves global impairment of many aspects of memory, judgment, and cognition. As it progresses, higher cortical functions (such as abstract reasoning, language and ability to follow directions) deteriorate. In contrast to the rapid onset of delirium, dementia has a slow, chronic, insidious onset. Often the level of consciousness is unimpaired until late in the course. Patients typically have a normal level of arousal. Both recent and remote memory are impaired. The speed of psychomotor actions is generally normal. There is less disruption of the sleep/wake cycle than in delirium.

Table 15.3 Symptoms of delirium*

- Rapid onset
- Usually lasts for several days to several weeks
- Clouding of consciousness, which is often fluctuating
- Patient may act bewildered or confused
- Activity level varies; the patient may be restless and hyperactive, psychomotorically slowed, or show changing activity level
- Prominent deficits in attention, distractible in thought
- Frequent perceptual disturbances, visual hallucinations, or illusions
- Alteration in sleep/wake cycle, may be drowsy
- Often disoriented to time, but may also be disoriented to place or person; orientation may fluctuate over time
- Marked impairment in memory, particularly for recent events
- Speech may be incoherent, confused, unintelligible, or unclear
- Changes of setting (including overstimulation or understimulation) can worsen the condition
- The patient may be acutely aware of their disorganization, but not always
- Can present at any age

*Adapted from Andreason NC and Black DW. *Introductory Textbook of Psychiatry*, 3rd edn. American Psychiatric Association Press, 2001. Gilder M (ed.). *New Oxford Textbook of Psychiatry*. Oxford University Press, 2000. Hales RI (ed.). *American Psychiatric Association Textbook of Psychiatry*, 3rd edn. American Psychiatric Association Press, 1999. Sadock BJ and Sadock VA. *Kaplan and Sadock's Comprehensive Book of Psychiatry*, 7th edn. Lippincott, Williams & Wilkins, 2000. Keltner NL and Folks DG. *Psychotrophic Drugs*, 3rd edn. Mosby, 2001.

Dementia is an acquired condition, and its incidence increases with age.[1-4]

- 1–6 percent of those 65 to 75 years of age have dementia
- 7–8 percent of those 75 to 85 years of age have dementia
- 18–32 percent of those over 85 years of age have dementia

Clinicians treating the elderly population should therefore be especially attuned to signs, symptoms (see Table 15.5), and evaluation of dementia.

Most dementias are chronic. Sixty-five percent of dementias are progressive, and because of its gradual onset dementia is often overlooked by patients and families. Some families would prefer not to identify that "grandpa is confused," and show considerable denial. The intellectual deterioration is often attributed to normal aging, particularly early in the course. The patient is often unaware of the loss of cognitive functions, or denies that changes are occurring.

As with delirium, *dementia indicates a serious underlying medical problem affecting the functioning of the brain*. Even though most are not treatable, searching for the underlying illness cause (see Table 15.6) is the most important issue for the clinician. Dementia patients are poor historians, and it is always essential to interview significant others and family to obtain valid historical information.

Table 15.4 Causes of delirium*

Causes within the brain

- Direct brain trauma
- Infections, including meningitis and encephalitis
- Brain tumors
- Vascular disorders
- Epilepsy and postictal states

Causes outside the brain

- Drug ingestion, including medication (both prescribed and street/recreational drugs) as well as poisons
- Drug withdrawal
- Drug side effects
- Endocrine dysfunction, including:
    - Hyper- and hypo-pituitarism
    - Hyper- and hypo-adrenalism
    - Hyper- and hypo-thyroidism
    - Hyper- and hypo-parathyroidism
- Liver disease (hepatic encephalopathy)
- Kidney disease (uremic encephalopathy)
- Hypoxia
- Congestive heart failure, arrhythmia and hypotension
- Vitamin deficiencies, including folic acid, B_{12}, and thiamine
- Hypoglycemia
- Systemic infections with fever and sepsis
- Electrolyte imbalance from any cause including dehydration
- Post-operative states

*Adapted from Andreason NC and Black DW. *Introductory Textbook of Psychiatry*, 3rd edn. American Psychiatric Association Press, 2001. Gilder M (ed.). *New Oxford Textbook of Psychiatry*. Oxford University Press, 2000. Hales RI (ed.). *American Psychiatric Association Textbook of Psychiatry*, 3rd edn. American Psychiatric Association Press, 1999. Sadock BJ and Sadock VA. *Kaplan and Sadock's Comprehensive Book of Psychiatry*, 7th edn. Lippincott, Williams & Wilkins, 2000. Keltner NL and Folks DG. *Psychotrophic Drugs*, 3rd edn. Mosby, 2001.

As the condition progresses, the person has few complaints of cognitive loss, and often appears unconcerned about his or her own condition. The patient may show wandering, pacing, repetitive or stereotypic behaviors, temper outbursts, and complaining. More aggressive actions, such as pushing, biting, scratching, or kicking, may also occur.

Management of delirium and dementia

Unless a patient is acutely disruptive, uncontrollable, or unsafe, medication should take fifth place in the treatment of delirium and dementia behind the following four considerations:

1 *Insure the safety of the patient.* If the patient remains out of the hospital, discuss safety issues with the family or caregivers. Include assessment of the risks in the residence, such as accessibility of medications/toxins/poisons, access to cooking appliances (stove/oven), and other dangerous items such as weapons or tools. Assess and discuss the patient's risk of wandering or getting lost, including at night. In the hospital, keep the patient near the nursing station. Have frequent orientation by consistent staff members, or have family members stay with the patient. If the behavior is more disruptive, the patient may need a sitter or be secluded/restrained.

2 *Perform a thorough medical evaluation* as described in Table 15.7, with appropriate neurological consultation. Serial mental status examinations will help to document the progression and course of the illness (see Appendix 1).

3 *If the dementia is due to drug intoxication or side effects, stop the offending agent.* If due to drug withdrawal, manage the withdrawal.

4 *Correct whatever medical problem is occurring* to whatever extent it is correctable.

Table 15.5 Symptoms of dementia*

- Subtle personality change – "He/she is not him/herself"
- Impaired social skills
- Decreased range of interests, loss of interest in hobbies
- Emotional lability and shallow affect
- Somatic complaints
- Gradual loss of intellectual functions
- Depression, which may occur prior to other symptoms

Late symptoms

- Increasing memory loss (recent memory is lost before remote memory)
- Confabulation (the making up of tales, or responding to questions without regard to fact)
- Increasing mood and personality change with exaggeration of previous personality traits
- Loss of orientation to person and place, in addition to loss of orientation to time
- Sleep problems
- Wandering – patient gets lost
- Impulsiveness and compromised judgment with little foresight and planning
- Psychotic symptoms, including hallucinations, illusions, delusions, and ideas of reference
- Language impairment, thought blocking, occasionally mute

*Adapted from Andreason NC and Black DW. *Introductory Textbook of Psychiatry*, 3rd edn. American Psychiatric Association Press, 2001. Gilder M (ed.). *New Oxford Textbook of Psychiatry*. Oxford University Press, 2000. Hales RI (ed.). *American Psychiatric Association Textbook of Psychiatry*, 3rd edn. American Psychiatric Association Press, 1999. Sadock BJ and Sadock VA. *Kaplan and Sadock's Comprehensive Book of Psychiatry*, 7th edn. Lippincott, Williams & Wilkins, 2000. Keltner NL and Folks DG. *Psychotrophic Drugs*, 3rd edn. Mosby, 2001.

Table 15.6 Causes of dementia*

- Brain tumors (both primary and metastatic)
- Brain trauma
- Chronic brain infection, including syphilis and AIDS
- Jacob-Creutzfeld disease
- Cardiovascular causes, including single or multiple infarctions ("multi-infarct dementia")
- Congenital or hereditary diseases, including Huntington's disease
- Epilepsy
- Normal pressure hydrocephalus
- Vitamin deficiencies
- Chronic metabolic disturbances
- Chronic anoxia
- Degenerative dementias, including
  - Alzheimer's disease
  - Parkinson's disease
  - Pick's disease
  - Wilson's disease
  - Progressive supranuclear palsy
- Demyelinating diseases, such as multiple sclerosis
- Intoxication and poisoning from various elements including alcohol, carbon monoxide, heavy metals, medications, or irradiation

*Adapted from Andreason NC and Black DW. *Introductory Textbook of Psychiatry*, 3rd edn. American Psychiatric Association Press, 2001. Gilder M (ed.). *New Oxford Textbook of Psychiatry*. Oxford University Press, 2000. Hales RI (ed.). *American Psychiatric Association Textbook of Psychiatry*, 3rd edn. American Psychiatric Association Press, 1999. Sadock BJ and Sadock VA. *Kaplan and Sadock's Comprehensive Book of Psychiatry*, 7th edn. Lippincott, Williams & Wilkins, 2000. Keltner NL and Folks DG. *Psychotrophic Drugs*, 3rd edn. Mosby, 2001.

Medication use in delirium and dementia

As emphasized earlier in this chapter, medication is not usually the first or second intervention for confused patients. Ensuring safety, a thorough medical evaluation, removing any intoxicating substances and treating any underlying medical causative factors are initially more important. Psychotropic medication *is* used for the patient who is confused and disorganized, however, in two circumstances:

- Medication for non-specific behavioral control (acute or chronic)
- Medication aimed at mediating one of the possible causes of the Alzheimer's type dementia.

Many, but not all, patients with delirium or dementia will show agitation and problematic disruptive behaviors. Agitation is a general term, akin to the terms fever or pain, and is not a diagnosis in itself. While the behaviors of some agitated patients may be signs of an underlying psychiatric disorder (for example,

Table 15.7 Medical work-up for delirium and dementia*

- Complete medical history, usually provided or supplemented by information from family or caregivers
- Thorough physical and neurological examinations
- Detailed standardized mental status examination (see Appendix 1)
- Laboratory studies, including complete blood count, serum electrolytes, serum glucose, calcium, albumin, magnesium, blood urea nitrogen, creatinine, liver function tests
- Screening for syphilis and HIV, thyroid function tests, vitamin B_{12} and folate levels, EKG, and chest X-ray
- Urinalysis and urine drug screen
- Arterial blood gases
- Baseline psychological testing may be helpful
- If the clinical condition warrants it, lumbar puncture, CT scan or MRI, EEG, blood cultures, lupus prep or antinuclear antibody levels

*Adapted from Trzepacz PT and Wise MG. Neuropsychiatric aspects of delerium. In: SC Yudofsky and RE Hales (eds) *American Psychiatric Press Textbook of Neuropsychiatry*. American Psychiatric Association Press, 1997, pp. 447–470.

psychosis or depression), these behaviors may be a result of social disinhibition or ignoring social norms and cues. These behaviors, while disturbing to caregivers, may not be reflective of specific underlying diagnoses. Such agitated behaviors may be purposeful but performed in an uncoordinated or erratic way, or appear purposeless to the observer. Some behaviors may have a stereotypical, repetitive quality, and others are random. If the behaviors are not clearly acutely dangerous, it may be most beneficial initially to observe the patient medication-free while undertaking the diagnostic evaluation. Some behaviors can be violent and harmful, however, when they are acute, persistent, self-directed, or directed at other persons or property. Specific medications have been used to attempt to control or manage these agitated behaviors, and are discussed by class. Anxiolytics, antipsychotics, antidepressants, and anticonvulsants have all been used beneficially in the agitated patient.

Whenever medication is used, the patient must be carefully monitored for signs of clouding of consciousness, worsening of disorientation, excess sedation, and fall risk. (See Chapter 12 for further discussion of medication treatment behavioral control for the elderly agitated patient.)

Anxiolytics

Benzodiazepines alone seldom control delirium and dementia. Acutely anxious patients may benefit from a short-acting benzodiazepine, however, particularly when used in combination with a traditional or atypical antipsychotic (see Chapters 5, 6, and 12). Longer-acting benzodiazepines should generally be avoided with cognitively impaired persons. Chronic or repeated administration of benzodiazepines can lead to further clouding of consciousness and worsening of attention problems. Benzodiazepines may, however, be the medication of choice for a delirium associated with seizures, or precipitated by withdrawal from alcohol or sedatives. The non-benzodiazepine anti-anxiety alternative to these drugs is buspirone; it does avoid some of the difficulties associated with benzodiazepine use and may be modestly useful. Because it requires a build-up over a period of time in order to be effective, however, buspirone is a poor choice for acute control of agitation.[5]

Antipsychotics

Antipsychotic medications have long been the mainstay of treating agitated patients, particularly in the elderly. Although the use of atypical antipsychotics is rapidly replacing conventional antipsychotics, the combination of 2–5 mg of haloperidol plus 1–2 mg of lorazepam remains a standard treatment in many institutional care facilities for agitation. Unfortunately, typical antipsychotics have been used rather indiscriminately for sedation and behavioral control, rather than being targeted to diagnosed *psychotic* patients. This has created significant problems when conventional antipsychotics have been used long term, because of their propensity to cause movement disorders and tardive dyskinesia. There is now ample evidence for the positive benefit of using atypical antipsychotics in agitated behavioral disturbances and confused patients. Although these agents, particularly risperidone, olanzapine, quetiapine, aripiprazole, and ziprasidone, have beneficial side-effect profiles, it remains to be seen whether they will be used as first line control in the treatment of agitation and confusion in the demented patient.[6-8] Starting doses of these agents are as follows:

- Respiridone 0.25–0.5 mg
- Olanzapine 2.5–5 mg
- Quetiapine 50–100 mg
- Ziprasidone 20–40 mg
- Aripiprazole 15–20 mg.

The use of these agents has been hampered by the lack of intramuscular preparations, although intramuscular ziprasidone and olanzapine are now available. Intramuscular risperidone and aripiprazole will likely be available in the USA soon.

Clozapine, because of its risk of agranulocytosis, hypotension, excess sedation, and anticholinergic side effects, is generally not a first-line choice for the agitated, demented elderly.

Antidepressants

Many of the newer antidepressants, including SSRIs, nefazodone, mirtazapine, bupropion, and the more traditional trazodone, have been found to be useful in treating depression in the elderly as well as, to some degree, for sedation and behavioral control. Sedative drugs such as mirtazapine, nefazodone, and trazodone are more beneficial for this latter purpose.[7]

Anticonvulsants

Valproic acid and carbamazepine, in smaller doses, have been useful for sedation and behavioral control. There are limited controlled data on the use of any other anticonvulsants.

Medications for dementia of the Alzheimer's type

Dementia of the Alzheimer's type is the most common form of dementia, affecting more than 4 million people in the USA, with a prevalence that has been estimated as high as 10 percent for individuals over 65 years of age.[9] The exact cause of this devastating illness is still being elucidated; however, there is ample evidence to suggest that there is degeneration in the cholinergic neurons, more rapidly and more consistently than in other neurotransmitter systems.[10] There is a prominent loss of cholinergic markers in the cortex and hippocampus, which are involved in cognition and memory. It is thought that the decrease of neurotransmission in these acetylcholine-dependent neurons leads to many of the functional deficits of Alzheimer's disease, including memory impairment, aphasia, apraxia, agnosia, and disturbance in executive functions (planning, organization, sequencing, and abstracting).

Cholinesterase inhibitors

Early efforts to increase the production of acetylcholine by providing precursors to acetylcholine formation were unsuccessful. More recent efforts in the past decade have been directed at blocking acetylcholinestrase, the enzyme that breaks down acetylcholine, thereby leading to a functional increase in acetylcholine levels. Tacrine, the first drug developed for this problem, was effective, but was hampered by severe liver toxicity and the necessity of giving four separate daily doses. Because of these disadvantages, it has fallen largely out of favor.

There are currently three cholinesterase inhibitors on the market in common usage: donepezil, rivastigmine, and galantamine. Donepezil and galantamine inhibit acetylcholinestrase, while rivastigmine inhibits both acetylcholinestrase and butyrylcholinestrase, which may provide a more broad-spectrum activity and increased efficacy. Each of these agents has shown benefits for Alzheimer's patients in improving overall assessments of behavior functioning, anxiety, aggression, agitation, and wandering from home. When the patient's memory, cognition and ability to maintain activities of daily living improve, confusion and agitated behaviors decrease.

It is generally thought that these cholinesterase inhibitors slow the progression of acetylcholine-dependent neurotransmission loss, thus delaying the intensification of Alzheimer's symptoms. There is evidence that in some patients there is an actual reversal of symptoms, although this effect is modest. There is no pharmacological cure for Alzheimer's disease. Differences in side-effect profile, frequency of dosing and effectiveness in more severe cases of Alzheimer's is being determined through multiple studies of these various drugs at the time of publication. The therapeutic effect of these medications in different patients can vary from mild to moderately significant.[11–13]

Psychiatric diseases that may present with confusion

While it is not the intent of this text to detail a full psychiatric differential diagnosis, or medication recommendations for psychiatric disease, some patients with major psychiatric disorders present with confusion or inattention as one of the symptoms. If delirium/dementia have been ruled out, and a psychiatric cause for the patient's disorganization is considered, some of the following additional symptomatic cues may be useful in making a tentative diagnosis and assessing the cause of mental confusion.

With *psychosis*, the patient often has the presence of hallucinations. Auditory hallucinations are common, but they may be visual, olfactory, or tactile. There may be delusions (fixed false beliefs that do not change despite factual information to the contrary). The patient's affect is often flattened. There may be a history of previous psychotic episodes.

In *mania*, in addition to mental disorganization and confusion there can be rapid, pressured speech, excess energy or physical motion, and a lack of need for sleep. The patient may be grandiose in ideation or plans. At other times there is little grandiosity and the patient is primarily angry or pressured, with intense irritability out of proportion to the circumstances.

Confusion and cognitive impairments associated with *depression* have the specific label of "depressive pseudodementia." The differentiation of pseudodementia from true dementia is often difficult. However, a depressed patient will often have sad, dysphoric or depressed affect. In addition, these patients have psychomotor slowing and, at times, suicidal thoughts or actions.

The intensely *anxious patient* who is also somewhat confused and distractible will often have other physical signs of anxiety, including pacing, sweating, tremor, or shaking. There may be a history of overt panic attacks.

In *attention deficit disorder* (ADD), acute confusion is not prominent, although a patient with ADD may have chronic difficulty with attending to details or memory. It is important to remember that ADD is a lifelong condition, present in all circumstances, and usually evident from early childhood. The patient will have difficulty with inattention and easy distractibility in most or all situations requiring close concentration. In general, ADD does not have an adult onset without symptoms in childhoood.

More detailed discussion of the diagnosis of psychiatric conditions can be found in any of the widely used, authoritative textbooks on psychiatry.[14–16]

References

1 Breteler MMB *et al*. Epidemiology of Alzheimer's disease. *Epidemiol Rev* 1992;14:59–82.

2   Aronson MK *et al*. Dementia. Age-dependent incidence, prevalence, and mortality in the old. *Arch Intern Med* 1991;151:989–992.

3   Canadian Study of Health and Aging Working Group. Canadian study of health and aging: study methods and prevalence of dementia. *Can Med Assoc J* 1994;150:899–913.

4   Bachman DL *et al*. Prevalence of dementia and probable senile dementia of the Alzheimer type in the Framingham Study. *Neurology* 1992;2:115–119.

5   Semla T, *et al*. *Geriatric Dosage Handbook, Including Monitoring, Clinical Recommendations and OBRA Guidelines*, 5th edn. Lexi-Comp, 2000.

6   Ellingrod VL *et al*. Comparison of respiridone with olanzapine in elderly patients with dementia and psychosis. *Pharmacotherapy* 2002;22(1):1–5.

7   Rawling JN and Verma S. Behavioral disturbances in older patients: guidelines for management. *Psychiatric Times* 2001; October: 72–74.

8   Blake L *et al*. Optimal management of psychosis and agitation in the elderly. Published on the Internet www.medscape.com/viewprogram/1706vnt

9   Kaschkow J. Cognitive enhancers for dementia: do they work? *Curr Psychiatry* 2002;1(3).

10 Katzman R. Alzheimer's disease. *New Engl J Med* 1986;314:964–973.

11 Zurad EG. New treatments for Alzheimer's disease: a review. *Drug Benefit Trends* 2001;13(7):27–40.

12 Borson S. New strategies for management of behavioral disturbances and psychosis in older patients. Presented at the American Association for Geriatrics Society 15th Annual Meeting, Orlando, Florida, February 2002.

13 Brandt MJ. Pharmacotherapy for dementias. Presented at the American Pharmaceutical Association 148th Annual Meeting, San Francisco, California, March 2001.

14 Gilden M (ed.). *New Oxford Textbook of Psychiatry*. Oxford University Press, 2000.

15 Hales RI (ed.). *American Psychiatric Association Textbook of Psychiatry*, 3rd edn. American Psychiatric Association Press, 1999.

16 Sadock BJ and Sadock VA. *Kaplan and Sadock's Comprehensive Textbook of Psychiatry*, 7th edn. Lippincott, Williams & Wilkins, 2000.

Part IV Medication Dilemmas and their Clinical Management

Chapter 16

Psychotropic medications and side effects

Any healthcare practitioner who is legally authorized to prescribe medication can write a prescription for a psychotropic. One of the distinguishing characteristics of the knowledgeable practitioner, who will maintain greater success with mental health patients, is the practitioner who can successfully manage the side effects of a medication. The manner in which a practitioner discusses side effects can have a major effect on whether the person takes the medication, or becomes a frightened, non-compliant patient. Some practitioners will ignore or fail to assess side effects because they don't know how to offer solutions if the patient admits to having them. This chapter will discuss the common and potentially uncomfortable side effects that occur with psychotropic medications, and how the astute clinician can manage them. Less common, but potentially more serious, adverse reactions are discussed in Chapter 17.

During the initial evaluation

For many patients, the risk of side effects is *a* major, or in some cases, *the* major issue in taking psychotropic medications. The popular press now describes many mental health medications in detail, including possible side effects. With the vast amount of information available on the Internet, patients often come to the office armed with a series of questions about what potential unwanted effects may be associated with a prescribed medication. If a patient brings up the issue of side effects early in the initial interview, it is wise to suggest that the evaluation first be completed to determine *if* medication is needed and *which* medication might be most helpful. The clinician should reassure the patient that side effect issues will be covered before treatment decisions are made.

Discussing the side effects of a medication

For the typical physically healthy individual, serious side effects with psychotropics are remarkably rare and the clinician can be genuinely optimistic that medications prescribed are unlikely to cause significant harm. For physically compromised patients, or for patients taking a complicated medical regimen, there may be some risk of adding a psychotropic. When present, these risk issues need to be individualized and discussed with each patient as their situation dictates. Table 16.1 lists some facts regarding psychotropics and side effects.

When it comes time to introduce the issue of side effects, toward the end of the initial evaluative session for a routine patient without special risk factors, the concept can be introduced as suggested here.

TALKING TO PATIENTS

"Most people take this medication without side effects, and that is what I expect for you. As with any medication, however, there can be some unwanted effects. Fortunately, if these unwanted effects occur, they are usually of the annoying, short-term variety, and are not serious or life-threatening. If anything is not mild or is not going away, I want you to call me so, together, we can decide how to proceed."

If patients have read about or heard of specific side effects, or are especially fearful of a particular adverse reaction, these possibilities must be addressed specifically. Many times the patient's concerns can be alleviated with simple reassurance, and in fact the side effect of concern may be of minimal likelihood with the medication to be prescribed. If the side effect the patient is concerned about *is* a possibility with the particular medication chosen, acknowledge this with:

TALKING TO PATIENTS

"Yes, that has been reported with some, but not most, patients. (Include any data or statistics to approximate the frequency, if known.) I know you are concerned about this and we will be watching for this possibility carefully. If it emerges as a problem, we will deal with it at that time. However, I do not believe the small possibility of the problem should stop you from beginning the medication. How do you feel about this plan?"

Table 16.1 Facts regarding psychotropics and side effects

- Most side effects of psychotropics are more annoying than serious
- Life-threatening or irreversible side effects are rare
- Many side effects are remediable or pass with time

Usually this is sufficient to have the patient begin treatment. If the patient does remain resistant or highly skeptical, the clinician should outline what, if any, other medication alternatives might be tried and the reasons the initial recommendation has been made. Often, having heard clinicians thinking and rationale, the patient can proceed with a trial of the first-choice medication. On occasion, a patient may insist on a second-line choice, even when its therapeutic potential is less, because it avoids or minimizes a particular side effect. As long as the clinician feels the choice has some reasonable chance of success, it is a good idea to form a contract to use a second choice of medication initially if it means the patient can be compliant. Of course, if because of side-effect fears a patient is requesting a clinically inappropriate medication, the clinician needs to discuss why he or she will not agree to this prescription.

Even if the patient brings no information about side effects, it is important to cover a few common side effects that might occur with any medication prescribed. The key to success is striking a balance between identifying some possible side effects while refraining from frightening the patient with a litany of possible, but unlikely, adverse consequences.

TALKING TO PATIENTS

For example, when prescribing an SSRI antidepressant you might say: *"Most people take these medicines without problem. If there are going to be any side effects, the most common ones tend to be upset stomach, diarrhea, headaches, sleepiness, agitation, or some interference with sexual arousal. If you get any of these problems and they are mild, bear with them because they will often pass within several days to a week. If the side effects are not mild or are not passing, be sure to let me know so that we can decide how to fix the problem."*

For a discussion of a side effect that is serious and carries significant risk for this patient, the representative presentations shown here can serve as models.

TALKING TO PATIENTS

To an elderly schizophrenic patient in the hospital who might be at risk for a fall:

"Mrs Fisher, I am going to prescribe (name of medication) *to help decrease the voices in your head that you have told me about. This medicine is a good choice for you. However, the medicine has the possibility of making you somewhat sleepy or lightheaded.*

Therefore, we will start with a small dose and evaluate how you tolerate it. I do not want you to fall or lose your balance. Please get up slowly when you have been lying down or sitting, or ask for assistance from the nursing staff. Also, tell them if you feel light-headed or dizzy."

When prescribing carbamazepine (which could lower the estrogen levels via P-450 enzyme induction – see Chapter 17) to a patient on birth control pills:

"In prescribing carbamazepine, there is a possibility that this medication may cause your body to break down estrogen more quickly and could lower the birth control protection from your low-dose estrogen pills. We have tried several other mood stabilizers without success, and your symptoms remain significant. I believe carbamazepine is now the best choice to help you feel more stable. I want you to contact your Ob/Gyn practitioner to change your birth control pill to one with a higher strength of estrogen before we begin this medication. If you like, I will call him/her to explain why I am suggesting this."

Side-effect assessment in follow-up visits

If a clinician does not ask about side effects and intervenes when necessary, the patient will stop the medication or drop out of treatment!

Asking the patient if he or she is experiencing any unwanted effects from the medicine is mandatory for each of the first several follow-up appointments, at least until such time as the patient is stabilized and is clearly tolerating the medicine without problem. *Do not assume that the patient will spontaneously volunteer side effect information.*

When the practitioner learns of any side effects, the following questions will help to identify a course of action and/or remedy:

- What changes, sensations or symptoms are you experiencing? (Have the patient first describe facts, not their own assessment, beliefs, or assumptions about the cause.)
- How often do you feel this?
- Is there any pattern to when this occurs?
- When, in relation to taking the medication, does the problem occur?
- Is the problem diminishing or intensifying with time?
- Does anything make the problem better or worse?
- How troublesome is this for you? (Use a 1–10 numerical scale.)

For example, if a patient complains of nausea, this fact alone is insufficient information. The clinician needs to know when the nausea occurs. Is it constant? Does it occur at specific times of the day? Does it occur within an hour or two of taking the pill, or at other times as well? Does it interfere with sleep, or occur in the middle of the night? Is it accompanied by vomiting? Have the patient's eating habits been affected by the nausea? Only with these data can the clinician decide to lower or split the dose, prescribe it at bedtime, add an antinauseant, or change the psychotropic medication.

How much of a problem is it?

With any given side effect, it is crucial to find out how severe and troublesome this particular side effect is to this particular patient. Individuals have very different tolerances for adverse effects of medication. For example, some people are remarkably tolerant of gastrointestinal side effects and others are intensely bothered. Likewise, headache, sexual interference and weight gain may be acceptable consequences for some individuals, and be absolutely intolerable, even when mild, to others. As discussed in Chapter 6, quantification of the patient's words is often helpful to the clinician in evaluating side effects as well.

CLINICAL TIP

It is useful to have the patient quantify the amount of the particular side effect on a scale of 0–10, with 0 being no side effects at all, 1 being minimal and 10 being maximal. Such clarification can help the clinician decide if a side effect is of a magnitude to require intervention or a change of medications.

TALKING TO PATIENTS

Ask the patient: *"On a scale of 0 to 10, where zero is 'I am never bothered by this problem' and 10 is 'I am extremely, intolerably bothered by this problem all the time,' how does this affect you?"* In general, side effects rated by the patient as a 4 or above will almost always require intervention. A patient rating of 1 to 3, particularly if the side effect is beginning to wane, is often tolerable, at least for a short time. Mentally, the clinician may adjust the patient's rating of a side effect up or down the scale depending on the clinician's assessment of the consequences of the side effect. For example, headache, fatigue, or sexual interference are bothersome, but usually do not have serious imminent sequelae for healthy patients. The clinician may mentally move the patient's rating down a bit, even though it is bothersome to the patient. The occurrence of a seizure, changes in blood cell counts, severely decreased or increased blood pressure, repetitive vomiting, marked changes of liver function, or the onset of tardive dyskinesia have potential serious outcomes and sequelae. The clinician may mentally move the rating of this type of side effect higher, even if the patient's rating is not particularly high (patients do not always appreciate the gravity of some side effects).

Other issues to consider in evaluating side effects

Just because a patient complains of a side effect that he or she believes is a direct effect of the medication, this may or may not be the case. Further detailed inquiry is essential. The clinician should first, look for other causes besides the prescription that may account for the unwanted effect, and then inquire about any recent medications prescribed by other practitioners, herbal or over-the-counter medications, food intolerances, or changes in sleep and/or activity schedules that correlate in time with the onset of the complaint.

The clinician should next consider possible indirect effects relative to the medication prescribed. For example, P-450 interactions may change the blood levels of other medications the patient is taking, and these blood level changes can result in the patient experiencing adverse effects without actually being a direct side effect of the medication prescribed (see Chapter 17).

Third, the practitioner should assess the frequency of the particular side effect described: Is it continuous or intermittent? Does it occur most or all days, or relatively infrequently?

Fact: Most psychotropic medication side effects are typically continuous or very frequent. Side effects that occur once a week or several times a month are often, at least in part, related to other causes, and are not solely due to the psychotropic. Side effects that occur for several days and then are totally absent for weeks or months are again much less likely to be related directly to the psychotropic.

Occasionally a psychotropic can predispose an individual to a side effect that can then be precipitated by a second independent cause. If this is the case, modifying the second external cause may allow the patient to continue taking the psychotropic without a need to change medication. For example, a psychotropic may cause loose bowel movements. While this may be tolerable in general to the patient, significant diarrhea occurs only when certain foods are eaten. Rather than discontinuing the psychotropic, the simple solution is to identify and temporarily avoid the offending food while the medication is being prescribed.

Fourth, the timing of the side effect in relation to ingestion should be assessed. Side effects that occur within 30 minutes to an hour after taking the pills are often related to a rapid rise in blood concentration to a high peak level. Symptoms such as an upset stomach, headache, nausea, or nervousness that only occur shortly after taking the pill may be minimized if the medication is taken at bedtime. As long as the side effect is not severe enough to awaken the patient, the problem may have diminished enough to be tolerable upon waking. Side effects from high peak blood levels can also be improved by lowering the total daily dose, or dividing the dose into two or more smaller quantities taken at different times of the day.

Changing medication due to side effects

A frequent dilemma facing a clinician is whether or not to change medications because of side effects. In addition to the severity of the side effect, the clinician should take into account:

- The patient's therapeutic response to the medication, so far
- The presence or absence of suitable alternatives
- The length of time that the patient has been on the medication
- The patient's individual concerns and wishes.

Severity of side effects

Side effects can be classified as mild, moderate, significant, or serious. The clinician's response will vary depending upon the classification. For *mild* side effects (1 to 2 on the scale previously mentioned), education and labeling the symptom as a side effect, along with reassurance, is all that is usually necessary. Sometimes a watch-and-wait approach will allow the symptom to disappear, but in any case the course of the side effect should be re-evaluated at follow-up visits.

For *moderately intrusive* side effects (3 to 5 on the scale), there may be ways to remedy the problem without actually changing medications. These may include splitting the dosage, taking the medication at a different time of day, changing to a long-acting formulation of the medication, or recommending changes in diet and/or exercise.

For more *significant* side effects, either because of the patient's discomfort or the clinician's assessment of possible risk (6 to 8 on the scale), it is absolutely essential that the side effects be addressed specifically and promptly. If not, the patient may drop out of treatment or, at the very least, stop the medication, sometimes without telling the clinician.

For *serious* side effects, again either because of the patient's discomfort or the clinician's assessment of risk (9 or 10 on the scale), it is imperative that the clinician responds quickly and decisively. For example, with the onset of a seizure or fainting episode leading to unconsciousness, it is essential to address the issue, discontinue the medication or significantly reduce the dosage. Specialty consultation with a neurologist or internist may be necessary to evaluate other causes for such symptoms. Other examples requiring prompt action would be serious abnormalities of laboratory testing, such as drops in white blood count (to less than 1500 absolute neutrophil count),[1] platelet count (below 100 000 per cubic millimeter) or a marked increase in liver function tests (above two or three times normal). The clinician needs to communicate the need for a prompt evaluation to the patient and, if appropriate, to the patient's family. These more serious risk issues will be covered in more detail in Chapter 17. Even if the medical risk of the side effect is small, when a patient rates a side effect at 4 or above on the basis of discomfort and/or frequency, the clinician should act promptly if compliance is to be maintained.

When serious side effects occur, the clinician's written records are crucial and provide documentation of his or her assessment, thinking and interventions. In the event of medicolegal action because of serious adverse consequences from medication, the written medical record provides the best defense. Such documentation should reflect:

- The onset of the symptoms/side effects, i.e. When did they start?
- When the clinician was made aware of these complaints

- Exactly what recommendations were made regarding remediation
- Any dosage changes instituted
- When, and if, the medication was recommended to be stopped
- Any specific behavioral precautions that were advised.

Side effects and clinical response

When the patient is receiving a strong positive therapeutic response to a medication and/or there are few or poor alternatives available, a mild to moderate side effect should generally be managed by watching and waiting, adding a non-prescription remedy, or adding a prescription remedy. Ultimately, if these interventions are unsuccessful, changing medications may be the only option, even if the alternatives are less desirable.

If, on the other hand, the patient is having a mediocre response and/or there are good alternatives for change, the clinician will likely change medications sooner. It is always possible to return to medication A, if medication B is tried unsuccessfully. If the patient is only having a mediocre or poor therapeutic response, changing medications may provide two benefits – engendering a more positive treatment response, as well as minimizing side effects. Therefore, with a mediocre response, changing medications should be tried before trying non-prescription or prescription remedies for the side effect itself. These alternatives were summarized in Table 6.1 in Chapter 6.

The novice clinician and side effects

If a patient complains of side effects, it is appropriate to empathize with the patient's discomfort without denial or defensiveness. The novice clinician may feel uncomfortable at having caused seeming harm or discomfort to the patient. Side effects are possible with the prescription of any medication, and the presence of side effects does not necessarily indicate bad practice or poor decision-making.

To recognize and manage side effects effectively, novice clinicians and non-mental health practitioners do well to become knowledgeable about one or two medications in each class of psychotropic. Understanding medication side-effect profiles for only several medications will form an effective knowledge base that can be broadened once the clinician has more experience. If, alternatively, at the outset of a career the novice clinician attempts to learn and prescribe, for example, eight different mood stabilizers, it will be difficult and confusing to remember the side-effect profile of each.

PRIMARY CARE

If you do not prescribe psychotropics commonly, it is better to know one or two medications from each class well, rather than attempting to be superficially familiar with the universe of psychotropics.

Is it a side effect or not?

The use of print, media, and Internet resources, as well as personal consultation from colleagues, are important ways to learn side effects. The *Physician's Desk Reference* (*PDR*), the USP formulary and package-insert prescribing information can be helpful in sorting out what may or may not be a side effect of a particular drug. Additionally, all pharmaceutical companies maintain telephone support lines for medication prescribers that can be useful sources of data about potential side effects of their products. These telephone numbers are listed by company at the beginning of the *PDR*. Ultimately, even with appropriate input, a clinician may not know whether a side effect or complaint is actually related to a medication. *At times, the only way to assess whether a side effect is related to a particular medication is to stop the medication and observe.*

When appropriate, the practitioner should not hesitate to admit lack of certainty about a particular drug fact or possible side effect. It is better for the practitioner to investigate the question and get back to the patient rather than attempt to appear assured when he or she is not, and guess.

Almost all side effects referable to psychotropic medications pass quickly and should be totally eliminated within 7–14 days of stopping the medication. If a patient continues to complain of side effects weeks or months after discontinuation of the medication, it is highly unlikely that such a side effect was related to the psychotropic, and other etiologies should be evaluated.

Side effects seen most frequently

The most common side effects of psychotropic medications are listed in Table 16.2. Assessment and remedies are discussed in the following text.

The first two sections focus on opposite side effects, namely sedation and overactivation. Both are common, but each presents different challenges to the prescriber. Sedation is usually a relatively simple and straightforward side effect.

Table 16.2 **Common side effects of psychotropic medications**

- Sedation
- Overactivation
- Nausea and other gastrointestinal problems
- Sexual dysfunction
- Weight gain
- Headaches
- Asthenia (weakness)
- Dry mouth
- Hair loss
- Skin reactions
- Prolactin elevation
- Hypotension

Overactivation is more complicated, and may have widely differing root causes with markedly differing remedies.

Sedation

When taking psychotropic medication, sedation (often perceived as sleepiness or grogginess) is one of the single most commonly reported side effects. Sedation that occurs when starting medication may or may not be related directly to the medication itself. When patients have been sleep deprived from their illness, sleeping longer than normal for up to a week may represent their "catching up" on lost rest. During the first week, even if patients interpret this pattern as sedation from the medication, a wait-and-watch approach is appropriate, as their normal sleep pattern may emerge.

Sedation, when present, is not always undesirable. In an agitated or anxious patient, some daytime sleepiness may contribute to calmness during the initial period of symptom resolution. This then becomes a specific application of the general principle mentioned above, which states that side-effect tolerance is very individualized for each patient. In this case, what may be intolerable for one patient may be tolerable and even desirable for another.

There are, however, patients with no history of sleep deprivation who become sleepy with psychotropics that cause daytime sleepiness at the outset or with dosage increase. If the sedation is medication-related and mild, allowing 7–14 days for accommodation is prudent and may allow patients to adjust satisfactorily.

Historically, patients were dosed with psychotropics throughout the day in the belief that this was necessary in order to achieve optimal therapeutic response. Current practice is that antidepressants, antipsychotic or mood-stabilizing response can usually be obtained with once-daily dosing.

CLINICAL TIP

The vast majority of psychotropic medications do not need to be given multiple times a day to be effective.

If medication doses taken during waking hours cause daytime sleepiness, a simple remedy may be to move all the medication to bedtime dosing. In this way, the sedative side effect may provide a useful sleep aid. For patients who require daytime dosing of potentially sedative medications, consider giving a smaller daytime dose and a larger bedtime amount. For example, a patient may tolerate 10–25 percent of their full dose in the morning and receive 75–90 percent at bedtime without daytime sleepiness. This plan can, however, present problems for the patient who complains of grogginess the morning after taking the larger dose of medicine at bedtime. Moving the evening medication dose to earlier in the evening, particularly if the sedative effect of the medication takes several hours to emerge, may minimize morning hangover. Taking the medication at 8 pm or at dinner often significantly decreases morning grogginess. As a last resort, for a medication that is very effective and for which there are not available alternatives, divide the total dose into three or four small doses throughout the day, having the patient tolerate a consistent mild to moderate amount of daytime sedation.

If a medication causes marked intolerable sleepiness, or after several weeks of attempts at accommodation without success, a change in medication should be undertaken. Fortunately, within each of the major classes of medications there are generally alternatives that will be less sedative to individual patients. It may take several trials to find a medication that is minimally sedative to each particular patient. Within the *antidepressants*, there are several choices that for most patients will be less sedative. These include bupropion, desipramine, fluoxetine, and venlafaxine. Within the *atypical antipsychotics*, ziprasidone may be a less sedating choice. Within the *traditional antipsychotic* class, molindone or loxapine may be less sedating. Within the *mood-stabilizer* category, each medication in general comes from a different chemical class and their tendency to promote sedation may vary greatly. Therefore, individual tolerances for the sedative effect of mood stabilizers may also vary, and it may be necessary to try several different medications to find a non-sedative option for a particular patient. Benzodiazepine *anti-anxiety medications*, as a class, offer no options that are "non-sedative." Here, patient tolerance becomes the crucial variable. Shorter half-life drugs such as lorazepam or alprazolam may sedate for less time than their longer acting cousins – diazepam, clorazepate, or chlordiazepoxide.

It should be noted that, *although these generalizations are made, individual sensitivity to the sedative effect of any particular medication can vary greatly.* Some patients may experience significant sleepiness on any of the medications listed above, even if that medication is less sedative in general.

Overactivation/anxiety

An overactivated response to psychotropic medication may show itself in a variety of forms, and may be signaled by different symptoms, including:

- Feelings of mental nervousness or agitation
- Internal restlessness
- Difficulty in falling or staying asleep
- Shakiness/tremor
- Feeling emotionally "out of control"
- Feeling mentally speeded/pressured or "unable to slow down."

Before automatically assuming that the cause of a complaint of overactivation is the medication the patient should be evaluated for other causes that are not directly related to the medication, such as:

- Excessive caffeine intake
- Ingestion of non-prescribed stimulants, including appetite suppressants, diet pills, and "energizing" herbs

- Use of recreational drugs, including cocaine and amphetamines
- Excessive work pressure, family, or life stressors.

If all these causes have been ruled out or are minimal, medication side effect should be suspected and the various possibilities considered separately.

The five potential causes of overactivation are shown in Table 16.3. These are each separate entities, and have markedly different solutions. In order to remedy overactivation satisfactorily, accurate assessment is essential to decide which cause is present.

Nervousness

A patient who is prescribed a psychotropic may complain of mental anxiety, of feeling agitated or being restless. The nervousness can be solely internal without external signs, or may show tremor and/or sweating externally.

Such nervousness is most commonly associated with non-sedating antidepressants (see above), but can also occasionally occur with mood stabilizers and antipsychotics. In general, if nervousness alone is present (without any of the other symptoms of overactivation, discussed in the following sections) and is mild, the patient should be reassured that this most likely will pass. If the symptom persists, decreasing the dose of the medication may, for some patients, make the regimen tolerable. As a last resort, addition of a small dose of a benzodiazepine (lorazepam 0.25–1 mg/day or clonazepam 0.25–1 mg/day) to the regimen for a several-week period of time may allow accommodation to the anxiety-causing medication.

For example, a patient on fluoxetine for depression may feel agitated and nervous. Using a small dose of a benzodiazepine for several weeks can allow the patient to accommodate to this nervousness, which will often pass with time. If the nervousness persists beyond the first several weeks when the benzodiazepine is withdrawn, switching antidepressants is the next alternative. On some occasions when switching is not desirable or possible, it may be necessary to continue taking the benzodiazepine for the entire period the patient is taking the offending primary psychotropic. While this is less desirable, if it allows a patient to take an antidepressant that is otherwise working well for depression it may be a satisfactory trade-off.

Anxiety and nervousness, as a side effect from medication, may not be mild and can present as frank panic attacks – either singly or in groups. This develop-

Table 16.3 Potential causes of overactivation side effects

- Nervousness
- Akathisia
- Hypomania
- Sleeplessness
- Tremor alone

ment may occur as a flare-up of previously quiescent panic attacks or occur *de novo* in a patient who has never previously experienced panic attacks. Panic attacks are acutely distressing and uncomfortable for the patient, and require a prompt response from the clinician. A PRN dose of a benzodiazepine (e.g. alprazolam, clonazepam, or lorazepam 0.5–1 mg) will usually quell the immediate symptoms, but the medicine causing this side effect should be decreased in dose or discontinued entirely.

While this reaction may occur in patients who have never experienced an anxiety attack, it is more commonly seen in patients previously prone to panic. These individuals may be acutely sensitive to SSRIs or other new generation antidepressants. A panic attack may occur with even the first dose. Should this occur, the medication should be decreased to a fraction of the usual starting dose and very gradually increased as tolerated by the patient. The patient usually accommodates to the slowly increasing dose with minimal discomfort.

There are rare patients who are exquisitely sensitive to antidepressants, and may react with excessive anxiety/panic to even a small amount. Such patients may be *very* slowly titrated on the medication using a liquid preparation, beginning with only a drop or two to start. Although it may take several months to reach a traditional therapeutic dose, the use of liquid medication does allow such depressed patients to be treated with an antidepressant. Patients who have previously experienced panic attacks with antidepressant medication therapy are understandably afraid of starting any antidepressant for fear it will again precipitate the attacks. Such patients benefit from being given wide latitude in when, and by how much, their antidepressant dosage is increased. With this sense of control, these patients develop confidence and proceed to a higher dose only when they are ready. Carrying a PRN "emergency" dose of benzodiazepine also provides extra assurance to these patients.

Akathisia

Akathisia, a sense of internal restlessness, is a common side effect with traditional antipsychotics, and may be perceived as overactivation. It is less typical with new generation antipsychotics, but still may occur. Some antidepressants, particularly fluoxetine, bupropion and some tricyclics, may also cause akathisia. Patients with akathisia often have difficulty in describing their condition clearly. They will feel uncomfortable, at times intensely so, but have trouble articulating the source of their discomfort. They have difficulty sitting still, may pace, and will become more agitated if they are not permitted to do so. They may describe the sense that their intestines are agitated or moving, even though no frank gastrointestinal symptoms are present. Such patients often present as fidgety in the office, and may have difficulty sitting in a chair throughout an interview. Persons with akathisia can be uncomfortable to the point of attempting drastic solutions to rid themselves of the feeling. Serious akathisia has been linked to attempted or completed suicide. It is critical for the clinician to have a high index of suspicion for akathisia with traditional antipsychotics. Immediate intervention is vital, since failing to diagnose this symptom can lead to fatal consequences.

Once akathisia is diagnosed, a reduction in dosage of the offending drug may help. Unfortunately this side effect may continue, even at a lower dose, and a change to another class of antipsychotic is indicated. Akathisia with a traditional antipsychotic may abate with a change to an atypical antipsychotic.[2,3,4] If the patient has a particularly positive response to a medication and the clinician is hesitant to alter positive results, the addition of a beta-blocker (for example, propranolol 20–80 mg), an anticholinergic (benztropine 1–2 mg) or a benzodiazepine (alprazolam 0.25–0.5 mg) may be a useful countermeasure to the akathisia.[5] In all cases, the patient should be closely monitored over time.

Hypomania

Antidepressants, atypical antipsychotics and even medications thought to be mood stabilizers can induce mania or hypomania (partial, mild manic symptoms). Hypomania can present with symptoms similar to other causes of overactivation discussed above, such as anxiety, panic attacks, internal restlessness, fidgeting, and pacing. Hypomania, however, is also usually accompanied by other symptoms, including rapid speech, increased speed of thought, inability to sleep, a lack of need to sleep, impulsive behavior, displays of unusual energy, or feelings of exceptional well-being.

The onset of such signs shortly after beginning an antidepressant points to a diagnosis of hypomania, although such mania may present at any time during the treatment with an antidepressant. Other classes of medications with antidepressant properties, including some "mood stabilizers" (for example gabapentin, lamotrigine, and topiramate) or atypical antipsychotics (ziprasidone, risperidone, olanzapine, and quetiapine), may also cause hypomania as a side effect. This is paradoxical, since the intent of these medications is to stabilize mood and reduce mania.

Once new or unexpected manic/hypomanic symptoms present, a reconsideration of the diagnosis may be required. Patients who may have been previously assessed as having unipolar depression or dysthymia often should now be given a bipolar or cyclothymic diagnosis. Although some clinicians consider mania that solely occurs in the presence of an antidepressant as a separate subcategory of bipolar disorder, most clinicians will respond to antidepressant-induced mania in the same way as they would treat other subtypes of bipolar disorder.

Beyond re-diagnosing the patient, the clinician can remedy the hypomanic response by:

- Decreasing the dosage of the antidepressant
- Discontinuing the antidepressant
- Adding a mood stabilizer to the current dose of antidepressant.

It should be noted that most (if not all) patients with an antidepressant response leading to hypomania will revert to depression when the antidepressant is withdrawn.

Sleeplessness as a side effect

Another common overactivation side effect to antidepressants, but which may occur with some mood stabilizers as well, is sleeplessness. Patients may complain of difficulty falling asleep, sleep continuity disturbance, or a worsening of a pre-existing sleep disturbance. If there are no other symptoms of akathisia or hypomania, sleeplessness alone may be treated in several ways. Moving the antidepressant dose away from bedtime to an earlier time in the day may minimize the sleep-disturbing effect. More often, however, some other remedy must be instituted. A sedative antidepressant, such as trazodone, mirtazapine, doxepin, nefazodone, or trimipramine, can be added at bedtime to promote sleep. Other sedatives/hypnotics, such as a benzodiazepine, zolpidem, or zaleplon, may be added briefly. A third option is to add valproic acid or an atypical antipsychotic (e.g. quetiapine) in small doses for the purposes of sleep alone. Particularly activating antidepressants may require some form of sleep medication frequently in the early stages of their use. Some depressed patients who are particularly sensitive to the sleep disruption may require sleep medication on a more chronic basis while they are treated.

Attention to sleep patterns is important, since adequate sleep is not just a comfort in patients with serious anxiety or depressive disorders; it is also healing and restorative. When an antidepressant is working well otherwise, it is reasonable to continue sleep medication on a longer-term basis if it is needed and if the alternative is sleep deprivation. (See Chapter 13 for further information about medication and sleep difficulties.)

Tremor

Some patients may interpret the presence of a tremor as suggestive of anxious overactivity, since it has been common in Western culture to assume that someone who shakes is anxious. While this may be true for some people, there are many patients with tremor who are minimally anxious or not anxious at all. Conversely, many anxious people will never experience tremor. Unaddressed, pronounced tremors may interfere with fine motor activities such as writing, eating, grasping objects, or serving food, and be of significant embarrassment to patients. Psychotropics that have been associated with tremors are listed in Table 16.4.

If a patient develops a tremor while taking psychotropic medication, his or her caffeine intake should be assessed. Many patients may develop tremors or have existing tremors worsened for several hours by the ingestion of caffeine.

If caffeine is not the culprit and a tremor is deemed to be medication-induced, small amounts of a beta blocker (e.g. propranolol 10–60 mg) or small amounts of a benzodiazepine (e.g., lorazepam or alprazolam 0.5 mg) can be considered. Since the anti-tremor effect of these remedies will only last from 3–6 hours, it may be necessary to repeat the dose several times to achieve control throughout the day.

Patients with tremor may not need to have the tremor controlled throughout a

Table 16.4 Medications used in mental health that can cause tremor*

- Lithium
- SSRIs and other new generation antidepressants
- Stimulants
- TCAs
- Thyroxine
- Traditional and atypical antipsychotics
- Valproic acid
- Verapamil

*Adapted from Conner GS. Essential tremor: mechanisms and management. *Proceedings of a Symposium of Southern California Neurological Society*. ILab Publications, Los Angeles, California, 2001, p. 30.

24-hour period. Many patients, for example, are only concerned about tremor during working hours, at times when their behaviors are observed, or on occasions when they feel self-conscious. A beta blocker or benzodiazepine for tremor may be needed only at certain times during the day, or on certain days of the week, in order to make the situation bearable for the patient. Some patients may only use anti-tremor medication during the work week and omit the medication on weekends. Still others may use the anti-tremor medication only sporadically and intermittently, when they feel the tremor would be a particular hindrance. Responsible patients can be given significant latitude on when, and how often, to use anti-tremor medication. Once-daily use of long-acting beta-blocker preparations (e.g. Inderal-LA 60 mg) may give satisfactory tremor control through most or all of the day without repeating the dose.

Careful questioning may reveal the patient to have had an "essential" or familial tremor that has worsened with the use of psychotropic medication. Such "essential" tremors may not respond to the above remedies, and a separate neurological evaluation is indicated to rule out potentially more significant neurological illness.

Nausea and gastrointestinal problems

Gastrointestinal (GI) side effects from gastric and bowel reactions to medications are common. They may present as upper gastrointestinal problems, such as:

- Nausea or upset stomach
- Dyspepsia
- Gastric pain
- Increased gas
- Vomiting
- Lower GI distress and cramps
- Diarrhea
- Constipation.

Except for vomiting, recurrent diarrhea and severe constipation, these symptoms are not in general dangerous; however, they are often quite uncomfortable for the patient. GI side effects may also result in changes in appetite, eating habits, and weight. Patients who, by history, tend to be concerned about bowel function may react strongly to even mild changes in bowel movement frequency or consistency.

Nausea

As noted earlier, when patients complain of nausea with medication it is important to assess *when* the nausea occurs in relation to taking the dose, *how long* it lasts, and when, if ever, it remits. Nausea that occurs shortly (30–90 minutes) after taking a dose of medication may result from an irritated stomach lining. In this situation, several remedies are useful:

- Take the medication with food
- Take the medication at bedtime; as long as the nausea does not disrupt sleep, it can disappear or be minimal by morning
- Split one larger dose of medication into several smaller doses
- Take over-the-counter antacids at the time of dosing.

If the nausea is severe, occurs throughout most of the day, or does not remit with the above treatments, the psychotropic medication should be changed.

Constipation

For patients who experience constipation with psychotropic medications the clinician must evaluate the medication in the context of the patient's lifestyle, including diet, activity level, and other medications/foods that could be contributing to the problem. Although not limited to older adults, constipation is common in this population, particularly when multiple constipating medications are taken simultaneously. A geriatric lifestyle may be sedentary, and dietary preferences for dairy products and cheese may add to hardened stools and decreased bowel motility. When constipation occurs with the initiation of a psychotropic, remedies include:

- Increased physical activity
- Increased fluid intake
- Increased dietary intake of fruits and vegetables
- Psyllium husk (Metamucil) or other generic bulk-promoting preparations
- Stool softeners such as bisacodyl
- Preparations of senna, 20–60 mg per day
- A cholinesterase inhibitor (donepezil 5–10 mg)

If constipation is severe or is unresponsive to the above remedies, a change of medication is necessary.

Diarrhea

Mild diarrhea (or looser than normal stools) is not uncommon after beginning many psychotropic medications. If this is mild and infrequent, it is prudent to wait for up to a week to determine if bowel habits normalize. A slightly altered bowel habit, including more frequent or looser bowel movements, is not physiologically a serious problem, and reassurance to such individuals may be sufficient. If diarrhea persists beyond a few days, wakes the patient in the middle of the night, or creates urgency resulting in fecal accidents, the patient's situation must be addressed promptly. Bulk preparations, while useful in constipation, may also be of some use in mild diarrhea. Over-the-counter antidiarrheal preparations such as loperamide hydrochloride (Imodium and others) may also be somewhat helpful for mild loose stools. A prescription medication such as diphenoxylate with atropine (Lomotil) is useful for short-term treatment for diarrhea. Such preparations, however, are not appropriate long-term remedies. If diarrhea persists despite these remedies, or if the diarrhea recurs anytime the remedy is withdrawn, a change of medications is usually necessary.

Sexual interference

As psychotropic medications have been used more commonly, their ability to interfere with sexual arousal, desire and performance has been well publicized. While previously sexuality may have been an unspoken issue between prescriber and patient, it is now clearly within the purview of prescribing clinicians to address sexual issues, and it is a necessary area to be discussed when prescribing psychotropics.

Serotonin specific reuptake inhibitor (SSRI) antidepressants, as well as other antidepressants, mood stabilizers (particularly lithium and carbamazepine), and traditional and atypical antipsychotic medications are well known for sexual interference.[6] Decrease in desire for sex, decrease in physical arousability (male erection, female vaginal lubrication), increased time to ejaculation/orgasm and impaired ability to orgasm are common possible side effects of various psychotropics. Ideally, a patient's sexual functioning should be evaluated and documented prior to starting any medication. Since a decrease in sexual functioning or arousability is common in depressed, anxious and psychotic patients,[7,8] it is useful to ask about a patient's level of sexual activity at the time of initial evaluation. Often because of time constraints, however, and, particularly if the patient did not complain of sexual problems, the details of the patient's sexual behavior may not have been assessed or recorded. If a patient complains of a change in sexual behavior after a medication is started, it is important to attempt to assess the patient's level of sexual functioning prior to the medication as well as currently.

Even when the change in sexual behavior coincides with beginning medication, the clinician should inquire about other qualitative changes in the patient's sexual relationships, since not all changes in sexual activity are directly related to the medication. As patients begin to experience the benefit of psychotropic medications, they may also change partners, change the frequency of sexual activity, or otherwise change their sexual behavior in a way that affects their arousability.

When evaluating potential sexual interference from medication, *the clinician must ask detailed, pointed questions about the frequency and quality of sexual activity, elucidating facts and behaviors rather than accepting broad statements.* Patients can often state: "This pill knocked the heck out of my sex life" or "I'm just not into sex anymore," or "I can't do it with my spouse anymore." The clinician's questions must then be specific and direct about what changes have occurred in the patient's mental interest or physical arousal, to determine the etiology and possible remedies for the problem. Such questions include the following

1 *For both males and females:*
   - Are you mentally not interested in engaging in sexual activity as much as before?
   - Are you mentally interested, but have difficulty achieving essential physical elements of arousal?

2 *For males:*
   - Can you gain and maintain an erection long enough for sexual intercourse? How long can you maintain an erection? Are you unable to ejaculate? How long does it take to ejaculate? If it takes more time to ejaculate than before, how much longer? Have you noticed a change in the quality of the ejaculatory sensation?

3 *For females:*
   - Have you noticed a change in ability to obtain vaginal lubrication? Are you able to reach orgasm? What percentage of the time do you reach orgasm? How long does it take to reach orgasm? Is this different than before medication? Has the quality of orgasm changed?
   - Is there any evidence to suggest a new or recent onset medical condition may be affecting sexual functioning? (Common medical and surgical conditions that can cause sexual dysfunction are listed in Table 16.5)
   - Has there been a recent introduction of a non-psychotropic medication that could be affecting sexual function (such as those listed in Table 16.6)?

If, after gaining the above information, it appears that there is no other obvious cause for the change in sexual drive or behavior, and if the timing is consistent with starting psychotropic medications, it is probable that the medications are having a direct effect on the patient's sexual functioning. When this occurs, it is often soon after starting the medication, but it may also occur at some later interval – particularly after a dosage increase.

If it is the clinician's assessment that the medication is interfering with sexual functioning, it is crucial to determine how important the interference is to *this* patient at *this* time. The clinician can never assume that his or her own level of concern about sexual interference is the same as the patient's. Particularly when patients are feeling better emotionally, it is not a problem for some individuals temporarily to undergo a limited amount of diminished capacity for sexual arousal. Other patients may simply not put a high priority on sexual activity, and for them this side effect is of minimal importance at this point in life.

Table 16.5 Medical and surgical causes of sexual dysfunction*

Medical illnesses associated with sexual dysfunction:

1   Cardiovascular
   - Atherosclerotic diseases
   - Hypertension
   - Myocardial infarction
   - Cardiac failure and angina

2   Renal
   - Chronic renal failure

3   Genitourinary
   - Pelvic-genital infection
   - Atrophic vaginitis
   - Endometriosis
   - Peyronie's disease
   - Testicular disease
   - Genital trauma

4   Endocrine
   - Diabetes mellitus
   - Hypogonadal states
   - Hyperprolactinemia
   - Pituitary dysfunction
   - Thyroid dysfunction
   - Adrenal disease

5   Neurological
   - Multiple sclerosis
   - Peripheral neuropathy
   - Central nervous system tumors
   - Stroke
   - Spinal cord disease
   - Substance use disorder

Surgical procedures associated with sexual dysfunction:
- Prostatectomy
- Mastectomy
- Vaginal surgeries
- Episiotomy
- Lumbar sympathectomy

*From: Keltner NL and Folks DG. *Psychotropic Drugs*, 3rd edn. Mosby, 2001, p. 349.

Table 16.6 Classes of medication that may affect sexual response

Drug	Sexual response
Antihypertensives	
Diuretics	Libido, erectile, ejaculation problems
Timolol (ocular)	Libido, erectile, low ejaculate problems
Central-acting adrenergic inhibitors	Libido, erectile, ejaculation problems
Peripheral-acting adrenergic inhibitors	Libido, erectile, ejaculation problems
Alpha-adrenergic blockers	Low incidence of sexual dysfunction
Combined alpha- and beta-adrenergic blockers	Erection, ejaculation, delayed detumescence problems
Angiotensin-converting enzyme (ACE) inhibitors	Worsening of sexual dysfunction
Hormones	
Androgens	Libido decreased, impotence, testicular atrophy
Anabolic steroids	Azoospermia
Estrogens	Decreased vaginal atrophy, decreased libido in males
Cancer agents	
Alkylating chemotherapy agents	Gonadal dysfunction in males and females
Other chemotherapeutic agents	Gonadal dysfunction in males and females with procarbazine and vinblastine; suppressed testicular and adrenal androgen synthesis with ketoconzaole
Carbonic anhydrase inhibitors	Libido, erectile problems
Antiepileptic drugs	
Carbamazepine, phenytoin	Decreased libido or erectile problems

*Adapted from Buffum J. Prescription drugs and sexual function. *Psyciatr* Med 2001;10:181.

The reverse is also true. There are many patients who cannot tolerate even small changes in sexual functioning. For them, sexual activity and prowess may be an extraordinarily important part of their day-to-day life, and any diminishment in functioning may have significant ramifications to their self-esteem and their relationship with their partner. Such individuals, if not dealt with sensitively, will discontinue medication very quickly, at even the earliest sign of sexual interference. A significant number of patients who prematurely terminate medication do so because of sexual side effects that are not evaluated by the clinician.

If the clinician decides that sexual interference is likely caused by medication, the elements of Phase I interventions should be instituted as in Table 16.7.

If the sexually offending drug is a short to medium half-life antidepressant (paroxetine, sertraline, venlafaxine, and possibly citalopram), a "drug holiday"

Table 16.7 Phase I: first responses to medication-induced sexual interference

The clinician should:

1 Clearly state that he or she believes the patient's sexual interference *is* likely connected to the medication. This information should also be given to the patient's partner by the patient or, with consent, by the clinician.

2 Tell the patient that initial medication-induced sexual interference may diminish and pass with time. When such accommodation occurs, it usually does so within several weeks to several months.

3 Clearly state that, even if the interference is due to the medication, there will be no permanent change in sexual functioning. When the medication is discontinued, the person's baseline level of sexuality will return.

4 Assess the patient's response to this information. If acceptable, agree on a timeframe for further observation after which, if the situation has not resolved, other action will be considered.

5 Consider "drug holidays"

---

may solve the problem. This is accomplished by having the patient omit the medication dosage on the morning before planned sexual contact, which permits the blood level of medication to drop over the ensuing 12–18 hours. The amount of medication in the body may be sufficiently low by evening to avoid significant interference in sexual functioning. The patient then takes the regular dose of medication the following morning. It is unnecessary to take the missed dose. Surprisingly, many patients can satisfactorily accomplish this without any serotonergic withdrawal syndrome, and without loss of antidepressant activity. While a drug holiday requires planning as to the time of sexual activity and minimizes sexual spontaneity, this remedy can be an effective and simple tool for some patients.

If the Phase I strategies are unsuccessful, or the patient is unwilling to comply, the clinician can go to Phase II, as shown in Table 16.8.

Sexual interference that persists despite waiting and education may respond to dosage change or a change of medication. Lowering the dose of the psychotropic may help some patients, but is seldom totally remedial. If the medication causing the problem is an antidepressant, a change to nefazadone, mirtazepine, bupropion or trazodone may be effective in lessening sexual problems.[6,9] Since the sexual interfering effects of antipsychotics or mood stabilizers are quite variable from patient to patient, any change of medication or category may, in some individuals, reverse medication-related sexual dysfunction. There are some data to suggest that medications that increase prolactin (notably traditional antipsychotics and risperi-

---

Table 16.8 Phase II: remedies for medication-induced sexual interference

- Lower the dose of the offending psychotropic
- Change to another psychotropic
- Stop all psychotropics, if clinically possible
- Add a pharmacological antidote

---

done) may cause a higher rate of sexual dysfunction than others. Beyond that, there are very limited data as to which specific antipsychotic and mood-stabilizing medications are consistently less sexually interfering. Therefore there is no one recommended change, and any change may or may not be useful.

When changing medications, the other important consideration is maintaining the desired antidepressant, mood-stabilizing or antipsychotic effect. When the medication is changed because of persistent sexual interference, any changes should, in general, be done gradually and with a graduated crossover method (as discussed in Chapter 6) to give the patient the highest likelihood of maintaining symptom remission.

When the previous remedies are inadequate and medication change is contraindicated (or has been tried and failed), use of pharmacological antidotes is the next step. Pharmacological remedies that have shown some usefulness in modulating or reversing psychotropic-induced (especially antidepressant-induced) sexual interference are shown in Table 16.9.

Unfortunately, with the exception of sildenafil for erectile problems (which can be effective in reversing antidepressant-induced erectile dysfunction by 75–90 percent[10]) and bupropion (50–70 percent improvement in orgasmic function in women),[9,11,12] each of the remaining antidotes, individually and collectively, is only effective for a limited number of patients. When sildenafil and bupropion are ineffective, switching medications may be a more successful strategy than trying repeated add-on pharmacological antidotes.

With an aggressive pharmacological approach, patients can often obtain both adequate anxiety/mood effect and satisfactory sexual functioning. There are, however, some patients who, despite all attempts and strategies, will have to make a choice between emotional health and full sexual response. While not desirable, emotional stability may have to take preference over sexual satisfaction for some severely ill patients. This is a marginally tolerable situation for some patients, and is totally intolerable for others.

Weight gain

Maintenance of reasonable body weight is a medical health and safety issue. Additionally, body image is an important matter of self-esteem for both men and women. From a cultural standpoint, staying slim is a virtual obsession for many people in Western society. From a medical perspective, obesity can lead to a worsening of hypertension, cardiovascular disease, diabetes and stroke. The issue of how a psychotropic medication may affect weight, particularly if it may cause weight gain, is a major concern for many patients.

Obesity is generally defined via the Body Mass Index (BMI), which is a person's weight in kilograms divided by his or her height in meters squared. A BMI of 30 or greater is a commonly accepted definition of obesity. A person is overweight when the BMI is between 25 and 29.9.[13]

Some patients will ask about possible weight gain even before a medicine is prescribed. Other patients will only raise the issue when, and if, they begin to gain weight on the medication. A smaller group of patients will be almost

Table 16.9 Drugs used to treat antidepressant-induced sexual dysfunction*

Drug	Symptom/indicator	Dosage
Bethanecol	Erectile dysfunction	10–40 mg PRN
Amantadine	Anorgasmia	100 mg PRN 1 h before sexual activity
	Erectile dysfunction	100 mg bid
	Hypoactive desire	100 mg bid
Bupropion	Anorgasmia	75–150 mg PRN 1–2 h before sexual activity
	Hypoactive desire	75–150 mg bid
	Arousal	75–150 mg bid
Buspirone	Anorgasmia	20–60 mg/day
	Hypoactive desire	20–60 mg/day
	Erectile dysfunction	20–60 mg/day
Cyproheptadine	Anorgasmia	4–16 mg PRN 1 h before sexual activity
	Hypoactive desire	4–16 mg/day
Dextroamphetamine	Anorgasmia	5–20 mg PRN
	Hypoactive desire	2.5–5 mg bid
Granisetron	Anorgasmia	1 mg PRN 1 h before sexual activity
Gingko biloba	Hypoactive desire	60 mg bid–qid
Methylphenidate	Anorgasmia	5–20 mg PRN
	Hypoactive desire	5–20 mg/day
	Arousal	5–20 mg/day
Pemoline	Anorgasmia	18.75 mg PRN
	Hypoactive desire	18.75–75 mg/day
	Arousal	18.75–75 mg/day
Sildenafil	Erectile dysfunction	50–100 mg/day; $\frac{1}{2}$–4 h before sexual activity
Yohimbine	Anorgasmia	5.4–10.8 mg PRN
	Hypoactive desire	5.4 mg/day to 5.4 mg tid
	Arousal	5.4 mg/day to 5.4 mg tid

*From Keltner NL and Folks DG. *Psychotropic Drugs*, 3rd edn. Mosby, 2001, p. 362.

oblivious to a possible connection between the medication and weight changes. Therefore, the issue of weight maintenance will be important for the clinician to discuss prior to prescribing any medication likely to cause weight gain.

Chronically mentally ill patients are already two to three times more likely to be obese than the general population.[14] Depression, schizophrenia, and bipolar disorder carry their own burden of increased obesity.[15–20] Therefore, the management of weight when prescribing antidepressant, antipsychotic, and mood-stabilizing medications becomes even more crucial.

For psychotropic medications with an "average" incidence of weight gain, the majority of patients either do not gain or lose weight, or gain small amounts. Most psychotropics have an "average" incidence of weight gain with the exceptions noted in Table 16.10.

Weight gain or loss with psychotropic medication is usually reported as the average or mean collected from a group of patients. When dealing with patients and psychotropics clinically, there can be considerable variability among individuals. Many patients will not gain weight on drugs that have a higher than average statistical weight gain; conversely, some individuals may gain weight on medications with low or moderate statistical averages.

When patients do gain weight from medications, leaner patients (with a lower BMI) statistically gain more weight than obese persons (with a high BMI).[21] Therefore, patients who are obese should not automatically be excluded from using medications with higher than average risk of weight gain if the medication is otherwise indicated.

The mechanism of psychotropic weight gain is unclear.[22] It may be related to increased appetite, a direct influence on calorie metabolism or, at least in part, from the development of insulin resistance, altered blood glucose levels or blood leptin levels.

TALKING TO PATIENTS

If a patient raises the possibility of weight gain when using medications of *"average" weight gain*, the clinician can discuss the issue in the following way: *"Most people on* (name of medication) *do not gain weight. I do not expect that to be a significant issue for you. There is, however, almost no mental health medication that has not been alleged for some people, at some time, to cause weight gain. I, too, am interested in making sure that you maintain a reasonable body weight. There are good reasons why we are prescribing this medicine at this time, and I believe that those reasons are more important than the slight risk of possible weight gain. We will, however, be monitoring this together. Please notify me if there is any significant change in your weight, and we will discuss our options at that time."*

TALKING TO PATIENTS

When selecting a medication that does have risk of higher than average weight gain, early attention and prevention is the key. Therefore, the discussion can proceed as follows: *"I am prescribing* (name of medication) *for you. I believe this is a good choice for you and that it can make a significant improvement in your symptoms. We know that one possible side effect of* (name of medication) *is an increase in appetite. It is important that, if possible, we avoid making future decisions about your medication based solely on this factor. Therefore, I want both of us to keep track of your eating*

Table 16.10 Psychotropics and weight gain

Antidepressants causing *higher* than average amount of weight gain:
- Paroxetine[1]
- Mirtazepine[1,2]
- TCAs[3]
- MAOIs[3]

Antidepressants causing *less than* average weight gain:
- Bupropion[4,5]
- Reboxetine (UK only)[6]

Mood stabilizers causing a *higher* than average weight gain:
- Valproic acid[3]
- Lithium carbonate[3]
- Gabapentin[7]

Mood stabilizers causing *less* than average weight gain and/or weight loss:
- Topiramate[8–10]

Antipsychotic medications causing *higher than* average weight gain:
- Clozapine[11]
- Olanzapine[11,12]
- Low potency traditional antipsychotics, such as thioridazine[11]
- Risperidone[7,12]
- Quetiapine[7]

Antipsychotics causing *less than* average weight gain:
- Ziprasidone[11]
- Molindone[7]

[1] Sussman N and Ginsberg D. Weight gain associated with SSRIs. *Primary Psychiatry* 1998; Jan: 28–37 (available at http://www.mvelectric.com/ssri)

[2] Fava M *et al.* Efficacy and safety of mirtazapine in major depressive disorder patients after SSRI treatment failure: an open label trial. *J Clin Psychiatry* 2001;62:413–420.

[3] *The Maudsley 2001 Prescribing Guidelines*, 6th edn. Martin Dunitz, 2001, p. 195.

[4] Gaddem J. New weight loss tool. *JAMA* 1999;281:24.

[5] Weisler RH. Comparison of bupropion and trazodone for the treatment of major depression. *J Clin Psychopharmacol* 1994;14(3):170–179.

[6] Thase M. Efficacy and Tolerability of Reboxetine: A Review. Presented at the American Psychiatric Association Conference, New Orleans, May 2001.

[7] Malhotra S and McElroy S. Medical management of obesity associated with mental disorders. *J Clin Psychiatry* 2002;63(suppl 4):26.

[8] Dursun SM and Devarajan S. Clozapine weight gain plus topirimate weight loss. *Can J Psychiatry* 2000;40:198.

[9] Privitera MD. Topirimate: a new antiepileptic drug. *Ann Pharmacother* 1997;31:1164–1173.

[10] Hussain MA *et al.* Topirimate as an anti-obesity agent. In: *New Research Abstracts of the 153rd Annual Meeting of the American Psychiatric Association, May 18 2000, Chicago, IL.* Abstract NR 709:249.

[11] Allison DB *et al.* Antipsychotic induced weight gain: a comprehensive research synthesis. *Am J Psychiatry* 1999;156:1686–1696.

[12] Ratzone G *et al.* Weight gain associated with olanzapine and risperidone in adolescent patients: a comparative prospective study. *J Am Acad Child Adolesc Psychiatry* 2002;41:337–343.

habits, exercise and weight. Be sure to maintain a nutritious, low calorie diet and minimize significant intake of fruit juices and full-calorie soda. Let's discuss the amount of physical activity that you now do." Then map a plan for physical exercise. Use a dietitian, if necessary, to discuss which foods are low and high calorie if the patient is not knowledgeable in these areas.

Even though weight gain may be the concern in the clinician's mind, notice that the clinician warns of increased *appetite*, not specifically increased *weight*. This presentation is often much more palatable to patients (who can then feel some control over the process) than specifically identifying that they will gain weight (over which they are likely to feel they have little control).

At the time of initial evaluation, the patient's baseline weight and BMI should be noted so that any changes in weight can be accurately correlated to their pre-medication weight.

"It must be the medication . . ."

Once a medication is prescribed, and if a weight increase is noticed, it is common for the patient quickly to suspect that the medication is the cause of the problem. However, although weight gain from medication is possible, patients often find medication an easy and convenient target to blame for possible weight gain when there may be other causes to consider. Rather than immediately accepting the patient's assumption that any weight gain is caused by medication, the clinician should ask and document responses to the following questions:

- What is your previous weight history over time?
- How has your weight fluctuated with your emotional state in the past?
- What exercise, if any, do you do? How often? For how long?
- Has your level of exercise changed since you began the medication?

In the interval until the next visit, the clinician should ask the patient to:

1 Weigh him- or herself twice a week until the next visit. Describe the most accurate method for obtaining weight, which is to weigh oneself first thing in the morning, after using the bathroom and before having anything to eat or drink.
2 Maintain a written, detailed history of food intake (a "food diary") that lists everything put into the mouth for a 10-day period, including all snacks and beverages. Have the patient bring the diary and record of weight measurements to the next visit.

With this information, there may be clear indications of possible factors contributing to weight gain:

- There may have been a marked increase in food intake once the patient began feeling better

■ The overall diet may be high in fatty or caloric items
■ The amount of exercise may be minimal or non-existent
■ An anxious or manic patient may have slowed the amount of physical activity to "normal." This may have led the patient's weight to increase from a sub-normal level to a more normal level now that the anxiety or mania is improving and physical overactivity is waning
■ Some depressed patients who lost appetite and have eaten poorly for weeks or months may be below baseline weight. After medication, patients become less depressed, and a weight gain to baseline is not only normal, but also a sign of return to health.

Some patients who lose weight because of their illness enjoy the weight loss that may have returned them to a more personally desirable level, reminiscent of weight when they were an adolescent or young adult. An increase in weight as they recover on the medication, however, moves them away from this idealized earlier weight, which they should be counseled may not be realistically achievable as an adult.

Intervention helps

If, on evaluation of the above data, no other primary cause is apparent and the patient's weight is increasing, the medication may be playing a role. A crucial clinical fact is that advice, intervention and monitoring of the patient's diet and activity level by the clinician can make a difference. Several studies[23–25] now conclude that if the clinician takes an active role in helping patients to manage their weight, results are significant. These interventions can occur as the patient starts a possible weight-gaining medication (and thus minimizing or preventing the gain), or after the weight gain has started. They include:

■ A thorough discussion of weight management and the possible effect of medication
■ Nutrition counseling – directly or through referral to a dietitian
■ Monitoring and reporting weekly weight
■ A gradual increase in vigorous physical exercise.

Approaches to medication-induced weight gain

When it is suspected that weight gain is due to the medication, the following remedies should be considered:

■ If the weight gain is minimal (1–5 lb; 0.5–2.5 kg), a wait-and-see approach combined with appropriate diet and/or exercise may be sufficient.
■ If the patient's diet is not healthy and/or the patient's exercise is minimal, a frank discussion about the connection between calorie intake, physical activity and body weight is necessary. If the patient is doing well on a medication and the clinician feels it should be continued, it can be useful to consider

forming a contract with the patient for appropriate lifestyle changes to allow for ongoing medication. For some patients the course of medication is time-limited and a minor weight gain can be tolerated, or even reversed, with appropriate diet and exercise during that time.

■ Lowering the dose of medication to the least possible amount that satisfactorily treats the mental health symptoms may decrease any appetite enhancement and/or weight gain. (This may not be an effective strategy for weight gain associated with antipsychotics.[21])

■ For new or significant weight gain which starts only after the patient has been taking medication for a substantial period of time, the clinician should consider whether it is time to discontinue the medication, even if it is earlier than initially planned. If the patient can safely taper off the medication, medication-induced weight gain may no longer be an issue.

■ If lowering of dose, appropriate diet, and increase in exercise cannot stem weight gain, and it would be premature to discontinue the medication, a change of medications and/or class of medications is indicated, considering the options presented in Table 16.10.

■ Group support programs for weight loss may also be beneficial. Commonly used weight loss support programs include: Weight Watchers (www.weightwatchers.com); Richard Simmons (www.richardsimmons.com); Overeaters Anonymous (Telephone: 505-891-2664); TOPS Club, Inc. (www.tops.org).

■ Use of eating manuals, diet/nutrition books. Some useful self-help books on diet and nutrition include:[26] *The McDougal Program for Maximum Weight Loss* (McDougall JA, Penguin Group, 1995); *Eat More, Weigh Less* (Ornish D and Brown JSE, HarperCollins, 2001); *Dr Shapiro's Picture Perfect Weight Loss* (Shapiro HM, St. Martin's Press, 2000); *Eating Well for Optimum Health* (Weil A, Alfred A Knopf, 2000).

Even when medications are changed, continued watchful diligence is required by both the clinician and patient. Monitoring is necessary, and weight should be regularly recorded.

Pharmacotherapy of weight gain

Appetite suppressants can be utilized in select patients on a time-limited basis. These include:

■ Phentermine (30 mg before breakfast)
■ Desoxyn (5 mg before each meal)
■ Sibutramine (10–15 mg in the morning).

Note that virtually all appetite suppressants are sympathomimetric stimulants or have stimulant properties. They are FDA scheduled drugs that can have the same habit-forming potential of other stimulants. In addition to their ability to decrease appetite, they can cause physical side effects such as agitation, insomnia, tremor, or anxiety. In some individuals they can have antidepressant effects, cause hypomania or aggravate psychosis, and they are contra-indicated for use with MAOIs. They are not generally used long term.

Other medications include *Xenical* (orlistat), which is a weight-loss medication that acts by an entirely different mechanism to stimulants, and does not include central nervous system activity. The medication is a reversible inhibitor of gastric and pancreatic lipases, which convert dietary fat into absorbable free fatty acids in the gut. When not transformed in this way, triglycerides are not digestable into the systemic circulation and, pass out through the feces, so calorie reduction results. The dose is 120 mg three times a day.

Topirimate, an anti-epileptic medication used for partial seizures, has mood-stabilizing properties. Because of its weight-reduction property, it may be useful in a regimen of bipolar or antipsychotic medications.[27–29] If there is clinical necessity for the use of multiple mood stabilizers, the weight-reduction effect can be maintained when topirimate is used as an add-on to other drugs The dose is 50–100 mg per day. Another new anticonvulsant with some antimanic properties, *Zonisamide*, may also be helpful as an agent in the treatment of weight gain in mood disorder patients, although the results are still preliminary.[30]

There are several small studies showing that amantadine (100–300 mg daily)[31,32] and H_2 antagonists nizatidine (300 mg twice daily)[33] may possibly be useful in reducing weight in patients taking antipsychotic medications. One study of the use of the oral hypoglycemic agent metformin (glucophage), 500 mg three times daily, showed significant weight reductions in children taking olanzapine, risperidone, quetiapine, and valproic acid.[34]

Old sayings are still true

Whether or not weight changes are due to medication, two adages apply to weight loss remedies: *"There is no such thing as a free lunch;"* and *"If it sounds too good to be true, it probably is."* Inexpensive, over-the-counter weight-loss preparations often do not work, or contain potentially harmful ingredients. Products that promise significant "amazing" weight loss "without dieting or exercise" are likely, at best, to have little solid research to support their efficacy. At worst they may contain ephedra (or *Ma huang*, a herbal form of ephedrine), which can interact problematically with prescription antidepressants, stimulants and other herbal products, such as St. John's Wort. Ephedra has been linked to hypertension, stroke, myocardial infarction, nephrotoxicity, and sudden death.[35,36] "Fad" or "crash" diets are seldom helpful, and may be metabolically dangerous. Even if a patient manages to lose a significant amount of weight in a short timeframe, the weight loss is seldom maintained and the patient will often regain weight rapidly when a crash diet is stopped.

Headaches

Headache have been reported with many psychotropic medications. Sometimes the headaches are migraine in type, with all the consequent sequelae of migraines, but at other times they may have non-migrainous qualities and patterns. Some patients who start psychotropics will notice a worsening of pre-existing headaches/migraines, while other patients will start headaches anew. Not all patients with pre-existing headaches will have them worsen, and some patient's headaches may improve with the addition of an SSRI antidepressant or lithium.[37]

When headaches do occur and they are mild, taking the medication at bedtime may allow the headache to occur during sleep, such that it is minimal during the day when the patient is awake. Headaches that emerge within an hour or two of taking the medication may benefit from splitting the dosage into two or three smaller amounts that are dosed throughout the day. Such smaller dosages may eliminate the headache altogether, or allow the patient to live with very mild pain. Over-the-counter pain relievers such as aspirin, ibuprofen, or aceta-minophen may be sufficient to treat milder headaches. If none of these remedies is effective, a change of medication is often necessary.

Patients with pre-existing migraine headaches that worsen with mental health medication can require close cooperation between the mental health prescriber and a neurologist, since many of the most useful psychiatric drugs can alter the frequency or intensity of headaches. Likewise, many medications used to treat headache can have significant mood effects or create psychiatric mood instability in the psychiatric patient.

Asthenia

Asthenia, or weakness, may occur, particularly with strongly serotonergic antide-pressants. Patients with normal mood can also develop a "frontal lobe-like" syn-drome characterized by apathy, lack of motivation, intermittent fatigue and mental dulling. Generally, this is thought to result from excess antidepressant dose and excess serotonergic stimulation. Decreasing the dosage of the SSRI may limit and improve the apathy and dulling. Adding a stimulant or bupropion, both of which increase norepinephrine and dopamine activity, may also increase motivation and minimize fatigue. If these remedies fail, changing the medication is often necessary.

Dry mouth

With strongly anticholinergic medications such as TCA's and traditional antipsy-chotics, dry mouth can be a considerable problem. In its mildest form, it is an annoy-ance. When more severe and persistent, however, dry mouth is quite uncomfortable, may make speech and swallowing difficult, and lead to increased dental caries.

The clinician should, whenever possible, decrease the anticholinergic load by choosing medications that may be less anticholinergic. Switching from a TCA to an SSRI or other new generation antidepressant, or switching from a traditional antipsychotic to an atypical antipsychotic, may help in this regard. Other reme-dies for this problem include asking the patient to use chewing gum or sugar-free candy, or to drink increased amounts of water. Lastly, a cholinergic agent such as bethanechol hydrochloride (10–20 mg per day) or a cholinesterase inhibitor (e.g. donepizil 5–10 mg per day) may modulate the dryness.

Hair loss

While statistically uncommon, hair loss (alopecia) has been reported with a wide variety of psychotropic medications. When it does occur it can be markedly distressing to the patient, and the clinician will be queried. The patient will complain of noticing increased amounts of hair on a hairbrush, or seeing hair in the drain when taking a shower or bath.

Surprisingly little research has been done on this side effect, and much of our information on the subject is anecdotal or is based on isolated case reports. It is helpful to explain to the patient important facts that we do know about hair, hair growth, and hair loss:

- Of the roughly 100 000 hairs on the scalp, loss of up to 150 strands per day is normal.[38,39]
- Twenty-five to fifty percent of a person's hair must be lost before it becomes clinically evident.[38,40]
- Patients unfortunately associate any discussion of psychotropic medication-related hair loss with cancer chemotherapy hair loss, which is not a valid comparison. Hair loss due to cancer chemotherapy is generally much more severe than that which occurs with psychotropic medications, and is a result of a different mechanism.[38–41]
- Mental health patients will report idiopathic hair loss even when they are not on any psychotropic medication.
- Drug-induced hair loss is actually hair breakage, or shedding at the scalp line. The patient's hair follicles remain intact, and new hair will grow back to replace that which breaks off.[38,42]
- Medication–induced hair loss is generally time-limited, and will resolve spontaneously within several weeks or months.[38,41,43,44]
- Hair lost due to psychotropic medications will grow back within 2–5 months after the offending medication is stopped.[38]
- The hair that grows back has been reported for some patients to be a different texture when the offending agent is lithium or valproic acid. This has not been reported with other medications.[45]

The strongest psychotropic medication offenders in causing hair loss are shown in Table 16.11.

Many other medications have had a low incidence of case reports of hair loss associated with their use. The medications are shown in Table 16.12.

On evaluation of hair loss, other causes must be considered besides medication-induced alopecia. Since hypothyroidism is a known cause of hair loss, a thyroid function panel and thyroid stimulating hormone (TSH) level should be obtained on any patient who makes this complaint. Trichotillomania (compulsive hair pulling) is another possibility.

Unfortunately, there is no definitively curative treatment for alopecia caused by medication. Since the hair loss is transient and self-limited, if the medication is significantly beneficial to the patient for mental health symptoms, encourage the

Table 16.11 Psychotropic medications causing hair loss with significant frequency*

- Lithium carbonate
- Valproic acid
- Fluoxetine

*Adapted from Gautem M. Alopexia due to psychotropic medication. *Ann Pharmacother* 1999;33:631–636.

Table 16.12 Psychotropic medications with at least one case of possible medication-related hair loss*

Amitriptyline	Methyphenidate
Bupropion	Maprotiline
Carbamazepine	Mirtazepine
Citolapram	Nefazodone
Clonazepam	Olanzapine
Silbutramine	Oxycarbazine
Desipramine	Paroxetine
Donepezil	Propanolol
Fluvoxamine	Risperidone
Gabapentin	Sertraline
Haloperidol	Topirimate
Imipramine	Tranylcypromine
Lamotragine	Venlafaxine
Loxapine	

*Adapted from *Physicians Desk Reference*. Medical Economics Company, 2002.

patient to continue taking the medication if possible. In mild cases, the patient may be willing to do this, and the condition will resolve spontaneously. Other remedies that have been recommended include taking oral selenium (100 μg/day) and zinc (15 mg/day). Application of a selenium-containing shampoo (for example, Selsun Blue) directly to the scalp can also be tried. With more significant hair loss, patients are often more reluctant to continue the medication, and the clinician should decrease the dose or change medicines.

Skin reactions

Many psychotropics have reported a modest incidence of skin rashes or skin reactions as potential side effects. These may be described as maculopapular rashes, dermatitis, skin itching, or exacerbation of acne. In general, the majority of these skin problems are annoying but minor, and the incidence is no greater than 1–2 percent for any given medication. It is difficult to interpret the literature to know how many of these skin rashes are associated with actual drug allergy, since a skin rash is such a prominent part of allergic drug reactions. Even though some of these rashes might be more accurately described as a side effect and not represent

Table 16.13 Psychotropic medications with an incidence of skin rash greater than 3 percent

Generic name (Brand name)

- Alprazolam (Xanax)
- Bupropion (Wellbutrin)
- Silbutramine (Meridia)
- Fluoxetine (Prozac)
- Lamotrigine (Lamictal)
- Naltrexone (Revia)
- Pimozide (Orap)
- Quetiapine (Seroquel)
- Sertraline (Zoloft)
- Tacrine (Cognex)
- Topirimate (Topomax)
- Valproic acid (Depakote)
- Venlafaxine (Effexor)
- Ziprasidone (Geodon)

a true drug allergy, the appearance of a rapidly spreading rash in a patient on medication should be treated as an allergy, and the principles outlined in Chapter 18 followed. Some compounds, however, have a higher incidence of skin problems, and these are listed in Table 16.13.

In contrast to the benign rashes at a fairly low incidence that occur with many psychotropics, there are three mental health medications that have significant, frequent and potentially serious skin complications: lithium, lamotrigine, and carbamazepine.

Lithium has long been known to be a medication that can cause skin irritation, skin rash, or other skin problems. In addition to a rash *per se*, lithium may cause dryness of the skin, pruritis, exacerbation of acne, and a worsening of psoriasis. Because of this propensity, lithium should be a third- or fourth-line choice of mood stabilizer for patients with existing psoriasis. In rare cases, psoriasis has been precipitated *de novo* by taking lithium on a regular basis.

Lamotrigine has a documented incidence of severe rash (classified as Stevens-Johnson syndrome, or toxic epidermal necrolysis) in a small number of patients. In addition, up to 10 percent of patients taking lamotrigine may have a benign rash, which often does not progress or relate to the more serious forms. Because the clinician may have difficulty in distinguishing the more benign rash from the more serious variety, any patient who develops a rash on lamotrigine should have the medicine discontinued unless there is a strong clinical indication for continuing. This is unfortunate, since upwards of 95 percent of these rashes will turn out to be benign, will eventually disappear, and do not progress to Stevens-Johnson syndrome. Several clinical facts have evolved regarding the incidence of rash with lamotrigine that have led to clinical guidelines. The incidence of serious rash is significantly higher in the pediatric population than in adults (1 percent in patients less than 16 years old, and 0.3 percent in adults greater than 16 years old). High initial dosage or rapid dosage escalation are also associated with increased risk of serious rash. Therefore, the following recommendations are used with lamotrigine:

- Lamotrigine should not be used in patients under 16 years of age
- Lamotrigine should not be started at more than 50 mg per day and dosages should be increased by modest amounts every week or two (see lamotrigine product information for further description of a normal dosing schedule)
- The presence of valproic acid will increase the blood level of lamotrigine, whenever the two are prescribed simultaneously. Therefore, a patient who is already taking valproic acid should have lamotrigine started at 25 mg every other day and the dosage increased gradually from there.
- Most lamotrigine-precipitated serious rashes occur in the first 2–8 weeks of administration; however, a few have occurred after 6 months of continuous use.

Carbamazepine also has a small, but well-known, incidence of severe dermatological reactions, including toxic epidermal necrolysis and Stevens-Johnson syndrome. Rarely, these syndromes have led to death, but most of these fatal reactions occurred in the past, during the first years of usage of this compound. Other skin reactions occurring with carbamazepine include pruritic and erythematous rashes, urticaria, photosensitivity reactions, exfoliative dermatitis, erythyma multiforme, and erythyma nodosum. Unlike lamotrigine, no other obvious precipitating factors leading to an increased incidence of rash have, to date, been uncovered. These serious skin rashes appear to be an idiosyncratic response in certain individuals.

Despite the known incidence of these serious skin conditions with these three compounds, it must be reiterated that their frequency is small – certainly less than 1 percent, and in many cases less than 0.1 percent. Therefore, it is not necessary for clinicians to avoid the usage of these otherwise valuable mood stabilizers.

Prolactin elevation

Prolactin, a hormone secreted from the anterior pituitary gland, is, as its name suggests, responsible for breast milk production, and also stimulates breast epithelial cell proliferation. It does have a number of other functions as well, related to menstruation, sexual functioning, and fertility. Several antipsychotic medications, specifically all traditional antipsychotics and risperidone, have been known to increase prolactin secretion, presumably through a mechanism of dopamine receptor blockade and dopamine D_2 receptor occupancy. Except for risperidone, the other five atypical antipsychotics – olanzapine, clozapine, quetiapine, aripiprazole, and ziprasidone – have no detectable prolactin elevation, or a minimal transient elevation lasting no more than a few hours.[46]

Studies suggest that when typical antipsychotics and risperidone are given to a patient there is an immediate and pronounced increase in prolactin level within 15–30 minutes, and in general women have a greater elevation than men.[47–50] When stopped, prolactin levels show a rapid decline, reaching normal levels within 3 days of stopping the offending medication.

The amount of prolactin secretion caused by the administration of these antipsychotics is significantly less than the amount of prolactin released through primary hyperprolactinemia or prolactin-secreting tumors. In general, the side effects due to the elevated prolactin levels from antipsychotics are also much less intense and less severe than in these medical conditions. In primary hyper-prolactinemia there are more severe manifestations of hypogonadism, leading to decreased serum testosterone levels and estrogen deficiency in women. These symptoms and the sequelae of these lowered gonadal functions have only been shown in other causes of elevated prolactin level, and have not been shown in medication-induced hyperprolactinemia.

The clinical side effects listed below in Table 16.14 are presumably caused by elevated prolactin levels, although the exact chemical connection has not been proven by research.

When any of the side effects mentioned in Table 16.14 present in a patient taking a traditional antipsychotic or risperidone, elevated prolactin should be considered a possible cause. The patient should be screened with a random, non-fasting serum prolactin level, and if evaluated, the following measures of treatment considered:

1 If it is time to stop the antipsychotic medication and clinically indicated, do so.
2 Reduce the dose of the offending medication to the lowest possible effective dose.
3 Switch the patient to a non-offending psychotropic including clozapine, olanzapine, quetiapine, aripiprazole, or ziprasidone.
4 If the offending medication cannot be stopped or switching medication has failed:[51]
   ■ If the prolactin level is high-normal or mildly elevated (< 50 mg/ml), watch and wait. Recheck the prolactin level in 3 months and periodically thereafter, as long as the offending medication is continued.

Table 16.14 Clinical effects of elevated prolactin

■ Menstrual irregularity, infrequent or lack of menstrual periods
■ Sexual side effects, including decreased libido, impaired arousal and erectile function, and possible ejaculatory and orgasmic dysfunction
■ Infertility
■ Gynecomastia (breast enlargement)
■ Galactorrhea (leaking of breast milk and breast tenderness)
■ Weight gain

*Adapted from Compton MT and Miller AH. Antipsychotic-induced hyperprolactinemia and sexual dysfunction. *Psychoparmacol Bull* 2002;36(1):153.

■ If the prolactin level is > 50 mg/ml, consider an endocrinological consultation and/or CT or MRI of the head (cone-down sella turcica).

■ If symptoms in Table 16.14 persist and treatment is necessary, treat with
bromocriptine 5–12.5 mg/day.

Whenever a switch of medications is made or treatment for the hyperprolactinemia is instituted, women patients should be educated about the possible increase in
fertility potential. Patients who have been infertile and perhaps become lax in using
contraception while on the offending medication may find themselves more fertile,
and pregnancy becomes an increased possibility when the medication is stopped.

Hypotension

Patients taking MAO inhibitors, TCAs, and traditional and some atypical
antipsychotics may show lowered systolic and diastolic blood pressure with consequent dizziness and lightheadedness. If the amount of lowering is not dramatic,
and does not lead to near-fainting or passing out, several remedies may be helpful
to allow the patient to live with the mild symptoms. Lightheadedness that only
occurs when getting up quickly from a seated or lying position occurs because of
blood pooling in the distensible veins of the legs. Before getting up, have the
patient clench the calf and thigh muscles to compress leg veins and then arise
slowly. If the dizziness is non-positional and occurs walking or standing, the
patient can also be instructed to wear support hosiery to compress leg veins continuously. In more severe cases, and when the offending drug cannot be changed,
the patient can be instructed to use a stimulant. A small dose of methylphenidate
or other stimulant several times a day will often boost blood pressure sufficiently
so that lightheadedness is a minimal problem.

References

1 Silverstein FS *et al*. Hematological monitoring during therapy with carbamazepine in children [letter]. *Ann Neurology* 1983;13:685–686.

2 Miller CH *et al*. The prevalence and severity of acute extrapyramidal side effects
in patients treated with clozapine, risperidone or conventional antipsychotics. In:
*New Research Program and Abstracts of the 149th Annual Meeting of the Amer-
ican Psychiatric Association, May 8 1996, New York*. Abstract NR542:217–218.

3 Rosebrush PI and Mazurek MF. Neurologic side effects in neuroleptic-naïve
patients treated with haloperidol or risperidone. *Neurology* 1999;52:782–785.

4 Kapur S *et al*. Clinical and theoretical implications of 5-HT2 and D2 receptor
occupancy of clozapine, risperidone and olanzapine in schizophrenia. *Am J Psychiatry* 1999;156:286–293.

5 Fleuschacher WW *et al*. The pharmacologic treatment of neuroleptic induced
akathisia. *J Clin Psychopharm* 1990;10:12–21.

6 Seagraves R. Antidepressant-induced sexual dysfunction. *J Clin Psychiatry*
1998;59(suppl 4):48–54.

7 Bartlik B *et al*. Sexual dysfunction secondary to depressive disorders. *J Gender-
Spec Med* 1999;2(2):52–60.

8 MacLean F and Lee A. Drug induced sexual dysfunction and infertility. *Pharmaceutical J* 1999;262(7047):780–784.

9 Clayton A. Roster presentation, presented at the American Psychiatric Association, May 2001. Summary available on the Internet at www.pslgroup.com/dg/fa56e.htm

10 Nurnberg HG *et al.* Sildenafil citrate in extension of a double-blind placebo controlled study for serotonergic reuptake inhibitor-induced sexual dysfunction: open-label results. Presented at the American Psychiatric Association Conference, 2001.

11 Ashton AK and Rosen RC. Bupropion as an antidote for serotonin reuptake inhibitor-induced sexual dysfunction. *J Clin Psychiatry* 1998;59:112–115.

12 Labbate LA *et al.* Bupropion treatment of serotonin reuptake antidepressant-associated sexual dysfunction. *Ann Clin Psychiatry* 1997;9:241–245.

13 Aquila R. Management of weight gain in patients with schizophrenia. *J Clin Psychiatry* 2002;63(suppl 4):33–36.

14 Coodin S. Body Mass Index in persons with schizophrenia. *Can J Psychiatry* 2001;46:549–555.

15 McElroy S *et al.* Correlates of overweight and obesity in 644 patients with bipolar disorder. *J Clin Psychiatry* 2002;63(3):207–213.

16 Weissenburger J *et al.* Weight changes in depression. *Psychiatry Res* 1986;17:275–283.

17 Pine DS *et al.* The association between childhood depression and adulthood body mass index. *Pediatrics* 2001;107:1049–1056.

18 Elmslie JL *et al.* Prevalence of overweight and obesity in bipolar patients. *J Clin Psychiatry* 2000;61:179–184.

19 Elmslie JL *et al.* Determinants of overweight and obesity in patients with bipolar disorder. *J Clin Psychiatry* 2001;62:486–491.

20 Allison DB *et al.* The distribution of body mass index among individuals with and without schizophrenia. *J Clin Psychiatry* 1999;60:215–220.

21 Kinon BJ *et al.* Long term olanzapine treatment: weight changes and weight-related health factors in schizophrenia. *J Clin Psychiatry*. 2001;69:92–100.

22 Casey DE and Zorn SH. The pharmacology of weight gain with antipsychotics. *J Clin Psychiatry* 2001;1:65(suppl. 7):4–10.

23 Litrell KH *et al.* Educational Interventions for the Management of Antipsychotic-Related Weight Gain. The Promedica Research Center, Tucker, Georgia, 2002.

24 O'Keefe C *et al.* Reversal of weight gain associated with antipsychotic treatment. Presented at the American Psychiatric Association Annual Meeting, May 2001, New Orleans.

25 Ball PM *et al.* A program for treating olanzapine-related weight gain, *Psychiatric Serv* 2001;52:967–969.

26 Maren M. Evaluating weight loss programs. Presented at National Conference of Nurse Practitioners, Baltimore, MD, November 2001.

27 Dursun SM and Devarajan S. Clozapine weight gain plus topirimate weight loss. *Can J Psychiatry* [letter] 2000;40:198.

28 Privitera MD Topirimate: a new antiepileptic drug. *Ann Pharmacother* 1997;31:1164–1173.

29 Hussain MA *et al.* Topirimate as an anti-obesity agent. In: *New Research Abstracts of the 153rd Annual Meeting of the American Psychiatric Association, May 18 2000, Chicago.* Abstract NR709:249.

30 Gadde KM *et al.* Zonisanude in obesity: a 16-week randomized trial. Presented at the American Psychiatric Association Meeting, Philadelphia, May 2002.

31 Correa N *et al.* Amantadine in the treatment of neuroendocrine side effects of neuroleptics. *J Clin Psychopharmacol* 1987;7:91–95.

32 Floris M *et al.* Effect of amantadine on weight gain during olanzapine treatment. *Eur Neuropsychopharmacol* 2001;11:181–182.

33 Breier A *et al.* Nizatidine for the prevention of weight gain during olanzapine treatment in schizophrenia and related disorders: a randomized controlled double blind study. Presented at the Meeting of the Colleges of Psychiatric and Neurologic Pharmacists; 23–26 March 2001, San Antonio.

34 Morrison JA *et al.* Metformin for weight loss in pediatric patients taking psychotropic drugs. *Am J Psychiatry* 2002;159(4):655–657.

35 Centers for Disease Control and Prevention. Adverse effects with ephedra containing products. December 1993–September 1995. *Morb Mortal Wkly Rep* 1996;45:689–692.

36 Sussman N and Ginsberg D. Weight gain associated with SSRIs. *Primary Psychiatry* 1998;Jan:28–37. Available at www.mvelectric.com/ssri

37 Saper JR *et al. The Handbook of Headache Management.* Williams and Wilkins, 1993, pp. 104–109.

38 Warnock JK. Psychotropic medications and drug-related alopecia. *Psychosomatics* 1991;32:149–152.

39 Azrin N *et al.* Drug causes of hair loss. *Drug Ther Bull* 1978;16:77–79.

40 Blankenship ML. Drugs and alopecia. *Aust J Dermatol* 1983;24:100–104.

41 Maguire HC. Drug-induced alopecia. *Am Fam Physician* 1979;19:178–179.

42 Gautam M. Alopecia due to psychotropic medication. *Ann Pharmacother.* 1999; 33:631–636.

43 Brodin M. Drug related alopecia. *Dermatol Clin* 1987;5:571–579.

44 Barth J and Dawber R. Drug induced hair loss [letter]. *BMJ* 1989;298:675.

45 Potter WZ and Ketter TA. Pharmacological issues in the treatment of bipolar disorder: focus on mood stabilizing compounds. *Can J Psychiatry* 1993;38(suppl. 2):S51–S56.

46 Compton MT and Miller AH. Antipsychotic-induced hyperprolactinemia and sexual dysfunction. *Psychopharmacol Bull* 2002;36(1):143–164.

47 Meltzer HY and Fang VS. The effect of neuroleptics on serum prolactin in schizophrenic patients. *Arch Gen Psychiatry* 1976;33:279–286.

48 Yasui N *et al.* Prolactin response to bromperidol treatment in schizophrenic patients. *Pharmacol Toxicol* 1998;82:153–156.

49 Kuruvilla A *et al.* A study of serum prolactin levels in schizophrenia: comparison of males and females. *Clin Exp Pharmacol Physiol* 1992;19:603–606.

50 Grunder G *et al.* Neuroendocrine response in antipsychotics: effects of drug type and gender. *Biol Psychiatry* 1999;45:89–97.

51 Family Practice Notebook, at www.fpnotebook.com/end145.htm

Chapter 17

Danger zones – areas of risk with psychotropics

Statistically, and in day-to-day clinical practice, most psychotropic medication side effects are uncomfortable and bothersome but do not present areas of serious risk to health and safety. As with all medications, however, there are some psychotropic medication interactions and certain clinical situations that present serious risk of morbidity or, rarely, mortality. This chapter will focus on these areas of more significant risk, their symptoms, prevention, and treatment.

The areas covered in this chapter include:

- P-450 interactions
- Serotonin syndrome
- Anticholinergic intoxication
- Lithium toxicity
- QTc interval issues
- Extrapyramidal symptoms and other movement disorders
- Neuroleptic malignant syndrome

! Tardive dyskinesia (TD)

! Monoamine oxidase inhibitor (MAOI) interactions

! Other interactions, including blood dyscrasias, hepatoxicity, and seizures.

Other than issues of P-450 interactions which are better understood in a different format, each condition will be further divided to address:

■ The syndrome and its cause
■ Signs and symptoms
■ Clinical situations of increased risk
■ Prognosis
■ Prevention
■ Treatment.

P-450 issues made easy

Virtually unknown to most mental health practitioners 10 years ago, P-450 enzyme interaction issues are now well known and are a potentially important clinical consideration when clinicians prescribe psychotropics, particularly antidepressants. Although P-450 interactions are not limited to antidepressants, the majority of such interactions that concern mental health prescribers involve this group of medications. Broadly, *P-450 interactions are those interactions that affect a drug's pharmacokinetics – that is, a drug's absorption, distribution, metabolism, or elimination.*

The P-450 enzyme system is a cytochrome enzyme system located primarily in the liver, but also present in the small intestine, lungs, and kidneys. The system got its name – cytochrome P-450 (CYP450) – because this enzyme makes a 'peak' at 450 nm when analyzed by spectrophotometry. The names used to identify each individual enzyme within the system include several numbers and letters. Some books will preface the numbers and letters with the abbreviation CYP, meaning cytochrome P-450 system. The first number indicates the family of the enzyme, the letter indicates the subfamily within that family, and the second number indicates the specific enzyme within that family. Therefore, CYP1A2 indicates the cytochrome P-450 enzyme of the first family, the A subfamily and the second enzyme in the A subfamily.

The P-450 enzyme system is involved in the breakdown and metabolism (through hydroxylation) of medications. At present over 34 such enzymes have been identified, although only a small number of them are important to the mental health prescribing clinician. Metabolism of many psychotropics occurs by hydroxylation, which becomes the 'rate limiting step' of medication breakdown; that is, when speed of hydroxylation is affected, the entire process of breakdown and excretion may either be accelerated or slowed. When the effectiveness of a P-450 enzyme is either inhibited or induced (see below), it affects the speed of metabolism of any medication broken down by that enzyme. This can lead to significant changes in the serum blood concentration of that specific medication in the body.

The author suggests that the most effective way to learn about and clinically manage P-450 enzyme interactions is to understand certain key definitions, understand the principles of enzyme interaction, and be familiar with some of the more common interactions in mental health prescription. Beyond this basic understanding, it is best to use a chart that documents known P-450 interactions, since memorizing the list is virtually impossible.

Important definitions

A *substrate* is the site where an enzyme works, i.e. a medication that will be acted upon or broken down by an enzyme.

An enzyme is *inhibited* if its activity is blocked or slowed, resulting in a *raised* blood level of any substrate medication that is metabolized by that enzyme. Enzyme *inhibition* occurs when two or more drugs compete for the same enzyme. It can be reversible or irreversible. Usually it begins after the first dose of the inhibitor; its maximum effect is reached at steady state (usually within four to seven half-lives).

An enzyme is *induced* if more of the enzyme is produced or its activity is increased, which results in a *lowered* blood level of any substrate medication that is metabolized by this enzyme. Enzyme *induction* usually occurs because of increased synthesis of an enzyme when exposed to particular drugs or substances. This usually begins within 2 days, but takes more than a week to reach its maximum effect.

The conveyor belt analogy

A useful analogy to the understanding of the pharmacokinetic interactions associated with the P-450 enzyme is that of a conveyor belt used by workers to remove boxes of product from a factory. In this analogy, the boxes of product are medications to be metabolized and excreted from the body (moved outside the factory). P-450 enzymes are the workers that package the product into boxes and place the boxes on the conveyor belt for exit from the factory. Once outside the factory, the boxes (medications) have been excreted. On a normal workday (when the patient is taking a steady dose of a psychotropic medication), there is a regular inventory of boxes put on the assembly line by the workers (enzymes) at a predictable rate that leads to a steady removal (metabolism and excretion). The workers (enzymes) work at a fixed speed, leading to excretion at a predictable rate. When a worker is inhibited (for example, if a ball and chain is put on his leg), he is unable to do his job as rapidly. Less product is packaged and placed on the conveyor belt, and therefore the inventory of boxes inside the factory grows and may become abnormally high. At times this excess inventory may become so large as to cause problems inside the factory (drug accumulation side effects or toxicity).

When a worker (enzyme) is induced (for example, by offering him higher pay), he works faster and more efficiently. More product is packaged and placed on the conveyor belt for exit (excretion). Inventory of product in the factory becomes low (substrate medication levels drop). Because of this low inventory in the factory (low blood levels of medication), the medication may become clinically less effective or stop working.

Common P-450 facts and principles

The following statements are some of the more prominent issues relevant to psychiatric prescription, taken from a long list of possible P-450 issues and interactions.

■ Two enzymes, 3A3/4 and 2D6, account for 50 percent and 30 percent respectively of all P-450 phase 1 metabolism. All other enzymes combined account for the remaining 20 percent. Of the remaining 30+ enzymes, only 1A2, 2C9 and 2C19 have clinically relevant interactions for the mental health prescriber.

■ The most common significant inhibitors of P-450 enzymes are antidepressants – fluoxetine, paroxetine, and bupropion (which inhibit 2D6), and nefazodone and fluvoxamine (both of which inhibit 1A2 and 3A3/3A4). Several newer antidepressants have minimal or no documented P-450 interactions. These include mirtazapine and venlafaxine.

■ Grapefruit juice blocks enzyme 1A2. *No medication should be taken with grapefruit juice.* This includes all forms of grapefruit and grapefruit juice – fresh, canned, or frozen. All other juices are safe and do not result in significant P-450 interactions.

■ Of the population, 10–20 percent have no 2D6 enzyme (7–10 percent of Caucasians and up to 15 percent of Asians). Because they have no 2D6, these persons may have an initial serum blood concentration of any medication metabolized by 2D6 (including all SSRIs and tricyclics) that is significantly higher than usual on a small oral dose. This is one of the explanations for a person who gets exaggerated side effects and/or clinical effects to what is otherwise a small dose of medication. Although no commercial test for this absent enzyme currently exists, a finger-stick test is in development.

■ Several minor inhibitors of a particular enzyme may result in a clinically significant reaction when taken simultaneously, even if any one inhibitor does not significantly block metabolism.

■ The most common psychotropic to cause enzyme induction is carbamazepine.

■ The metabolism of estrogen and oral contraceptives is accomplished primarily via 3A4. Potent inducers of 3A4 (such as carbamazepine and lamotrigine) may accelerate the metabolism of estrogen and diminish the effectiveness of hormone replacement therapy or oral contraceptives.

■ Cigarette smoking and eating charbroiled meats induces enzyme 1A2, and may therefore decrease blood levels of all psychotropics metabolized by 1A2 (such as clozapine, fluvoxamine, haloperidol, imipramine, olanzapine and theophylline).

■ Medication with a narrow therapeutic index (a small difference between therapeutic serum levels and toxic serum levels) may result in clinically significant problems from P-450 interactions. Common drugs with a narrow therapeutic index include tricyclic antidepressants, cardiac anti-arrhythmics, and prescription pain medications.

Using blood levels to assist with P-450 interactions

If a substrate medication subject to a P-450 interaction is measurable through serum blood level monitoring (for example, TCAs, carbamazepine and clozapine), use of blood levels is helpful in readjusting the dose of these medications. A clinical example will illustrate. If paroxetine (a known inhibitor of 2D6) is added to a stable regimen of imipramine (a TCA metabolized by 2D6), the clinician can expect inhibition of the enzyme and decreased metabolism of the imipramine – leading to higher blood levels of imipramine. To prescribe safely in this situation and avoid toxicity, the clinician should obtain a blood level of imipramine before the paroxetine is started, then add paroxetine and prescribe only half of the current imipramine dose. The imipramine serum level should be rechecked in 4–7 days. Based on the result, the imipramine dose may be increased (or decreased), checking the blood level with each adjustment until a therapeutic imipramine level is achieved.

If the combination is started in reverse order (i.e. the imipramine added to a stable paroxetine dose), the imipramine should be started at half the usual starting dose, the serum blood level checked (expecting it to be higher than usual for this dose), and the imipramine dosage readjusted to reach a therapeutic level based on the serum blood level results. Several adjustments and serum level rechecks may be necessary.

Use of a chart

In the 2002 *PDR*, over 3200 prescription drugs are listed. This results in a potential 2.8×10^{15} combinations of medications. With each new drug approved, another 4.4 trillion possible multiple drug combinations become available.[1] While many of these interactions are clinically insignificant, it is clear that attempting to learn all of them is impossible.

Since it is not possible to memorize all P-450 enzyme interactions, and new interactions are being discovered almost monthly, beyond the common interactions noted in this section the clinician should utilize a chart that is current and keep a copy of this chart on hand in the office for consultation during medication prescription. A particularly helpful website that is actively updated and contains a number of possible P-450 interactions is maintained by Dr David Flockhart at the University of Indiana. The website address is http://medicine.iupui.edu/flockhart/. An example of a list of clinically relevant P-450 interactions, available at this website, is shown in Table 17.1. A more detailed list, including less common interactions, is also available for download at that site.

Further detailed information on P-450 interactions can be seen in review articles.[2,3]

Table 17.1 Drugs metabolized by known P-450s*

1A2	2B6	2C19	2C9	2D6	3A
Clozapine	Bupropion	Amitriptyline	Celecoxib	Amitriptyline	Alprazolam
Cyclobenzapine	Cyclophosphamide	Citalopram	Diclofenac	Carvedilol	Buspirone
Fluvoxamine	Ifosfamide	Diazepam	Flurbiprofen	Clomipramine	Calcium channel blockers
Haloperidol		Imipramine	Ibuprofen	Codeine	Carbamazepine
Imipramine		Lansoprazole	Losartan	Desipramine	Cyclosporine
Mexiletine		Nelfinavir	Naproxen	Dextromethorphan	Efavirenz
Olanzapine		Omeprazole	Phenytoin	Fluoxetine	Haloperidol
Tacrine		Phenytoin	Piroxicam	Metoprolol	HIV protease inhibitors
Theophylline		Pantoprazole	Torsemide	Nortriptyline	Statins
Zileuton			Tolbutamide	Oudaasetrun	(not pravastatin)
Zolmitriptan			Warfarin	Oxycodone	Midazolam
				Paroxetine	Nevirapine
				Propafenone	Tacrolimus
				Risperidone	Triazolam
				Timolol	Zolpidem

Inhibitors

1A2	2B6	2C19	2C9	2D6	3A
Cimetidine	Thiotepa	Cimetidine	Amiodarone	Amiodarone	Andodarone
Ciprofloxacin		Felbamate	Fluconazole	Chlorpheniramine	Dilliazem and verapamil
Fluvoxamine		Fluoxetine	Fluoxetine	Fluoxetine	Grapefruit juice
Levofloxaein		Fluvoxamine	Fluvostatin	Haloperidol	HIV protease inhibitors
		Isoniazid	Metronidazole	Indinavir	Hraconazole
		Ketoconazole	Paroxetine	Paroxetine	Ketoconazole
		Lansoprazole	Zafirlukast	Ritonavir	Macrolide antibiotics
		Omeprazole		Terbinatine	(not azithroycin)
		Ticlopidine		Ticlopidine	Nefazodone

Table 17.1 (Continued)

Inducers				
Carbamazepine	Phenobarbital	Carbamazepine	Phenobarbital	Carbamazepine
Chargrilled meat	Phenytom	Rifampin	Rifampin	Efavirenz and nevirapine
Rifampin	Rifampin			Rifabutin and rifampin
Tobacco				Ritomavir
				St. John's Wort
		Absent in 15–30% of Asians	Absent in 7% of Caucasians	

* From: Flockhart DA. Drugs metabolized by known P-450s. Available at *http://medicine.iupui.edu/flockhart/*

Another way to slice the pie

Although P-450 interactions are best learned by understanding the definitions and principles and then using a chart, as outlined above, some clinicians may find it helpful to look at selected P-450 data and important interactions by particular medication class and specific medication. Therefore the next two sections are organized in that way, and are included to assist those who prefer this style.

Antidepressants

Much of the data on P-450 interactions has been obtained from the usage of anti-depressants. The P-450 effects are substantially different from class to class, and within each class.

SSRIs

Fluoxetine is an inhibitor of 2D6. Therefore, all 2D6 substrates may be elevated when fluoxetine is added. TCAs are in this group of substrates. The potential dra-matic increase in TCA blood levels (which has led to toxicity and potential death) by the addition of fluoxetine is one of the classic examples of P-450 interactions.

Paroxetine is also a potent inhibitor of 2D6, and would likewise affect blood levels of tricyclics and other 2D6 substrates.

Sertraline is a relatively weak inhibitor of 2D6 and 3A4. In moderate doses its effect on 2D6 substrates is minimal; however, at high doses it may have inhibitory effects and similarly affect blood levels of tricyclics and other 2D6 substrates.

Fluvoxamine is a potent inhibitor of 1A2 and 3A4. Therefore it will block the metabolism of clozapine, TCAs, theophylline, alprazolam and triazolam. When fluvoxamine is added to a steady regimen of any of these medications, substantial blood level increase of the substrate can be expected.

Citalopram is a relatively weak inhibitor of 2D6, and in general is thought not to affect tricyclic blood levels, although there is one reported case of elevated con-centrations of desipramine and clomipramine when citalopram was added. The exact mechanism of this interaction is unclear.

Other new generation antidepressants

Bupropion is a potent inhibitor of 2D6, and will elevate the blood levels of tri-cyclic antidepressants and other 2D6 substrates.

Nefazodone is a potent inhibitor of 3A4, and will increase the concentration of 3A4 substrates including triazolam, alprazolam, and protease inhibitors used in HIV therapy.

Mirtazepine has insignificant interactions, with specific cytochrome P-450 enzymes, and is thought not to cause meaningful interactions.

Venlafaxine has minimal interactions with 2D6, 3A4, or other cytochrome enzymes; however, it has been reported to increase plasma concentrations of haldol by up to 70 percent and desipramine up to four-fold by unknown mechanisms.[4]

Monoamine oxidase inhibitors (MAOIs), although they have another set of potential interactions that will be discussed later in this chapter, do not have known P-450 interactions.

Mood stabilizers

Lithium has many medication interactions that are summarized later in the chapter under lithium toxicity, but no specific P-450 interactions are known.

Carbamazepine is both a substrate of CYP 3A4 and an inducer of 3A4. These characteristics lead to the phenomenon of "auto-induction," where the concentration of carbamazepine is gradually diminished over time as the body's ability to metabolize it is increased by induction of more 3A4 enzyme. As a potent inducer of 3A4, carbamazepine can reduce the concentrations of alprazolam, triazolam, clonazepam, cyclosporine, lovastatin, protease inhibitors, verapamil, estrogen, and oral contraceptives. Carbamazepine also decreases the concentration of lamotrigine by up to 40 percent by a different mechanism.

Oxcarbazepine, which is structurally similar to carbamazepine, can also induce metabolism of estrogen and oral contraceptives, and decrease lamotrigine levels by other mechanisms.

Valproic acid has multiple potential drug interactions with other anticonvulsants, particularly lamotrigine; however, these are not thought to result from P-450 interactions. The addition of carbamazepine to valproic acid may decrease valproic acid concentrations.

Lamotrigine can have decreased concentration caused by the addition of carbamazepine, and increased concentration by the addition of valproic acid, but neither of these is related to P-450 interactions.

Topirimate has its concentration decreased by carbamazepine, but not by a P-450 interaction.

Gabapentin is not primarily metabolized through the liver, and has no significant P-450 interactions.

Stimulants

Methylphenidate has caused increased tricyclic levels suggestive that there may be a P-450 interaction; however, this has not been specifically documented. When stimulants are added to a steady tricyclic regimen, it is prudent to decrease the tricyclic dosage.

Anti-anxiety medication

Benzodiazepines, particularly alprazolam, triazolam and, to some degree, diazepam, can have their metabolism inhibited via the 3A4 system when nefazodone, fluvoxamine, or erythromycin is added – each of which is a potent 3A4 inhibitor. This may lead to increased sedation and side effects from these anti-anxiety medicines.

Buspirone may have its concentration increased by 3A4 inhibitors such as nefazodone or fluoxamine, grapefruit juice, or ketoconazole.

Antipsychotics

Haloperidol's metabolism has been studied for many years, but is still somewhat unclear. There is evidence that 2D6, 3A4 and 1A2 may all be involved to various degrees in its metabolism. Nefazodone and fluvoxamine (3A4 inhibitors) may raise the blood level of haloperidol. The addition of haloperidol to tricyclics may show mutual metabolic inhibition, necessitating a reduction in doses of both drugs.

Clozapine has shown interaction with 1A2, 3A4 and, to some degree, 2D6. Addition of 3A4 inhibitors, such as fluvoxamine and nefazodone, increases plasma concentrations of clozapine. 2D6 inhibitors, such as fluoxetine and paroxetine, have also increased concentrations of clozapine. Additionally, ery-thromycin, a potent 3A4 inhibitor, has raised clozapine doses.

Risperidone, although metabolized primarily via 2D6 and, to some degree, by 3A4, has not shown clinically significant interactions in a number of studies, and may have a relatively benign P-450 profile.

Olanzapine is principally metabolized via 1A2, although clinical interactions via the P-450 system have not currently been shown.

Quetiapine is primarily metabolized via 3A4. In theory, inducers of 3A4 could decrease its plasma concentration, although clinical reports have not been noted.

Ziprasidone, although metabolized primarily via a non-P-450 enzyme (alde-hyde oxidase) and to a limited degree by 3A4 and 1A2, has shown little inter-action with major P-450 enzymes.

Serotonin syndrome

The syndrome and its cause

Serotonin syndrome is a hyperserotonergic state caused by the addition of two or more medications that increase serotonin (5-hydroxytryptamine) concentrations in the brain. This leads to hyperstimulation at serotonin receptors of the brain-stem and spinal cord, particularly the 5HT1A sub-receptor.

Signs and symptoms of serotonin syndrome

Symptoms of serotonin syndrome fall under five symptom clusters:

1 Mental status changes
2 Motor abnormalities
3 Cardiovascular changes
4 Gastrointestinal symptoms and
5 Miscellaneous other symptoms.

Specific symptoms that could occur in the context of the recent addition of a strongly serotonergic medication or a precursor of serotonin synthesis (such as L-tryptophan) are listed in Table 17.2.

Table 17.2 Symptoms associated with serotonin syndrome

1	Mental status changes	■ Confusion
		■ Restlessness
		■ Coma
2	Motor abnormalities	■ Myoconus (recurrent muscle twitching or spasm)
		■ Hyperreflexia
		■ Muscle rigidity
		■ Restlessness
		■ Tremor
		■ Ataxia and incoordination
		■ Shivering
3	Cardiovascular changes	■ Sinus tachycardia
		■ Hypertension
4	Gastrointestinal problems	■ Nausea
5	Other symptoms	■ Diaphoresis
		■ Unreactive pupils
		■ Fever

Medical situations of risk

Although the majority of cases of serious serotonin syndrome have occurred when monoamine oxidase inhibitors are combined with SSRIs, L-tryptophan, lithium or other strongly serotonergic medications, there are a number of psychotropics and other medications that have also been implicated. These are listed in Table 17.3.

Serotonin syndrome and neuroleptic malignant syndrome (NMS – see below) share many symptoms/clinical features, and are thought to exist on a continuum of the same disorder. NMS, however, is an idiosyncratic drug reaction, whereas serotonin syndrome is an effect of drug toxicity. Patients with NMS have higher fevers and pronounced extrapyramidal signs with muscle rigidity. In general, patients with serotonin syndrome have lower fevers, gastrointestinal dysfunction, and myoclonus.

Prognosis

Mild to moderate cases of serotonin syndrome usually resolve within 24–72 hours.[5] Most cases can be treated, and are completely resolved within a week, although some patients can become acutely and severely ill. Hospitalization, admission to intensive care and mechanical ventilation may be necessary in such cases. Mortality associated with severe cases of this condition is estimated to be 11 percent.[6]

Table 17.3 Drugs that affect serotonin levels and have been implicated in serotonin syndrome*

Effect	Drug
Increase serotonin synthesis	L-tryptophan
Decrease serotonin metabolism	Isocarboxazid Phenelzine Selegiline Tranylcypromine
Increase serotonin release	Amphetamines Cocaine Reserpine
Inhibit serotonin uptake	Amitriptyline Amphetamines Clomipramine Cocaine Desipramine Detromethorphan Doxepin Fluoxetine Fluvoxamine Imipramine Meperidine Nefazodone Nortriptyline Protriptyline Paroxetine Sertraline Trazodone Venlafaxine
Direct serotonin receptor agonists	Buspirone Lysergic acid diethylamide (LSD) Sumatriptan
Non-specific increase in serotonin activity	Lithium
Dopamine agonists	Amantadine Bromocriptine Bupropion Levodopa Pergolide Pramipexole

*Adapted from Mills K. Seratonin syndrome. *Am Fam Physician* 1995;52:1475–1482.
Sternbach H. The serotonin syndrome. *Am J Psychiatry* 1991;148:705–713.

Prevention

The most important element of preventing serotonin syndrome is knowing which medications are strongly serotonergic, and avoiding combinations of multiple strongly serotonergic medications. If combinations of strongly serotonergic medications are clinically necessary, it is important to start with small doses and make any dosage increases gradually.

Serotonin syndrome can occur even after a patient has stopped a drug if its clinicial effect persists, or if a long-lasting metabolite remains in the body. This especially applies to MAOIs and fluoxetine. When stopping MAOIs, a 2-week "wash out" period should be maintained before beginning another strongly serotonergic medication. When stopping fluoxetine and beginning an MAOI, a 4–5-week "wash-out" period should be allowed before beginning the MAOI, since a long-lasting metabolite (norfluoxetine) may still be present for that period of time.

Treatment

For most mental health practitioners, the most important elements of treatment are *recognition* of the syndrome and *discontinuation of one or more of the suspected serotonergic agents*, including any over-the-counter medications (e.g. dextromethoraphan, pseudoephedrine, or phenylpropanolamine). However if the patient is severely ill, referral for hospitalization is appropriate. While in intensive care, supportive measures including a cold blanket to reduce hyperthermia, antihypertensive medications for elevated blood pressure, and mechanical ventilation may be used. Pharmacological countermeasures include short-acting benzodiazepines or dantrolene for myoclonus and resulting hyperthermia, Cyproheptadine, propranolol or methysergide can be used if the symptoms persist.[7,8]

Anticholinergic intoxication

The syndrome and its cause

Anticholinergic intoxication (alternately referred to as anticholinergic psychosis, "toxic delirium," anticholinergic syndrome or "atropine psychosis") is an acute delirium caused by the ingestion of excessive amounts of medications with strong anticholinergic properties. There are over 600 different legal and illegal plants, various chemicals, and psychotropic medications that can have anticholinergic properties.[9-11] Ingestion may occur from iatrogenic polypharmacy, when the clinician prescribes multiple medications with highly anticholinergic properties (e.g. a traditional antipsychotic plus an anticholinergic agent for EPS and an antihistamine for cold symptoms).

The patient may precipitate anticholinergic intoxication through intentional or accidental overdose of anticholinergic agents. Anticholinergic drugs have been overused for recreational purposes and to potentiate the effects of other psychoactive substances (most notably heroin). Acute overdose is likely to occur more frequently in populations that abuse anticholinergic medication. The syndrome can also result from chronic overusage of anticholinergic medications for purposes of abuse.[12] Some schizophrenic patients have been observed to overutilize anticholinergic drugs in preference to an antipsychotic because of what they perceive as stimulant or euphorigenic properties of anticholinergics, using them orally, intravenously, or by smoking the drug.

Signs and symptoms

After ingestion of moderate amounts of medications or substances with strong anticholinergic properties, a patient will, within 20 minutes to 3 hours, develop the following signs:[13–16]

1 Agitation or euphoria
2 Mental confusion or obtundation
3 Paresthesias of fingers and toes
4 Motor incoordination
5 Mild drowsiness.

In cases of more severe intoxication, the patient will show:

■ Hot dry skin or hyperthermia
■ Urinary retention
■ Aggressive, paranoid or delirious behavior
■ Visual and or auditory hallucinations
■ Muscle spasms
■ Progressive central nervous system depression, tachycardia
■ Blurred vision
■ Dried mucosal services.

Gastrointestinal disturbances, including abdominal pain, nausea, vomiting, and constipation, occur occasionally and may vary in severity, but at times may be acute. Elderly patients with cerebrovascular disease are particularly prone to develop anticholinergic confusional states, even when taking therapeutic doses of medications with anticholinergic properties.

The signs and symptoms of anticholinergic intoxication have been incorporated into a mnemonic that has many variations when taught in different geographic locales. One of the more common versions describes the patient with anticholinergic intoxication as "Mad as a Hatter, blind as a bat, red as a beet, and hot as a pistol."

Clinical situations of risk

Situations particularly likely to lead to anticholinergic intoxication include:

1 Simultaneous prescription of strongly anticholinergic medications from various classes. This can include any of the medications shown in Table 17.4.

Table 17.4 Medications that have strongly anticholinergic properties

- TCAs
- Traditional antipsychotics
- Antihistamines
- Cycloplegics (medications that temporarily paralyze the ciliary muscle of the eye for dilation)
- Antispasmodics
- Antiparkinsonian medications
- Belladonna alkaloids
- Some H_2 blockers (for example, cimetidine or ranitidine) have also produced a syndrome indistinguishable from anticholinergic intoxication, particularly in high doses

2 Schizophrenic patients who abuse anticholinergic medications on a short-term or long-term basis.
3 Persons who ingest significant amounts of plants with anticholinergic activity, such as: Datura (Jimson weed, angel's trumpet), Atropa belladonna (deadly nightshade), Hyoscyamus niger (henbane), and Mandrogana officiarum (mandrake).

A useful chart, reproduced as Table 17.5, shows the approximate anticholinergic equivalent of various medications to trihexyphenidyl. For example, 75 mg of imipramine has the same anticholinergic effect as 10 mg of amitriptyline and 1 mg of Cogentin, 50 mg of Benadryl and 2.5 mg of trihephenidyl. Using the chart can give the clinician an approximation of the "anticholinergic load" occurring with the prescription of various medications.

Prevention

Prevention of this anticholinergic intoxication involves knowledge of which medications are strongly anticholinergic, and, whenever possible, avoiding their combination. Clinicians treating patients in a geriatric setting must be particularly alert to the sensitivity of this group to anticholinergic side effects. Likewise, clinicians who treat chronically psychotic and schizophrenic individuals need to be aware of anticholinergic intoxication when using multiple neuroleptics and/or anticholinergic medications for side effects. This patient group is also at high risk for abuse of anticholinergics. In vulnerable populations, consider using atypical antipsychotics that have less anticholinergic activity. When using anticholinergics or antihistamines for side effects, discontinue them whenever possible to observe whether they are still necessary. If an antidepressant is needed in someone already on a strong mix of anticholinergic medications, consider an SSRI or other new generation antidepressant rather than a TCA.

Table 17.5 Anticholinergic effect of commonly prescribed psychotropic drugs compared with trihexyphenidyl*

Drug	Equivalent (in mg)	Typical use
Atropine	0.5	Given before surgery
Benztropine (Cogentin)	1.0	Antiparkinsonism
Trihexyphenidyl (Artane)	2.5	Antiparkinsonism
Biperiden (Akineton)	1.0	Antiparkinsonism
Amitriptyline (Elavil)	10	Antidepressant
Doxepin (Sinequan)	30	Antidepressant
Nortriptyline (Pamelor)	60	Antidepressant
Imipramine (Tofranil)	75	Antidepressant
Desipramine (Norpramin)	150	Antidepressant
Amoxapine (Asendin)	600	Antidepressant
Clozapine (Clozaril)	15	Antipsychotic
Thioridazine (Mellaril)	50	Antipsychotic
Chlorpromazine (Thorazine)	370	Antipsychotic
Diphenhydramine (Benadryl)	50	Antihistamine

*From Keltner NL and Folks DG. *Psychotropic Drugs*, 3rd edn. Mosby, 2001, p. 436.

Prognosis

Mild anticholinergic intoxication can usually be managed by stopping the offending agents. In most cases, the condition will resolve on its own without pharmacological management. Even if the patient has developed significant sensory changes or psychosis, these conditions will usually clear within 36–48 hours of stopping the causative agents.

Treatment

The first and most important element of treatment is to *recognize the source of anticholinergic load* (medications or plants) *and stop the offending agents.* Patients experiencing an acute psychotic episode or other strong symptomatology after a significant overdose of anticholinergic drugs may require constant supervision for several days to prevent accidental injury or aspiration of vomitus, and to control hyperthermia (particularly in children).

Physostigmine, a cholinesterase inhibitor, has both central and peripheral *cholinergic* actions, and can be used specifically to counteract the *anticholinergic* symptoms.[15,17] Generally, the patient is given a slow 2 mg test dose intravenously over 2 minutes. Because physostigmine has a short duration of action, the patient's symptoms may recur and repeated doses may be necessary every 30–60 minutes.

If the cause of intoxication is overdose, management also includes the usual modes of treatment, such as gastric lavage, cathartics, and activated charcoal. When medication is necessary for control of agitation or delirium because of the overdose, traditional phenothiazine antipsychotics should be avoided as they increase anticholinergic load. A benzodiazepine, orally or by injection, may be helpful for behavioral control, and is less cholinergic.

Lithium toxicity

The syndrome and its causes

Lithium is commonly used for a variety of psychiatric and medical conditions, including:[18]

- Acute and prophylactic treatment of bipolar affective disorder
- As an augmentation agent with antidepressants for depression
- To treat rage reactions
- As a prophylactic agent for chronic cluster headache
- As a therapeutic agent to treat thyrotoxicosis.

Lithium toxicity (also referred to as lithium intoxication or lithium poisoning) is one of the more common of the potentially serious psychotropic side effects. Lithium toxicity occurs with some frequency because lithium has a narrow therapeutic index (a small difference between safe levels and toxic levels) and a number of common interactions that cause increased blood levels of lithium.

Lithium is 95 percent excreted in the urine, 4 percent in the sweat and 1 percent in feces. Eighty percent of the lithium filtered in the kidney is reabsorbed in the proximal tubules and is not reabsorbed in the distal tubules. By antagonizing the effects of antidiuretic hormone, the patient's urine output may increase, leading to dehydration. To compensate for this, proximal tubular reabsorption of water increases, along with increased reabsorption of lithium and consequent further toxicity.[18] Therefore, once started, lithium intoxication may begin a vicious cycle of increasing toxicity.

Signs and symptoms

Early signs of lithium toxicity include:[19]

1   Vomiting
2   Diarrhea
3   Coarse tremor
4   Sluggishness or sleepiness
5   Vertigo
6   Poor coordination
7   Dysarthria with slurred and indistinct speech.

Untreated or ignored, further elevation of lithium levels leads to:

- Muscle twitching and hypertonia
- Confused sensorium or coma

- Asymmetrical deep tendon reflexes
- Seizures
- A grayish hue to the skin.

Medical situations of risk

A variety of medical situations/causes may lead to lithium toxicity, including:

1 A single large overdose of lithium with suicidal intent
2 An accidental overdose (often by a manic patient with a wish to "improve quickly")
3 A decrease in renal lithium clearance without a corresponding reduction in dose, which may occur in the presence of:
   - Kidney disease
   - Sodium deficiency
   - Water deprivation
   - Medication interactions leading to elevated lithium levels.

Common clinical circumstances that lead to the above problems for a patient on lithium include:

- The initiation of a low-salt/no-salt diet
- A weight-reduction diet (without the addition of extra salt) and reduced fluid intake
- Use of diuretics
- Fever and excessive sweating
- Vomiting and diarrhea from gastrointestinal illnesses
- Prescription of inappropriately high oral doses of lithium
- Failure to regularly follow serum blood levels of lithium
- Use of concomitant non-steroidal anti-inflammatory agents (20 percent of patients using non-steroidals when on lithium will have increased lithium levels; 80 percent will have no change in levels).

Most lithium toxicity occurs at serum levels of > 2 meq per liter; however, it is possible that patients will have some symptoms of toxicity at lower levels. Some patients will have symptoms of mild lithium intoxication even at technically "therapeutic" levels (below 1.5 meq per liter). It has been estimated that serious toxicity occurs at levels between 2.5 and 3.5 meq per liter, and that life-threatening toxicity occurs at serum levels > 3.5 meq per liter. This latter level can result from an acute overdose of as few as twenty 300-mg pills.[20]

Prognosis

Patients with mild lithium toxicity will generally completely recover without after-effects.[20] Patients with moderately severe or life-threatening lithium toxicity, however, can have residual neurological signs, including ataxia, broad-based gait, lack of coordination, tremors, and nystagmus. Also reported with extensive lithium toxicity are cognitive damage, poor short-term memory, and dementia. If the signs continue for 6 months or longer, they are generally permanent.[21] In general, the seriousness of the syndrome as well as the likelihood of residual symptoms occurs in proportion to the elevation of blood level and the length of time the patient is exposed to the toxic dose.[22]

In the past, mortality rates in acute lithium overdosage have been estimated to be between 25 and 33 percent.[22,23] With better recognition and treatment, including the use of dialysis, this figure has been dramatically lowered to < 1 percent.[24]

Prevention

Keys to preventing lithium toxicity include patient education, clinician vigilance to potential situations of risk, and regular monitoring of serum blood levels.

All patients started on lithium should be thoroughly educated about the early signs and symptoms of lithium toxicity and possible medication interactions that could raise their serum lithium level. The signs of mild lithium intoxication can be often conceptualized for patients by telling them that the signs are similar to those that a person may experience from drinking too much alcohol and waking up hung over. These include:

- Nausea and vomiting
- Tremor
- Slurred speech or " thick tongue"
- Difficulty with walking or gait.

If patients notice any of these signs or symptoms, they must be instructed to withhold further lithium doses and contact the clinician at once. The clinician will order a serum lithium level and adjust the dosage downward.

The other elements of education include the identification of common medications or conditions that may increase lithium level, with particular focus on the concomitant use of diuretics or non-steroidal anti-inflammatory agents, gastrointestinal illnesses leading to diarrhea or vomiting, and the initiation of a low salt diet.

Regular lithium levels should be followed in all patients, but particularly in patients at risk, including geriatric patients, medically fragile patients, or patients with a complicated medication regimen. For long-term patients on a stable lithium regimen and who have had consistent lithium levels, these levels can be monitored every 3–6 months. More frequent levels should be monitored in patients at higher risk for toxicity, such as those who have a fluctuating salt and fluid balance, those who are prone to be non-compliant with medication, geriatric patients, patients with neurological or cognitive illness, and patients prone to dehydration. If any of the early warning signs of lithium toxicity occur, the patient's lithium level should be checked immediately and, if elevated, the dosage lowered.

Treatment

Treatment should be individualized depending on the extent of toxicity. Regard-less of the level of intoxication, when signs of toxicity are seen or suspected, *all lithium treatment should be temporarily stopped* until a blood level result is reported and the clinical signs are beginning to wane.

In the event of acute overdosage, gastric lavage or induced emesis should be used to remove unabsorbed lithium. Repeated lithium levels should be followed to insure that the serum level is diminishing. In severe overdose, hemodialysis is the treatment of choice.[25] It is highly effective in removing lithium from the body with the goal of reducing the level to < 1 meq per liter 6–8 hours after dialysis.[26]

In general, when the acute symptoms are minimal and the clinical situation dictates continued lithium therapy, the patient is gradually restarted on the lithium, leading to a target therapeutic dose within 24–72 hours. Usually the target dose is less than that which caused the toxicity, unless there were extenuat-ing circumstances (e.g. GI illness or dietary change) that will not reoccur.

QTc interval issues

Another example of a potential serious side effect that was virtually unknown to most practicing mental health practitioners 10 years ago, but is now of significant importance, is the QTc interval and its effect on heart rhythm. With current under-standing of the nature of this problem, we may now be able to explain some of the instances of sudden unexplained death from the use of psychotropics, particularly antipsychotic medications, in the past. Because of documented concerns regarding cardiac safety, certain psychiatric and non-psychiatric medications have been appropriately withdrawn from the market because of concerns about their ability to severely alter the QTc interval. It has also become a pharmaceutical company marketing message to identify a medication's propensity to lengthen QTc interval, as a reason for or against prescribing a particular medication.

The syndrome and its causes

As shown in Figure 17.1, cardiac rhythm begins with depolarization of the heart ventrical (the Q-wave) and ends with completion of repolarization (the T-wave). The time interval between the Q-wave and T-wave is the *QT interval*, measured in milliseconds. The QT interval varies with heart rate, and therefore has been "corrected" for changes in heart rate, thus leading to the term "QT interval cor-rected" or, more commonly "QTc interval." Normal QTc intervals run from 400 to 450 milliseconds.

A lengthened QTc interval can lead to an increased risk of ventricular arrhyth-mias, most notably *torsades de pointes* (literally meaning twisting of the points, from the appearance of the EKG of individuals with this serious and potentially fatally arrhythmia). *All known cases of* torsades de pointes *have been associated with QTc intervals of over 500 milliseconds.* QTc intervals of over 450 ms are considered to be of some concern since they are approaching the 500 ms barrier,

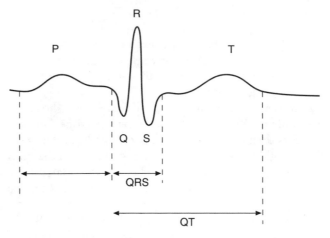

Figure 17.1 **QT interval**

but QTc intervals between 450 and 500 ms have no documented direct incidence of arrhythmias or *torsades de pointes*.

There are several factors that can cause changes in QTc intervals, thereby increasing the risk of a cardiac arrhythmia. These include:

■ Genetic predisposition (so-called "long QT syndrome")
■ Electrolyte imbalance
■ Cardiac disease (see medical situations of risk below)
■ Drug-induced lengthening.

QTc interval concerns may involve a psychotropic medication itself or a non-psychiatric medication that has accumulated in the body because a psychotropic is also taken – usually due to P-450 enzyme interactions. In this latter case, the QTc lengthening occurs from the excessive dose of the non-psychotropic drug, although the psychotropic may be the precipitating factor. This situation has led to the withdrawal from the US market of several non-psychotropic medications, including terfenadine (Seldane), astemizole (Hismanal), grepafloxacin (Raxar), and cisapride (Propulsid). One antipsychotic, Sertindol (Serlect), was also denied marketing in the USA because of its intrinsic propensity to lengthen the QTc interval. Two other antipsychotics, thioridizine (Mellaril) and mezoridizine (Serentil), received a "black box warning" for their ability significantly to lengthen the QTc interval. Ziprasidone (Geodon in the USA and Zeldox outside the USA) also modestly increases the QTc interval, necessitating a warning in its product information. To be clear about the proportionate risk, the average amount of QTc lengthening should be noted for each of these antipsychotics. Thioridizine and mezoridizine lengthen the QTc interval by approximately 30 ms, Sertindol (which was not marketed) by an average of 22 ms and ziprasidone by 9 ms.

Within our current scope of knowledge, a long QTc interval does not directly cause or lead to *torsades de pointes*. The longer interval is only a statistical marker that *torsades* is more likely. Interestingly, therefore, there are several non-psychotropic medications that cause a lengthened QTc interval but have not been shown to give an increased incidence of *torsades*.

Signs and symptoms

The lengthening of the QTc interval can be seen on an electrocardiogram (EKG) performed before or after a medication is started. Generally, a cut-off of 500 ms is used by most cardiologists, above which there is increased risk of arrhythmia and *torsades de pointes*.[27] No significant increased arrhythmia frequency has occurred in the range between 450 and 500 ms. It is important to note that a QTC interval of between 450 and 500 ms is not, in and of itself, a direct concern, but is a potential warning sign that the 500 ms cut-off could be reached by the addition of an offending medication.

Clinical signs that could alert the patient or clinician that an arrhythmia may be occurring include dizziness, lightheadedness, unexplained syncope, or seizure.

Medical situations of risk

In addition to the genetically inherited causes of long QT interval and the acquired risk with ingesting certain medications, there are other risk factors for a lengthened QTc interval.[28] These include:

1 Low blood levels of potassium or magnesium
2 Female gender
3 Increased age
4 Alcohol and illicit drug usage that may lead to electrolyte abnormalities
5 History of recent myocardial infarction or uncompensated heart failure.

In general, patients with any of these risk factors should have serum magnesium and potassium levels drawn and a baseline EKG performed prior to starting a medication that lengthens the QTc interval. Since 85 percent of congenital long QTc interval is familial, anyone with a family history of this condition or sudden unexplained fainting spells should also have a baseline EKG.

Table 17.6 lists medications that have been potentially associated with prolongation of the QTc interval and a tendency to induce *torsades de pointes*.

Prognosis

Patients may have a mildly prolonged QTc interval (in the 450–500 ms range) without any incidence of clinically significant or serious arrhythmias. When *torsades de pointes* occurs, *it is potentially fatal* (so far only documented in persons with QTc > 500 ms).

Table 17.6 Drugs that prolong the QT interval and/or induce *torsades de pointes**

Drug (Brand name®)	Drug class (clinical usage)	QT TdP comments
Amiodarone (Corarone, Pacerone)	Anti-arrhythmic (abnormal heart rhythm)	QT TdP F > M
Arsenic trioxide (Trisenox)	Anti-cancer (leukemia)	QT TdP Cases in Lit
Bepridil (Vascor)	Anti-anginal (heart pain)	QT TdP F > M
Chlorpromazine (Thorazien)	Antipsychotic/anti-emetic (schizophrenia/nausea)	
Cisapride (Propulsid)	GI stimulant (heartburn)	QT TdP F > M
Clarithormycin (Biaxin)	Antibiotic (bacterial infection)	Cases in Lit
Disopyramide (Norpace)	Anti-arrhythmic (abnormal heart rhythm)	QT TdP F > M
Dofetilide (Tikosyn)	Anti-arrhythmic (abnormal heart rhythm)	QT TdP
Dolasetron (Anzemet)	Anti-nausea (nausea, vomiting)	QT
Droperidol (Inapsine)	Sedative/anti-nausea (anesthesia adjunct, nausea)	QT TdP Cases in Lit
Erythromycin (EES, Erythrocin)	Antibiotic/GI stimulant (bacterial infection; increase GI motility)	QT TdP F > M
Felbamate (Felbatrol)	Anticonvulsant (seizure)	TdP
Flecainide (Tambocor)	Anti-arrhythmic (abnormal heart rhythm)	QT TdP Association not clear
Fluoxetine (Prozac, Serafem)	Antidepressant (depression)	QT TdP Association not clear
Foscarnet (Foscavir)	Antiviral (HIV infections)	QT
Fosphenytoin (Cerebyx)	Anticonvulsant (seizure)	QT
Gatifloxacin (Tequin)	Antibiotic (bacterial infection)	
Halofantrine (Halfan)	Antimalarial (malaria infection)	QT TdP F > M
Haloperidol (Haldol)	Antipsychotic (schizophrenia, agitation)	QT TdP
Ibutilde (Corvert)	Anti-arrhythmic (abnormal heart rhythm)	QT TdP F > M

Table 17.6 (Continued)

Indapamide (Lozol)	Diuretic (stimulate urine and salt loss)	QT Cases in Lit
Isradipine (Dynacirc)	Antihypertensive (high blood pressure)	QT
Levofloxacin (Levaquin)	Antibiotic (bacterial infection)	TdP Association not clear
Levomethadyl (Orlaam)	Opiate agonist (pain control, narcotic dependence)	QT
Mesoridazine (Serentil)	Antipsychotic (schizophrenia)	QT TdP
Moexipril/HCTZ (Uniretic)	Antihypertensive (high blood pressure)	QT
Moxifloxacin (Avelox)	Antibiotic (bacterial infection)	QT
Naratriptan (Amerge)	Serotonin receptor antagonist (migraine treatment)	QT
Nicardipine (Cardene)	Antihypertensive (high blood pressure)	QT
Octreotide (Sandostatin)	Endocrine (acromegaly, carcinoid diarrhea)	QT
Paroxetine (Paxil)	Antidepressant (depression)	TdP
Pentamidine (NebuPent, Pentam)	Anti-infective (pneumocystis pneumonia)	QT TdP F>M
Pimozide (Orap)	Antipsychotic (Tourette's tics)	QT F>M, Cases in Lit
Procainamide (Procan, Pronestyl)	Anti-arrhythmic (abnormal heart rhythm)	QT TdP
Quetiapine (Seroquel)	Antipsychotic (schizophrenia)	QT
Quinidine (Cardioquin, Quiniglute)	Anti-arrhythmic (abnormal heart rhythm)	QT TdP F>M
Risperidone (Risperdal)	Antipsychotic (schizophrenia)	QT
Salmeterol (Serevent)	Sympathomimetic (asthmas, COPD)	QT
Sertraline (Zoloft)	Antidepressant (depression)	QT TdP Association not clear
Sotalol (Betapace)	Anti-arrhythmic (abnormal heart rhythm)	QT TdP F>M

Table 17.6 (Continued)

Drug (Brand name®)	Drug class (clinical usage)	QT TdP comments
Sparfloxacin (Zagam)	Antibiotic (bacterial infection)	QT TdP
Sumatriptan (Imitrex)	Serotonin receptor agonist (migraine treatment)	QT
Tacrolimus (Prograf)	Immunosuppressant (immune suppression)	Cases in Lit
Tamoxifen (Nolvadex)	Anti-cancer (breast cancer)	QT
Thioridazine (Mellaril)	Antipsychotic (schizophrenia)	QT TdP
Tizanidine (Zanaflex)	Muscle relaxant	QT
Venlafaxine (Effexor)	Antidepressant (depression)	QT
Ziprasidone (Geodon)	Antipsychotic (schizophrenia)	QT
Zolmitriptan (Zomig)	Migraine treatment	QT

Key:
QT: Prolongation is mentioned in the FDA-approved labeling as a known action of the drug.
TdP: The FDA-approved labeling includes mention of cases or a risk of *torsades de pointes* (TdP)
Cases in Lit: There are case reports of TdP in the medical literature.
F > M (Females > Males): Substantial evidence indicates a greater risk (usually > two-fold) of TdP in women.
Off market: This drug has been removed from the US market because of drug-induced TdP.
* From: Woosley RL. Drugs that prolong the QT interval and/or induce *torsades de pointes*. www.qtdrugs.org (used with permission).

Prevention

Prevention of lengthened QTc interval and *torsades de pointes* involves clinician vigilance and knowledge about the causes of elongation. When risk factors are present, baseline blood electrolyte levels and EKGs are useful, as well as follow-up EKGs to measure any changes in QTc interval after medication is added.

Treatment

Even though a direct causative connection cannot be proven between increased QTc interval and arrhythmia, current wisdom suggests that if a patient's QTc intervals exceed 500 ms, the medication regimen should be changed. This usually involves switching to another medication that does not lengthen QTc interval or, in cases where the medication had been particularly useful and no other alternatives are available, to a lower dose. (The incidence of arrhythmias and *torsades de pointes* is dose-related for almost all drugs.[29]) Patients with baseline QTc intervals over 450 ms should not be placed on medications that may further lengthen the

QTc interval, unless there is clear clinical necessity. For clinical reasons, when a decision is made to utilize a drug that has the possibility of prolonging the QTc interval in a patient who is already at risk, written informed consent should be obtained and the possible risks explained.

Extrapyramidal symptoms, neuroleptic malignant syndrome, and tardive dyskinesia

The following three syndromes – extrapyramidal symptoms, neuroleptic malignant syndrome, and tardive dyskinesia – are constellations of symptoms almost totally associated with traditional antipsychotic neuroleptics. Since the use of traditional antipsychotics is gradually decreasing, the incidence of these syndromes will also likely decrease and eventually, in large measure, fade from the clinical landscape entirely. However, since traditional antipsychotics are still in common use in various parts of the world or are required in clinical situations where the patient is intolerant of (or non-responsive to) atypical antipsychotics, clinicians must still be knowledgeable about these conditions. They represent areas of significant risk, discomfort and, rarely, mortality to patients. These three syndromes are divided into early-onset syndromes (extrapyramidal symptoms and neuroleptic malignant syndrome) and a late-onset syndrome (tardive dyskinesia).

Extrapyramidal symptoms

The syndrome and its causes

The term "extrapyramidal symptoms" (EPS) covers three separate conditions – dystonia, akathisia, and parkinsonism (also called pseudoparkinsonism). Each is a discrete syndrome involving movement and motor activity associated with initiation of traditional antipsychotics. Dystonia and parkinsonism, as they occur in mental health prescribing, will be discussed in this chapter. Akathisia has already been covered as one possible cause of "overactivation" in Chapter 16.

The pyramidal system in the brain mediates voluntary movements such as walking or sitting. The *extra*pyramidal system is responsible for coordination and for fine-tuning the many involuntary muscle activities necessary to performing these tasks, and is modulated by dopaminergic and cholinergic neurons.

Dopinaminergic neurons are generally inhibitory and cholinergic neurons generally excitatory to normal motor function. It has been suggested that functional alteration of the extrapyramidal system is caused by a disruption of this normal balance between dopaminergic and cholinergic neurons.[30] When traditional neuroleptics are introduced, they block dopaminergic neurons, leading to a decrease in dopamine and a relative increase in cholinergic activity, disrupting the balance. The disruption of the normal balance between these neurotransmitters then leads to the loss of certain motor functions and their smooth coordination. This explanation most closely accounts for dystonia and pseudoparkinsonism, but does not clearly explain akathisia.

Dystonia

Dystonic movements (dystonias) are the involuntary contractions of striatal muscle groups. Although any muscle group may be involved, the commonly affected muscle groups are those of the face, head, extremities, neck, and back. These reactions are not under voluntary control and may appear suddenly (within minutes or hours of initiation of an offending agent), or may come on in a sporadic fashion over several days or weeks. In general the symptoms, which wax and wane over time, are made worse by emotionally upsetting experiences, and generally disappear during sleep. Dystonias usually end within a short period of time after discontinuation of antipsychotic medication, but in some cases it may take days or weeks for them to pass. The symptoms are often quite uncomfortable and anxiety-producing for the patient, and distressing to family members. The incidence varies greatly with the presence of risk factors (see below), and can be anywhere from 2–95 percent.[31,32]

Depending on which muscle group is involved, some dystonic EPS symptoms have specific labels such as:

- *Oculogyric crisis* (a rolling back and upward of the eyes toward the back of the head)
- *Trismus* (involuntary jaw clenching)
- *Torticollis* (twisting of the neck secondary to involuntary neck muscle contraction)
- *Carpopedal spasm* (involuntary contraction of the hand or foot musculature, leading to dorsiflexion of the toes and inward contraction of the hands, fingers and wrists)
- *Opisthotonos* (contraction of the back and neck muscles leading to a backwards arching of the back, spine and neck).

Parkinsonism

Drug-induced parkinsonism (or pseudoparkinsonism, as it is sometimes called) is another set of primarily motor symptoms that occurs weeks to months after the onset of dopamine blocking agents such as typical antipsychotics. In general parkinsonian symptoms are bilateral, although on occasion they are more pronounced on only one side of the body. Symptoms include:

- Muscle rigidity
- Tremor (often in the hands, and referred to as a "pill rolling" tremor)
- Bradykinesia (slowed motor movements) with difficulty in starting voluntary muscle activities
- Akinesia (lack of motor movement in general)
- Abnormal, shuffling gait
- Dysarthric speech
- Dysphagia (difficulty swallowing)
- Micrographia (cramped handwriting)

- Decreased motor movements in the facial muscles with lessened facial expression (often referred to as "mask-like facies")
- Cog-wheel rigidity (a ratchet-like loss of smooth fluid motion of joints), which may be elicited on examination of the elbows, wrists, knees, or neck.

Prognosis

Dystonias are often self-limited within 7–10 days of onset. For some patients they may persist indefinitely without treatment if the offending agent is continued. Despite their time-limited nature, they are sufficiently uncomfortable to the patient and distressing to family members that treatment is often initiated relatively quickly after onset.[33,34] When they occur acutely and strongly, as in oculogyric crisis, acute torticollis and opisthotonos, urgent interventions are necessary to relieve painful symptomatology and the resulting grotesque motor postures. Parkinsonism, once established, tends to persist or worsen with time if the offending medication continues to be taken.

Prevention

Prevention consists of minimizing the use of traditional neuroleptics. Whenever antipsychotic medication activity is required, utilization of atypical antipsychotics will dramatically lessen the incidence of EPS, akathisia, and parkinsonism. Because of the possibility of these side effects, it is particularly important, when possible, to avoid the use of traditional antipsychotics for non-psychotic symptoms (e.g. as a hypnotic, for affective disorders which are not psychotic, or as treatment for general behavioral control in delirious or demented patients). When it is necessary to use typical antipsychotic medication, the clinician should prescribe the lowest possible dose and be alert to the onset of any extrapyramidal symptoms in the first week of treatment (90 percent of all EPS occur within the first 4 days after initiation of the antipsychotic).[31]

Known high-risk statistical predictors of EPS include:

- Lower age (< 35 years)[35]
- Male sex[36]
- Use of high potency antipsychotics (haloperidol, fluphenazine)[37,38]
- Use of neuroleptics in a patient with an affective disorder
- Patients with a previous history of EPS
- During rapid tranquilization or after large dosage increases.

A useful preventative strategy involves the prophylactic use of anticholinergic medications in patients at high risk for EPS.[39] Benztropine 1–2 mg daily can be started simultaneously with the initiation of a traditional neuroleptic in those patients who are at high risk for EPS (e.g. a young male patient in whom a high-potency neuroleptic is being started at a relatively high dose). When prophylaxis is used, the patient's anticholinergic medication should be gradually discontinued after several weeks. In up to 50 percent of clinical situations, the patient will no longer need the anticholinergic and the EPS will not re-emerge. If the symptoms do re-emerge, the anticholinergic medication can be reinstated.

Treatment

When starting traditional antipsychotics, patient education about the benign course and nature of these side effects is essential to prevent excessive fear and overreaction. Patients and their families should be alerted to the possible signs of early EPS so that, if they occur, treatment can be instituted promptly.

When using a traditional antipsychotic and EPS emerge, the prescriber should switch to an atypical neuroleptic or, if the traditional antipsychotic is to be continued, change to a lower potency neuroleptic (e.g. chlorpromazine or thioridazine), or minimize the dose to the lowest possible therapeutic amount.[33,34] Use of the atypical antipsychotic agents olanzapine, ziprasidone, quetiapine, and clozapine will show a marked decrease in the incidence of EPS compared to typical antipsychotics.[40,41] Risperidone also has a lower incidence of EPS than traditional neuroleptics, if the total daily dose is kept below 4 mg per day.[42]

Pharmacological treatment of dystonia and parkinsonism involves the use of several medication groups, including:

- *Anticholinergics*, which decrease the availability of acetylcholine and therefore partially restore the dopamine–choline balance (benztropine, trihexphenidyl and others)
- *Antihistamines* (diphenhydramine and others) that have central anticholinergic effects and fewer peripheral effects than anticholinergics
- *Benzodiazepines* (lorazepam, diazepam, clonazepam, and others) are useful, particularly for akinesia or akathisia
- Drugs that enhance the release of dopamine and increase its availability at the synapse (e.g. *amantadine*) will modulate EPS symptoms
- Direct stimulators of dopamine receptor activity (e.g. *bromocriptine*) are used in NMS and parkinson's disease, but not typically for routine EPS.

Benztropine 1–2 mg per day will control modest levels of EPS sympatomatology.[43] Up to 6 mg per day may be necessary for severe symptoms. Parkinsonism may also be at least partially improved by the use of similar doses of benztropine[44,45] and amantadine.[46] In the inpatient setting, diphenhydramine (50 mg i.m. or i.v.), amantadine (200–400 mg per day)[47] and diazepam (5 mg i.m. or i.v.)[48] can be equally effective in reversing and preventing dystonias. For dystonias, anticholinergic medication may be given orally if the symptoms are mild and gradual in onset. If acute or intense dystonic symptoms occur rapidly, intramuscular and intravenous dosing of the anticholinergic will give more prompt symptom relief. Parenteral administration also avoids the problem of difficulty swallowing oral medication, which may be part of the dystonic picture.

When using medication to treat EPS, the treating remedy should be gradually withdrawn after 4–6 weeks to see if its continued use is necessary.

Neuroleptic malignant syndrome

The syndrome and its causes

Although the rarest of the serious adverse reactions to typical antipsychotics (with an incidence of 0.2 percent), neuroleptic malignant syndrome (NMS) is significantly important because it is life-threatening if unrecognized and untreated. This syndrome is neither specific to any one psychiatric diagnosis, nor limited to mental health patients. It can be seen in any patient where the brain is exposed to medication that induces dopamine-2 receptor blockade resulting in sudden decrease in brain dopamine levels. Even when dopamine-blocking medications are used for other non-psychiatric purposes (such as prochlorperazine, promethazine and droperidol, which can be used for blocking emesis, promoting peristalsis, or as anesthesia/sedative), NMS can occur. Although most of the cases of NMS have been reported with traditional antipsychotics (neuroleptics), the actual incidence of NMS with the use of *atypical* antipsychotics remains unclear[49] (there have been six reported cases involving clozapine and two with quetiapine).

The symptom complex includes:[50]

1 Muscle rigidity (often referred to as "lead pipe" rigidity) with cogwheeling, myoclonus and coarse tremors
2 Mental status changes, including delerium, stupor, and coma
3 Hyperthermia (> 38 °C) with profuse sweating
4 Autonomic activation and instability, with changes in blood pressure and tachycardia
5 Rapid and labored breathing
6 Drooling, incontinence
7 Laboratory test abnormalities, including:
   ■ Elevated serum creatine phosphokinase (CPK), sometimes increased to extraordinary levels, reflecting significant muscle necrosis (rhabdomyolysis);
   ■ Metabolic acidosis, hypoxia, low serum iron and electrolyte abnormalities.

The syndrome can occur within the first 24 hours after beginning neuroleptic treatment, and two-thirds of all cases occur within the first week. Once symptoms develop, progression is quite rapid and symptoms reach peak intensity within 72 hours. NMS does not generally result from an overdose of neuroleptic medication, and usually occurs when medication dose is within the therapeutic range.[51]

Medical situations of risk

Although many factors have been evaluated as potential risk factors for NMS, the evidence is neither extensive nor convincing for any one risk factor, other than the recent initiation of a dopamine-blocking agent. There is some evidence to support increased risk with high potency traditional antipsychotics, high ambient temperatures, male sex, genetic predisposition, and possibly an association of concomitant usage of lithium with the neuroleptic. The bottom line, however, is that any medication that blocks dopamine in the brain may precipitate NMS. Patients with a previous history of NMS are at increased risk for future episodes.

Prognosis

Once traditional neuroleptic medication is discontinued NMS is generally self-limiting, with most patients recovering in 7–10 days.[51,52] Nearly all patients recover within 30 days, and most patients who survive make a full recovery. The course of NMS may be prolonged if the precipitating agent is a long-acting depot neuroleptic.[51] The mortality rate is approximately 5 percent, but has much improved in the last two decades.

Prevention

Clinician vigilance and lowered usage of strong dopamine-blocking agents has already lessened the incidence of NMS in recent years. The wider use of atypical antipsychotic agents will likely further decrease its incidence.

Rechallenging a patient with a neuroleptic after a history of NMS has been a matter of some debate. Current estimates are that approximately 30 percent of patients who recover from NMS will have a recurrent episode following traditional neuroleptic rechallenge. The majority of patients can be rechallenged, however, if done so in very gradual doses, no sooner than 2 weeks following recovery. It is prudent to consider the use of an atypical antipsychotic or a lower potency traditional neuroleptic if a rechallenge is going to be undertaken. When retrying a typical antipsychotic, the patient should be given a small test dose and carefully monitored for signs of NMS.

Treatment

Specific treatments for NMS include:[53]

- Cessation of any dopamine-blocking drugs
- Supportive medical/nursing care including fluid replacement, fever reduction, use of cooling blanket, and support of cardiac, respiratory and renal function
- With moderate symptoms, use of dopamine agonists can reverse the dopamine blockade. The following agents have been shown to be useful: amantadine 100 mg p.o. via NG tube every 8 hours; bromocriptine 2.5–5 mg p.o. via NG tube every 8 hours; or dantrolene 1–2.5 mg/kg i.v.
- High-dose benzodiazepines such as lorazepam 1–2 mg i.m./i.v. every 8 hours can also be helpful
- Electroconvulsive therapy (ECT) remains the definitive treatment for those patients with a syndrome severe enough to be admitted to an intensive care unit.[54,55] The average number of ECT treatments is 10, and response is usually seen after four treatments.

Tardive dyskinesia

The syndrome and its causes

Tardive dyskinesia (TD) literally translated means abnormal involuntary movements of late onset. It is one of several late-onset movement disorders associated with dopamine-blocking agents such as traditional antipsychotics (neuroleptics). *Tardive akathisia* and *tardive dystonia* can also occur after months or years of neuroleptic usage; however, the incidence of these latter syndromes is significantly less frequent than tardive dyskinesia, on which most of the clinical investigation has been focused. The signs, symptoms and treatment of late-onset tardive dystonia and tardive akathisia are similar to their early-onset counterparts discussed previously.

The essential element of tardive dyskinesia is brain exposure to drugs that result in strong central dopaminergic blockade, particularly at the dopamine-2 receptor.[56] Although most cases of TD have been related to traditional antipsychotics, other non-psychiatric medications such as levodopa, prochlorperizine (Compazine), amphetamine and metoclopramide (Reglan, Maxelon – UK only) have also been associated with TD. The antidepressant agent amoxapine, which itself blocks dopamine, and Triavil, which contains perphenazine (a dopamine-blocking traditional antipsychotic agent), can also lead to significant dopamine blockade and TD.

Essential to the diagnosis is exposure to the dopamine-blocking agent for at least 3 months (1 month if the patient is greater than 60 years old). Usually this syndrome emerges gradually over a number of months, but on occasion it will occur relatively quickly when dopamine antagonists are decreased in dosage or withdrawn altogether (withdrawal dyskinesia).

Although exposure to dopamine-blocking agents is thought to be essential to tardive dyskinesia, it is clear that many elderly patients have a spontaneous incidence of dyskinesia. *Schizophrenic patients and patients with dementia may have a higher incidence of spontaneous dyskinesia than the general population, even without exposure to dopamine-blocking agents.* Therefore, estimates of the prevalence rate of tardive dyskinesia have been quite variable. It is currently estimated that TD occurs in 15–30 percent of patients exposed to traditional antipsychotics.[57] Risk of TD has been shown to be considerably lower with use of atypical agents compared to traditional antipsychotics.[58] Although there are some abnormal movement problems, clozapine and olanzapine are associated with very low TD rates.[59–63] Risperidone, with lower rate of EPS than traditional neuroleptics, should also have lower rates of TD,[64] although there are several case reports of risperidone's association with TD.[65]

Although research evidence can be at times contradictory, several factors do emerge as clear risk factors for an increased incidence of TD.[66] These include:

- Advancing age
- Higher doses of a typical antipsychotic
- Longer duration of exposure to the antipsychotic

- Female sex
- Smoking
- Diabetes
- Previous history of neuroleptic-induced parkinsonism
- Diagnosis of affective disorder or dementia when compared to a diagnosis of schizophrenia.

Signs and symptoms

The symptoms include hyperkinetic, involuntary movements in a variety of body parts including:

1 Orofacial dyskinesia with
   - Exaggerated movements of the tongue and mouth
   - Grimacing and chewing movements
   - Bulging or puffing of the cheeks
   - Vermiform ("worm-like") movements of the tongue
   - Increased blinking and blepharospasm
2 Choreoathetoid (slow, writhing) movements of the hands, arms, legs, feet
3 Rocking and swaying of the trunk and pelvis.

Because of the involuntary movements, patients may have trouble in eating, speaking, or using their hands with dexterity. Occasionally, the patient will make grunting sounds or have difficulty breathing. The movements may be worse during periods of emotional stress and when the patient's attention is distracted away from the movements. Movements usually disappear during sleep.

Since orofacial dyskinesia is the most common presentation of TD, it is important not to misidentify TD in a patient who simply has ill-fitting dentures. Be sure to ask about the presence of dentures in the evaluation process for TD. The AIMS (Abnormal Involuntary Movements Scale), developed by the National Institutes of Mental Health Psychopharmacology Research branch, is the standard tool for evaluation of movement disorders (see Appendix 6).

Situations of medical risk

A patient who is treated with any dopamine-blocking agent is at risk for tardive dyskinesia, particularly if the exposure continues for extended time. Therefore, vigilance on the part of the clinician is always essential when this group of medications is used. Based on the risk factors identified above, any elderly female diabetic who is a smoker is especially at risk for developing TD. Patients with affective disorders are also a high risk, and strong dopamine-blocking agents should be avoided in their care whenever possible.

Prognosis

Although early wisdom suggested that many cases of tardive dyskinesia were irreversible, further evidence suggests that a large percentage of persons with TD will show remission once the offending agent has been removed for a long period of time. This is particularly true if the length of exposure to the medication was short and the patient is young. The exact persistence rate of TD, once it becomes evident, is difficult to estimate. Most recent studies, however, show that if a long-term timeframe (2–5 years) is used to evaluate the patient after discontinuation of the antipsychotic, 50–90 percent show improvement of at least 50 percent on AIMS ratings.[67] Sixty percent of patients have TD symptoms disappear or improve greatly in the course of 2–3 years. Nevertheless, 30 to 40 percent of patients who develop TD will continue with TD symptoms on a chronic basis. Direct mortality from TD has not been reported; however, the patient's lifestyle, functional behavior and self-care ability may be significantly hampered.

Prevention

Because treatment options are, at best, of only limited success, prevention of TD is the most significant area for clinicians to consider. This involves minimizing exposure to strong dopamine-blocking agents, both in dose and duration. Of particular importance is avoiding the use of traditional neuroleptics for non-psychotic purposes, such as sedation, anxiety or behavioral control in non-psychotic patients. Whenever possible, atypical antipsychotic medication or other medication groups should be used in preference to traditional antipsychotics.[59,68]

Involvement in precipitating TD through the use of traditional antipsychotics has long been an area of medicolegal risk for mental health prescribers. Even though the use of these agents is decreasing, it continues to be important that a patient placed on a strong dopamine-blocking agent signs an adequate informed consent document. The alternatives available and the possibility of the emergence of TD should be explained to the patient if he or she is competent; if this is not the case, such risk should be explained to the family or legal guardian.

A patient who is placed on a traditional neuroleptic should have the medication regimen re-evaluated periodically for ongoing necessity. When possible, supplementary agents including lithium, valproic acid, carbamazepine, benzodiazepines, or atypical antipsychotic agents should be used to augment antipsychotic activity and allow minimization of the dosage of traditional neuroleptic.

Treatment

There is no one accepted treatment for tardive dyskinesia, and remediation is based primarily on preventing the onset of the condition.[68] Once diagnosed, treatment strategies include:

■ Discontinuing the offending antipsychotic or switching the patient to an atypical antipsychotic.

■ When traditional antipsychotics are necessary, lowering the dose to the least amount necessary for clinical response and maintaining the exposure for the shortest period of time.

■ Pharmacological treatments have included trials with amine-depleting agents, dopamine antagonists, cholinergic agents, GABA agonists, anxiolytics, anticholinergics, vitamin E, and beta-adrenergic blocking agents. No one treatment has shown significant clinical response, although there is anecdotal evidence for some modest benefits from using vitamin E, levodopa, benzodiazepines (particularly clonazepam), botulinum toxin, and reserpine.[59,68]

Raising the dose of the offending dopamine-blocking agent will temporarily mask or alleviate TD symptoms. While this may provide some short-term benefit it is obviously not a useful long-term strategy, and is not considered part of good treatment.

Unfortunately, the concept of "drug holidays" – stopping the dopamine-blocking agent medication for days or weeks at a time – does not provide significant protection against the emergence of TD. While logical in concept and appealing in that it minimizes neuroleptic exposure, rigorous evaluation has found that it is not of benefit, and may actually aggravate the symptoms of TD.[69,70]

If the patient is being withdrawn from a traditional neuroleptic because of the onset of TD, this should be done in a gradual fashion to avoid a flare-up of TD (withdrawal dyskinesia) and also to prevent a rapid, florid worsening of the psychosis. The only exception to this gradual tapering principle would be the patient with TD who also develops neuroleptic malignant syndrome, which itself is an emergency, and for which the neuroleptic should be withdrawn immediately.

Monoamine oxidose inhibitor reactions

Monoamine oxidase inhibitors (MAOIs) have been used since the 1960s, and are useful antidepressants for bipolar depression, treatment-resistant depression and so-called "atypical depressions" (patients with mood reactivity, hypersomnia, leaden paralysis, hyperphagia and rejection sensitivity). In twenty-first century psychopharmacology, MAOIs represent fourth- or fifth-line choices for most patients because of dietary restrictions and problematic medication interactions. Because of the possibility of strong, sudden and serious interactions, these medications engender apprehension on the part of patients and, at times, clinicians. Nevertheless, certain patients respond to MAOIs when all other medication groups have failed. Understanding their possible interactions is necessary to prescribing or monitoring any patient who is taking them. These interactions occur with *irreversible* MAOIs such as phenelzine, tranylcypromine and selegiline – the only three currently available in the USA. A *reversible* MAOI meclobemide (Manerix) is available in a number of European and Latin American countries, as well as in Canada. Because of its improved safety profile and the lack of dietary restriction that is necessary for irreversible MAOIs, meclobemide has had some popularity in these regions, although there has been some question about its efficacy compared to irreversible MAOIs. Currently, a transdermal delivery system of an irreversible MAOI is in testing. Since this system bypasses the enteric–hepatic circulation, it will not require dietary restrictions. If successfully tested, it may trigger a resurgence of MAOI usage.

The syndrome and its causes

Problematic interactions with irreversible MAOIs are two-fold:

1 Serotonin syndrome
2 Hypertensive crisis

Serotonin syndrome, which occurs when strongly serotonergic medications are combined with MAOIs, was discussed earlier in the chapter. Those psychotropic medications with strongly serotonergic properties, which are contraindicated in patients taking irreversible MAOIs , are listed in Table 17.7.

The second set of interactions with MAOIs involves markedly elevated blood pressure (*hypertensive crisis*) when MAOIs are combined with certain medications and foods. This occurs because the MAOI blocks monoamine oxidase, the enzyme that breaks down monoamines in the body. When an irreversible MAOI is taken consistently, monoamine oxidase is irreversibly blocked for up to 2 weeks. During this time, if the patient ingests foods that contain pressor monoamines, these cannot be metabolized, and will accumulate in the body and raise blood pressure. The most common such amine implicated in these reactions is tyramine. Therefore, when irreversible MAOIs are used the patient should be cautioned to avoid eating or drinking foods that are potentially high in tyramine. Substances that are likely to be high in tyramine are listed in Table 17.8.

If an MAOI is stopped, dietary restrictions should still be maintained for 2 weeks. This is because the monoamine-blocking effect may last for up to 14 days after discontinuation of an MAOI.

Elevated blood pressure and hypertensive crisis can also be precipitated by the combination of an MAOI with various medications. These include over-the-counter cough and cold medications, diet pills, certain street drugs, prescription stimulants, narcotics, and centrally acting antihypertensives (see Table 17.9).

In the past, the combination of a tricyclic antidepressant and an MAOI was thought to be risky and was contraindicated. It has been shown more recently that this combination can be tolerable for certain patients if the combination is instituted simultaneously and the TCA used is doxepin, amitriptyline, or trimipramine.[71,72] It is contraindicated to add a TCA to an ongoing regimen of an MAOI or to use imipramine as the TCA.

Table 17.7 Strongly serotonergic psychotropics prohibited in conjunction with MAOIs

- All SSRIs, including fluoxetine, paroxetine, sertraline, citalopram and fluvoxamine
- Venlafaxine
- Nefazodone

Table 17.8 Dietary restrictions for patients taking irreversible MAOIs*

Foods to avoid completely

- Aged cheese (all cheeses *except* cottage, farmer, ricotta, and cream cheese)
- Pickled or aged meats (fermented and dry sausage, pepperoni, salami), aged poultry or fish (herring), caviar
- Spoiled meat, poultry, or fish (such as that left in the refrigerator too long)
- Fava (broad) bean pods
- Concentrated yeast extracts (Marmite or brewer's yeast tablets; yeast used in baking is safe)
- Sauerkraut
- Soy sauce and soy-bean condiments
- Tap beer, red wine, sherry, Chianti, liqueurs
- Liver from beef or chicken (fresh beef or chicken meat is safe)
- Banana peel

Foods to avoid in large quantities

- White wine, bottled or canned beer, vodka, gin
- Ripe avocados
- Anchovies
- Chocolate
- Meat tenderizers
- Beverages containing caffeine

*NB: Dietary restrictions should be maintained for 2 weeks after stopping an MAOI.
From: Current status of monoamine oxidase inhibitors in psychiatric practice. *Essent Psychopharmacol* 1997;1(3):255–272.

Signs and symptoms

Patients who ingest one of the prohibited foods or medications while taking an irreversible MAOI will, within 15–90 minutes, begin experiencing:

1 Severe headache, usually occipital and temporal ("like the top of my head is going to come off")
2 Sweating
3 Elevation of systolic and diastolic blood pressure
4 Mydriasis (dilated pupils).

If the headache and other symptoms do not occur within 2 hours after ingestion of a prohibited compound, it is unlikely that they will occur subsequently. Rarely, during a strong reaction, intracerebral hemorrhage and death can occur.

Medical situations of risk

Given proper prescriptive habits and appropriate education about problematic interactions, the most likely situations in which a patient could still experience a hypertensive crisis or serotonin syndrome are:

Table 17.9 Drugs contraindicated for patients receiving irreversible MAOIs*

Over-the-counter cold and cough medications
- Ephedrine
- Pseudoephedrine
- Phenylephedrine
- Dextromethorphan
- Phenylpropanolamine

Stimulants
- Methylphenidate
- Dextroamphetamine

Diet pills
- Prescription
- Over-the-counter

Street/recreational drugs
- Cocaine
- "Speed" (amphetamines)

Narcotics
- Meperidine is most risky
- Morphine is less dangerous
- Codeine is generally safe

Centrally acting antihypertensives
- Reserpine
- Guanethidinene
- α-methyldopa

Serotonergic agents/SSRIs
- Clomipramine
- Venlafaxine
- Nefazodone
- Fenfluramine
- Dexfenfluramine
- Sumatriptan (Imitrex)

Anesthetics containing pressors

* From: *Essent Psychopharmacol* 1997;1(3):264.

1 When the patient *accidentally* ingest one of the prohibited foods
2 When *inappropriate medication combinations* are prescribed by a clinician who is unaware that the patient is taking an MAOI.

Ingestion of prohibited foods most often occurs when patients are outside their usual eating routine, or are unaware of the ingredients in what they are eating. At a restaurant or when ingesting food prepared by someone else, they may unknowingly eat a prohibited ingredient.

Dangerous medications could accidentally be simultaneously prescribed when patients come to the emergency room unconscious, and do not have an ID bracelet or other indication that they are taking an MAOI. The unsuspecting clinician may prescribe a hazardous combination of medications inadvertently.

Prognosis

In general, if small amounts of the prohibited substance are ingested, the patient experiences a severe headache, sweating, and moderately elevated blood pressure, but recovers within several hours without ongoing sequelae. Serious consequences of a hypertensive crisis, specifically cerebrovascular accident and death, have had markedly reduced incidence over the last decade. This is due in part to better education about the possible problematic interactions, and lessened usage of MAOIs.

Treatment

Instruct patients that if they experience any symptoms of hypertensive crisis, particularly a severe headache, they are immediately to seek emergency medical evaluation and care. Although many hypertensive crises will pass without treatment, patients cannot be assured of how much of the prohibited substance they may have ingested, and how high their blood pressure will rise. In the past, patients were instructed to use an "emergency pill" of nifedipine or another blood pressure lowering agent to prevent severe hypertensive reactions while they were *en route* to the emergency room. However, this practice led to further complications from severely lowered blood pressure, and has been discontinued.[73]

After arrival at the emergency room, when proper medical care is available, a blood pressure lowering agent such as nifedipine can be given, the effect of which lasts 4–6 hours. Usually, by the end of that time, the crisis has passed and blood pressure will normalize without further treatment. If large amounts of a prohibited substance have been ingested, however, repeat doses may be necessary to maintain a safe blood pressure.

Prevention

The most important preventive measure is ongoing education to the patient about prohibited foods and medications. The patient is strongly urged to be diligent about avoiding ingestion of any prohibited substances *without experimentation*. Each patient taking an MAOI should carry documentation of this fact at all times (e.g. an ID card in the wallet or purse, and/or a medical ID bracelet).

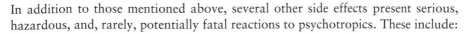

Other potentially dangerous side effects

In addition to those mentioned above, several other side effects present serious, hazardous, and, rarely, potentially fatal reactions to psychotropics. These include:

- Blood dyscrasias
- Liver toxicity
- Seizures.

Blood dyscrasias (abnormalities of blood cell parameters)

Abnormalities of blood parameters with psychotropics usually involve changes in white blood cell count or platelet count. The most serious of these is an extremely low neutrophil count or agranulocytosis (defined as an absolute neutrophil count of 100 per microliter or less). The presence of very low numbers of white blood cells leaves the patient open to frequent severe infections or sepsis.

Although many cases of incipient agranulocytosis are heralded by gradually decreasing neutrophil counts, some are precipitous and sudden. If a patient has a neutrophil count of under 2000, a hematological consult should be obtained and serious consideration given to switching medications. Those medications associated with the incidence of agranulocytosis are listed in Table 17.10.

A baseline level of blood parameters drawn via a complete blood count (CBC) should be done prior to instituting any of these agents. Follow-up monitoring is as follows:

- For carbamazepine, CBCs should be done 4–6 weeks after initiation and then every 3 months for the first year. There is some evidence that a rash with carbamazepine may be a precursor of a blood dyscrasia.[74] A patient who develops a significant rash with ongoing carbamazepine therapy should have close monitoring of blood count for possible drops in neutrophil count.

Table 17.10 Medications known to have some risk of agranulocytosis
Antipsychotic medications
Chlorpromazine*
Clozapine*
Prochlorperazine
Thioridizine*
Trifluoperizine*
Mood stabilizers
Carbamazepine*
Miscellaneous
Desipramine
Chlordiazepoxide

*Worst offenders.
Adapted from Distenfeld A. *Agranulocytosis*, at www.emedicine.com/med/topic82.html

■ For clozapine, the patient's blood count is monitored once weekly for the first 6 months and every other week thereafter.

Clinical symptoms that may indicate a lowered white blood cell count include:

■ Frequent, recurrent infections, particularly recurrent sore throats and ulcers, infections of the oral mucosa, gums, skin, and sinuses
■ Fever
■ Sepsis.

Thrombocytopenia (low platelet count) may occur with carbamazepine or valproic acid. In general, normal platelet counts are between 150 000 and 450 000 per cubic millimeter. Platelet counts from 100 000 to 150 000 per cubic millimeter, even though technically in the "low" range, are not worrisome unless unusual or abnormal bleeding is occurring. When platelet counts are lowered, the clinician should be particularly alert to complaints of unusual bleeding, bruising or petechiae. If any of these clinical signs emerge, a CBC should be drawn and the patient's clinical condition monitored more carefully. When platelet counts drop below 100 000 per cubic millimeter, a medication change is usually wise. With valproic acid, there are reports of abnormal bleeding that may occur even with normal platelet levels, due to interference with normal platelet function. When using valproic acid, therefore, evidence of abnormal bleeding may raise a concern even in the face of normal platelet levels.

Hepatotoxicity

Most psychotropics are metabolized through the liver. Some medications may cause gradual hepatotoxicity and increasingly abnormal measures of liver functions over time. Other psychotropics may show an acute fulminant hepatitis with rapidly rising liver enzymes and a clinical picture that resembles viral hepatitis. Rarely, this leads to liver failure.

Psychotropics known to have a significant incidence of liver toxicity are listed in Table 17.11.[75–77]

Although there is a low but measurable incidence of hepatotoxicity with virtually all antidepressants, the frequency is relatively small for most SSRIs and other new generation antidepressants. The known exception is nefazodone, which has been shown to have an increased incidence of hepatitis with hepatocellular injury in a small number of patients. Traditional antipsychotics, clozapine, carbamazepine, valproic acid and MAOIs have long been known to be potentially hepatotoxic, and should be used with caution in persons with liver disease.

The clinical management of most potential hepatic effects from psychotropics initially involves drawing a baseline set of liver functions prior to instituting medications that have a high incidence of hepatotoxicity (as listed in Table 17.11). A follow-up set of liver functions should be drawn 4–6 weeks after beginning the medication, and every 3–6 months thereafter for the first year. In general, small increases in liver function test values (two to three times normal) are not

Table 17.11 Psychotropics associated with liver toxicity

Antipsychotics
- All traditional typical antipsychotics (neuroleptics)
- Clozapine

Antidepressants
- Nefazodone
- Irreversible MAOIs
- Clomipramine

To a lesser degree:
- Mianserin
- Lofepramine (UK only)
- Trazodone
- Fluvoxamine

Mood stabilizers
- Valproic acid
- Carbamazepine
- Lamotrigine

necessarily an indication that the medication must be stopped, although it would be prudent to monitor liver functions more frequently in such patients. If the values continue to rise, discontinuation may be necessary. When liver function elevations reach three times normal, changing medication is almost always necessary. In mild hepatocellular injury, there may be minimal or no observable external clinical signs of hepatocellular disease, other than the laboratory test abnormalities.

Although the serious forms of hepatotoxicity are rare, they are idiosyncratic. Unfortunately, laboratory monitoring is a poor indicator of these rare toxic episodes. Serious hepatic toxicity can occur after repeated laboratory monitoring showing normal or only minimally elevated liver enzymes. Such serious toxicity is often heralded by physical signs and symptoms as shown in Table 17.12. When these occur, liver function tests are markedly abnormal.

Seizures

The rate of unprovoked seizures in the general population is 0.07 to 0.09 percent.[78] In large studies, the rate of seizure occurrence during use of therapeutic doses of most commonly used antipsychotics and antidepressants ranges from 0.1 to 1.5 percent. Because of methodological differences in research, however, the data are confusing. The exact range is hard to specify, the variability is large, and precise differences between drugs is hard to discern.[78] Although an absolute increase in risk is measurable, the clinical risk of seizure in the non-epileptic, non-head-injured patient when using psychotropics is small. Medications that have relatively low risk of causing a *de novo* seizure in an otherwise healthy patient are shown in Table 17.13.

Table 17.12 Clinical symptoms of liver toxicity

- Jaundice
- Fever
- Ascites
- Nausea
- Vomiting
- Lethargy
- Confusion
- A change in blood-clotting ability

Table 17.13 Psychotropics with a low risk of seizure*

Antidepressants
- Fluoxetine
- Paroxetine
- Sertraline
- Venlafaxine
- Trazodone
- Phenelzine
- Tranylcypromine

Antipsychotics
- Risperidone
- Haloperidol
- Fluphenazine
- Pimozide

*Adapted from Pisani F *et al*. Effect of psychotropic drugs on seizure threshold. *Drug Safety* 2002;25(2):91–110.

Use of anticonvulsant mood stabilizers and benzodiazepines (which can raise seizure threshold and make seizures *less* likely) are even less problematic. Patients who, at baseline, are more at risk for seizures are those with:

- A history of head injury
- A history of seizure or epilepsy
- Bulimia
- An overdose of medications
- Alcohol/street drug use, abuse, and withdrawal
- A strong family history of seizure disorder.

Some of the more common mental health scenarios potentially leading to seizure include:

- A bulimic patient whose vomiting decreases intracellular fluid volume such that the epileptogenic effect of medications may be increased. This is particularly noticeable with bupropion.

■ Patients who take large doses of benzodiazepines, either chronically or in overdose, then have a precipitous drop in benzodiazepine blood level due to suddenly stopping the medication. Short half-life benzodiazepines create a greater risk than long half-life compounds for seizure in this situation.
■ Precipitous alcohol withdrawal from high chronic usage
■ Accidental or intentional overdose of large doses of medication or mixed overdose.

Except for drug overdose (in which the rate of seizures may be as high as 30 percent), such at-risk patients show only a small absolute risk of a psychotropic causing a new or increased frequency of seizure. Several studies now show that if a psychotropic is introduced at low doses, with slow, gradual increases, the targeted mental health condition improves with minimal change in seizure threshold. In up to one-third of studied patients, the frequency of seizures actually improves.[78–80]

Other clinical guidelines for psychotropic prescription in patients at risk for seizure include maintaining the minimal effective dose, since the frequency of seizures is dose proportionate. Also, complex polypharmacy should be avoided.

There are some psychotropics associated with higher than average incidence of seizure. These are listed in Table 17.14, and should be considered second-line choices in patients at higher baseline risk for seizures.

For purposes of illustration, it is useful to look at absolute percentages within this table. While the incidence of seizures with bupropion is greater when compared to other antidepressants, its total incidence of seizures (0.4 percent when the dosage is less than 400 mg per day) is still small compared to the seizure incidence of clozapine, which has a 1–2 percent incidence of seizures at doses less than 300 mg; 3–4 percent at doses between 300 and 600 mg; and 5 percent incidence of seizures at doses over 600 mg.[80] Therefore, at typical doses, clozapine is over 10 times as likely to induce a seizure than is bupropion.

If a patient has a seizure when taking a psychotropic

If a patient has a first seizure during psychotropic prescription, it is almost never clear without further evaluation whether or not the medication is absolutely

Table 17.14 Psychotropic medications associated with higher than average seizure risk

1 Antidepressants
   ■ Maprotiline
   ■ Clomipramine
   ■ Bupropion
2 Antipsychotics
   ■ Clozapine
   ■ Traditional antipsychotics, particularly chlorpromazine

implicated. Therefore, in the event of seizure, the patient should be referred for urgent medical evaluation and psychotropic medication doses should be held until such evaluation is begun. This evaluation, consisting of neurological consultation, EEG and imaging studies, may or may not reveal the cause of the seizure, but should be accomplished as promptly as possible. If it is imprudent or clinically risky to stop medication totally, half doses should be used until further information is obtained.

If neurological disease, head trauma, substance withdrawal or epilepsy is discovered, any decisions about restarting psychotropic medication must be made in concert with the medical/neurological treators. If no other obvious cause for the seizure is found, it still does not prove the psychotropic is the cause but suspicion is raised, particularly if the patient:

- Has been recently started on the psychotropic
- Has been on high doses
- Has had the dose recently increased
- Is on one of the medications listed in Table 17.14.

If continued psychotropic medication is clinically necessary, it is generally wise to change medications and, when possible, change to a medication with a low potential for seizure induction. If no alternative exists, or other alternatives are clinically ineffective, the clinician may have no choice but to restart the potential offending medication. If so, begin at low doses, increasing slowly. If possible, the clinician should aim for a lower final target maintenance dose, at least for several months, to observe for further seizure activity. If no further seizures occur within 90 days and the lower maintenance dose is clinically insufficient, the dose can gradually be raised to the previously effective level. In this clinical situation, written informed consent must be obtained from the patient, describing the acknowledged risk of seizure. In the chart, the clinician should document the lack of available alternatives and the clinical decision-making process.

References

1   Preskorn SH *et al*. Physician perceptions of drug–drug interactions and how to avoid them. *J Psychiatric Pract* 2002;8(2):112–115.

2   DeVane CL and Nemeroff CB. 2002 guide to psychotropic drug interactions. *Primary Psychiatry* 2002;9(3):28–57.

3   Strouse TB. Interactions between psychotropics and other prescription medications: a focus on antidepressants. *Essent Psychopharmacol* 2001;4(1):1–22.

4   Ogasawara H *et al*. Simultaneous measurement of venlafaxine and its major metabolite. *Clin Chem* 1999;47:1061–1067.

5   Martin TG. Serotonin syndrome. *Ann Emerg Med* 1996;28:520–526.

6   Mills K. Serotonin syndrome. *Am Fam Physician* 1995;52:1475–1482.

7   Brown T *et al*. Pathophysiology and management of serotonin syndrome. *Ann Pharmacother* 1996;30:527–532.

8 Lappin RI and Auchincloss EL. Treatment of the serotonin syndrome with cyproheptadine. *N Engl J Med* 1994;331:1021–1022.

9 Shader RI and Greenblatt DJ. Belladonna alkaloids and synthetic anticholinergics; uses and toxicity. In: RI Shader (ed.) *Psychiatric Complications of Medical Drugs*. Raven Press, 1972, pp. 102–147.

10 Shader RI and Greenblatt DJ. Clinical implications of benzodiazepine pharmacokinetics. *Am J Psychiatry* 1977;134:642–645.

11 Tune L. Serum levels of anticholinergic drugs in treatment of acute extrapyramidal side effects. *Arch Gen Psychiatry* 1980;37:293–297.

12 Hidalgo HA and Mowers RM. Anticholinergic drug abuse. *Ann Pharmacother* 1990;24:40–41.

13 Adcock EW. Cyclopentolate (Cyclogyl) toxicity in pediatric patients. *Pediatr Pharmacol Ther* 1971;79:127–129.

14 Ananth JV and Jain RC. Benztropine psychosis. *Can Psychiatr Assoc J* 1973;18:409–414.

15 Granacher RP and Baldessarini RJ. Physostigmine: its use in acute anticholinergic syndrome with antidepressant and antiparkinson drugs. *Arch Gen Psychiatry* 1975;32:375–382.

16 Greenblatt DJ and Shader RI. Anticholinergics. *N Engl J Med* 1973;288:1215–1219.

17 Duvoisin RC and Katz R. Reversal of central anticholinergics syndrome in man by physostigmine. *JAMA* 1968;206:1963–1965.

18 Aggrawal A. Lithium toxicity – a review. *Anil Aggrawal's Internet Journal of Forensic Medicine and Toxicology* 2000;1(2).

19 At http://www.vh.org/providers/conferences/CPS/32.html

20 Haddad LM and Winchester TF. *Clinical Management of Poisoning and Drug Overdose*, 2nd edn. WB Saunders, 1990, p. 658.

21 Groleau G. Lithium toxicity. *Emerg Med Clin North Am* 1994;12:511.

22 Hansen HE and Amdisen A. Lithium intoxication (report of 23 cases and review of 100 cases from the literature). *Q J Med* 1978;47:123.

23 El-Mallakh RS. Acute lithium neurotoxicity. *Psychiatric Dev* 1986;4:311–328.

24 Krishel S and Jackimczyk K. Cyclic antidepressants, lithium, and neuroleptic agents. Pharmacology and toxicology. *Emerg Med Clin North Am* 1991;9:53.

25 Kech PE and McElroy SL. Clinical pharmacodynamics and pharmacokinetics of antimanic and mood stabilizing medication. *J Clin Psychiatry* 2002;63(suppl. 4).

26 Thomsen K and Schou M. Renal lithium excretion in man. *Am J Physiol* 1968;215:823–827.

27 Glassman A and Bitter JT. Antipsychotic drug: prolonged QTc interval, torsades de pointes and sudden death. *Am J Psychiatry* 2001;158:1774–1782.

28 Gelenberg A. Ziprasidone (Geodon). *Biol Ther Psychiatry* 2001;24(6):21–22.

29 Woosley RL. Drugs that prolong the QT interval and/or induce torsades de pointes. www.qtdrugs.org September 2002. Used with permission.

30 Marsden CD and Jenner P. The pathophysiology of extrapyramidal side-effects of neuroleptic drugs. *Psychol Med* 1980;10:55–72.

31 Ayd FJ. A survey of drug-induced extrapyramidal reactions. *JAMA* 1961;175:1054–1060.

32 Tarsy D. Neuroleptic-induced extrapyramidal reactions: classification, description, and diagnosis. *Clin Neuropharmacol* 1983;6:9–26.

33 Gelenberg AJ. Treating extrapyramidal reactions. *Biol Ther Psychiatry* 1983;6:13–16.

34 Gelenberg AJ. Treating extrapyramidal reactions: some current issues. *J Clin Psychiatry* 1987;9(suppl.):24–27.

35 Addonizio G and Alexopoulos GS. Drug-induced dystonia in young and elderly patients. *Am J Psychiatry* 1988;145:869–871.

36 Swett C. Drug-induced dystonia. *Am J Psychiatry* 1975;132:532–534.

37 Sheppard C and Merlis S. Drug-induced extrapyramidal symptoms: their incidence and treatment. *Am J Psychiatry* 1967;123:886–889.

38 Man PL. Long-term effects of haloperidol. *Dis Nerv Sys* 1973;34:113–118.

39 Boyer WF *et al.* Anticholinergic prophylaxis of acute haloperidol induced acute dystonic reactions. *J Clin Psychopharmacol* 1987;7:164–166.

40 Miller CH *et al.* The prevalence and severity of acute extrapyramidal side effects in patients treated with clozapine, risperidone or conventional antipsychotics. *New Research Program and Abstracts of the 149th Annual Meeting of the American Psychiatric Association, May 8, 1996, New York.* Abstract NR542:217–218.

41 Rosebush PI and Mazurek MF. Neurologic side effects in neuroleptic-naïve patients treated with haloperidol or risperidone. *Neurology* 1999;52:782–785.

42 Kapur S *et al.* Clinical and theoretical implications of 5-HT$_2$ and D$_2$ receptor occupancy of clozapine, risperidone and olanzapine in schizophrenia. *Am J Psychiatry* 1999;156:286–293.

43 Donlon PT and Stenson RL. Neuroleptic induced extrapyramidal symptoms. *Dis Nerv Sys* 1976;37:629–635.

44 Chouinard G *et al.* Long-term effects of l-dopa and procyclidine on neuroleptic-induced extrapyramidal and schizophrenic symptoms. *Psychopharmacol Bull* 1987;23:221–226.

45 Friis T *et al.* Sodium valproate and biperiden in neuroleptic-induced akathisia, parkinsonism and hyperkinesias. *Acta Psychiatr Scand* 1983;67:178–187.

46 Fann WE and Lake CR. Amantadine versus trihexyphenidyl in the treatment of neuroleptic-induced parkinsonism. *Am J Psychiatry* 1976;133:940–943.

47 Borison RL. Amantadine in the management of extrapyramidal side effects. *Clin Neuropharmacol* 1983;6(suppl.):S57–S63.

48 Gagrat D *et al.* Intravenous diazepam in the treatment of neuroleptic-induced acute dystonia and akathisia. *Am J Psychiatry* 1978;135:1232–1233.

49 Caroff SN *et al.* Atypical antipsychotics and neuroleptic malignant syndrome. *Psychiatric Ann* 2000;30:314–321.

50 Velamoor VR *et al.* Progression of symptoms in neuroleptic malignant syndrome. *J Nervous Mental Dis* 1994;182:168–173.

51 Caroff SN and Mann SC. Neuroleptic malignant syndrome. *Med Clin North Am* 1993;77:185–202.

52 Caroff SN and Mann SC. Neuroleptic malignant syndrome. *Psychopharmacol Bull* 1988;24:25–29.

53 Neuroleptic Malignant Syndrome Information Service, at www.nmsis.org/general_information.shtml

54 Davis JM *et al*. Electroconvulsive therapy in the treatment of the neuroleptic malignant syndrome. *Convulsive Ther* 1991;7:111–120.

55 Serfertova D. Treatment of the neuroleptic malignant syndrome by electroconvulsive therapy. *Biol Psychiatry* 1997;42:1835.

56 Brasic JR and Borenson B. Tardive dyskinesia. Published on the Internet eMedicine Journal 2002;2(2), at www.emedicine.com/neuro/topic262/html/

57 Goetz DG. Tardive dyskinesia. In: RL Watts and WC Koller (eds), *Movement Disorders: Neurologic Principles and Practice*. 1997, pp. 519–526.

58 Sherr JD. The prevention and management of tardive dyskinesia in the elderly. *Psychiatric Ann* 2002;32(4):237–243.

59 Beasley CM *et al*. Olanzapine versus placebo: results of a double-blind, fixed dose olanzapine trial. *Psychopharmacology* 1996;124:159–167.

60 Ereshefsky L *et al*. Clozapine: an atypical antipsychotic agent. *Clin Pharm* 1991;8:691–709.

61 Lieberman JA *et al*. Clozapine guidelines for clinical management. *J Clin Psychiatry* 1989;50:329–338.

62 Safferman AZ *et al*. Update on the clinical efficacy and side effects of clozapine. *Schizophrenia Bull* 1991;17:247–261.

63 Safferman AZ *et al*. Clozapine and akathisia [letter]. *Biol Psychiatry* 1992;31:749–754.

64 Cohen LJ. Risperidone. *Pharmacotherapy* 1994;14:263–265.

65 Chouinard G *et al*. A Canadian multicenter placebo-controlled study of fixed doses of risperidone and haloperidol in the treatment of chronic schizophrenic patients. *J Clin Psychopharmacol* 1993;13:25–40.

66 Casey DE. Tardive dyskinesia and atypical antipsychotic drugs. *Schizophrenia Res* 1999;35:561–566.

67 Driesens F. Neuroleptic medication facilitates the natural occurrence of tardive dyskinesia. A critical review. *Acta Psychiatr Belg* 1998,88:195–205.

68 Alexander B and Lund B. Tardive dyskinesia. Published on the Internet Virtual Hospital 1999, at www.vh.org/providers/conferences/CPS/08.html

69 Jus A *et al*. Epidemiology of tardive dyskinesia, part 2. *Dis Nerv Syst* 1976;37:257–261.

70 Kane JM *et al*. Tardive dyskinesia: prevalence, incidence and risk factors. *J Clin Psychopharmacol* 1988;8:52S–56S.

71 Graham PM *et al*. Combination monoamine oxidase inhibitor/TCA interaction. [letter]. *Lancet* 1982;2:440.

72 White K and Simpson G. The combined use of MAOIs and tricyclics. *J Clin Psychiatry* 1984;45:67–69.

73 Grossman E *et al*. Should a moratorium be placed on sublingual nifedipine capsules given for hypertensive emergencies and pseudoemergencies? *JAMA* 1996;276:1328–1331.

74 Cates M and Powers R. Concommitant rash and blood dyscrasia in geriatric psychiatry patients treated with carbamazepine. *Ann Pharmacother* 1998;32(9);884–887.

75 Garcia-Pando AC *et al*. Hepatotoxicity associated with new antidepressants. *J Clin Psychiatry* 2002;63(2):135–137.

76 *The Maudsley 2001 Prescribing Guidelines*, pp. 120–124.

77 *British National Formulary* 43rd edn. British Medical Association, 2002, p. 189.

78 Pisani F *et al*. Effect of psychotropic drugs on seizure threshold. *Drug Safety* 2002;25(2):91–110.

79 Janicak TG *et al. Principles and Practice of Psychopharmacotherapy*, 2nd edn. Williams & Wilkins, 1997, p. 195.

80 Gross A *et al*. Psychotropic medication use in patients with epilepsy: effect on seizure frequency. *J Neuropsychiatry Clin Neurosci* 2000;12(4):458–464.

81 Davidson J. Seizures and bupropion: a review. *J Clin Psychiatry* 1989; 50:256–261.

Chapter 18

Medication allergies

Although allergic responses to psychotropic medications are fundamentally no different to allergic responses to any other medication, it is helpful to review the management principles of allergic reactions as they present to the prescriber of mental health prescriptions.

An allergic reaction to a medication can occur:

■   With **ANY** medication,
■   At **ANY** time,
■   With **ANY** practitioner.

Such reactions can occur regardless of the purpose for prescribing, the dosage, the length of time the patient has been taking the medication, or the practitioner's skill level. Therefore, the clinician always must be aware of the possibility of allergic reactions when medications are being prescribed.

While allergic reactions often occur within the first 30 days of usage, allergic responses can occur at a much later date, even after several years of treatment. Although allergic responses are more likely to occur when medication dosages are increased, they may also occur when doses have not changed. Unfortunately, allergic responses may occur when the medication is helping the patient considerably, although they also occur when there is little therapeutic response.

Identification of allergic responses

Patients will both underestimate and overestimate the occurrence of an allergy. While often believing they know what an allergy is and how it might present, patients are not always correct and may overlook a true allergy unless it is identified for them. There are also many individuals who have a heightened sensitivity to allergies and assume that any adverse effect that occurs from a medication is an "allergy." A commonly mistaken example is often found with traditional antipsychotics. Patients who experience extrapyramidal symptoms (EPS) have often labeled themselves as being "allergic" to traditional antipsychotics, when in fact they are not allergic at all. They have experienced a significant and unpleasant side effect, but it is not an allergic reaction. Distinguishing a side effect from an allergy is significant in that side effects can be managed and may be temporary, permitting the patient to continue taking the medication. Most allergies, however, do not resolve with time, and, when severe, may present life-threatening symptoms. Therefore, when a patient is experiencing a true medication allergy, that patient should discontinue the medication and, in general, not be rechallenged.

Some patients do have true multiple drug and food allergies. For those patients who are, in fact, allergic to many different medications, a gradual institution of small doses of medications will lessen the likelihood of a dramatic allergic reaction that might ensue if a full dose is given initially. Other individuals have labeled themselves "allergy prone," and will often describe a long list of allergies in the initial evaluation interview. Even if it is the clinician's assessment that many of these "allergies" are really side effects, such patients are anxious about starting a medication. Generally, they are reassured if any new medication is started in very small doses. By doing so, the clinician recognizes the patient's sensitivities to medications.

Typical medication allergy symptoms are listed in Table 18.1.

The core allergic symptom is a rash. It is often itchy and reddened and may or may not be raised. Drug allergies typically begin centrally, that is on the trunk, and spread to the extremities. The spread of the rash may occur over several hours or several days. Typically, the rash does not remain confined to one extremity or one area. Rashes that affect only a small area of the skin and do not spread are often of another cause. Similarly, a rash with a sharply defined circumscribed pattern may not be a true drug allergy (for example, a rash that occurs

---

Table 18.1 Common allergy symptoms

- Rash – starts centrally and spreads
- Itchiness
- Reddened skin
- Urticaria (hives)
- Swelling/edema
- Respiratory distress, in more serious allergic reactions

only in those areas exposed to sunlight may be a sun sensitivity, not an allergy). Rashes confined to an area solely covered by clothing may be the result of allergy to soap products or to the material in the clothing.

In addition to a rash, the patient may have urticaria or hives. Hives are large blotchy spots that itch, may have variable diameters, and may be present with or without a finer rash.

Swelling and edema of various body parts often accompanies a rash and urticaria. Such swelling can occur around the eyes and face, and there may be dependent edema in the ankles.

Certain patients, sometimes fueled by practitioners who specialize in "allergic problems" or "environmental sensititivity," will believe that allergies are the cause for behavioral symptoms, psychiatric illness or mental reactions. While true allergies may not be totally ruled out, if the patient's symptoms do not include at least one of those identified in Table 18.1, the presence of a true medication allergy should be highly suspect. In general, within our current state of knowledge, mental health symptoms and syndromes are not primarily allergic in origin.

Management of allergy symptoms

The practitioner's response to possible allergy symptoms is summarized in Table 18.2.

Of primary importance is that the practitioner be able to observe directly the rash and/or urticaria. Based on the previous discussion, it may be relatively apparent, when seen, whether or not the rash is likely a drug allergy. The patient should be seen as soon as possible by the practitioner, particularly if he or she is telephoning with complaints suggestive of an allergic response. Small or very circumscribed rashes can often be ruled out as being unlikely to be due to drug allergies simply by inspection. On the other hand, significant and spreading rashes, which can occur from a drug allergy, can also be highly suspected solely through observation. When in the office, the patient should be asked to disrobe only sufficiently to allow the practitioner to see some of the affected areas. If the rash is present on the breast, groin or buttocks areas in either sex, and these areas need to be observed, it is safest to have another staff member present when the observation is made.

Table 18.2 Drug allergy assessment and treatment

- Examine the rash directly
- If a drug allergy is a likely cause, stop the offending medication as soon as possible
- Give diphenhydramine (Benadryl) 25–100 mg daily by mouth. An alternative would be Loratadine (Claritin) 10 mg/day
- Suggest a tepid bath or damp cloth soaks and, if necessary, a topical steroid cream for the rash
- Do not start any replacement medication until the allergy symptoms are resolved, unless the mental health target symptoms create an emergency

---

Other issues of evaluation when allergy is suspected

At the time of the observation of the rash, the patient should be questioned about any changes in foods, and about other over-the-counter preparations, prescription medications or lifestyle changes within the several weeks prior to the emergence of the rash. Even when a drug allergy is likely identified, it may turn out that it is not the psychotropic medication prescribed that is the cause. Other substances to which the patient is exposed – fabrics, detergents, colognes, foods, new over-the-counter compounds, or prescriptions written by other practitioners – may also be responsible for the allergy diagnosed.

The patient should also be specifically questioned about the presence of shortness of breath, wheezing, or difficulty breathing.

DANGER
Any breathing difficulties observed by the clinician or described by the patient constitute a potential emergency. *Such patients should be sent directly to the emergency room for assessment of breathing capacity, and need for oxygen and/or mechanical ventilation.*

While the rash and urticaria may be uncomfortable, the potentially lethal outcome in an allergic reaction is respiratory arrest. While respiratory problems from medication allergy are not routine, when present they are of immediate concern.

Stopping the offending medication

If it is the assessment of the practitioner that a drug allergy is present, the medication should be stopped immediately. Strong, uncomfortable rashes, large areas of urticaria, and/or breathing problems mandate that any offending medication be stopped, even from a relatively high dose, risking the possibility of rebound symptoms. If the symptoms are minimal, tolerable, no breathing problems are present, and the medication is one that could precipitate a discontinuation syndrome (see Chapter 8), a rapid taper can be somewhat more comfortable for the patient. In any case, the medication should be stopped quickly.

If allergy symptoms are questionable, assume it is a drug allergy until proven otherwise. From a medicolegal viewpoint, it is much safer for a practitioner to stop a medication on the assumption that an allergy is present, and discover later that it was not. The riskier course would be to continue a medication only to learn that a patient is truly allergic and have possible serious symptoms ensue.

Allergic reactions will subside within several days to a week. Even the most severe allergic reaction should be totally resolved within a 10-day period. Many patients require little or no treatment during this period, other than having the offending medication removed. For some patients, however, itchiness can be quite uncomfortable and can disrupt sleep. For these patients, the use of 25–100 mg diphenhydramine or another antihistamine daily will minimize the discomfort. *Tepid* baths or tepid, moist cloth soaks on areas of urticaria and rash will also diminish the itchiness. Hot baths or soaks will likely aggravate the rash. For particularly uncomfortable rashes, betamethasone 0.5% topical cream or a similar agent may be used.

What else to do

Documentation of the allergy, and of the practitioner's response to it, is crucial to good medical practice and may prevent any allegation of mismanagement. The clinician should document, in writing: *the symptoms described* by complaint and/or on examination; *when* the patient *made* the clinician *aware* of these symptoms; *when* the patient was *seen in person* and *by whom*; and *what recommendations* were made regarding treatment and/or further assessment.

Following an initial evaluation in which medication allergies are suspected or confirmed, the clinician should be in contact with the patient within several days to ask whether the symptoms are improving, and document the follow-up contact. If it is not convenient to have a face-to-face follow-up evaluation and the allergic reaction is mild, a telephone assessment is satisfactory as long as documentation is completed.

If the clinician assesses that a drug allergy to his or her prescription has occurred, the patient should be clearly informed that this was a drug allergy and advised that this medication should not be taken again. The appropriate portion of the patient's chart should be labeled for future reference. Some facilities or practitioners will paste a brightly colored stick-on to the front of the chart noting any allergies. Another useful tool is to make a list of patient allergies on the patient's medication list. Thus, when going to document any new medication or prescription, it is easy for the clinician to glance at these medicines to which the patient is allergic and avoid. Although resolution of the allergic symptoms with discontinuation does not prove the connection, it is usually assumed to be true.

In unusual circumstances (e.g. another more likely cause than the psychotropic is discovered for the symptoms, or the clinician feels the patient must be re-tried on this medication for lack of viable alternatives), a rechallenge with the suspected offending agent may be tried. If attempted, the drug should be re-introduced very gradually, with frequent clinical re-evaluation for the onset of rash, urticaria or respiratory difficulties. If the symptoms recur, the rechallenge is generally abandoned.

Pills contain more than just the active ingredient

Some patients are allergic to dyes, additives, food coloring, flavoring or preservatives used in the preparation of capsules or pills, but not to the psychoactive compound. A particularly common allergy is to tartrazine (FD&C yellow #5). A recent study[1] showed that approximately 3.8 percent of patients exposed to tartrazine-containing compounds developed allergic reactions. These allergic reactions subside within 24–48 hours after stopping the tartrazine and none of these patients showed allergy to non-tartrazine containing brands. A history of aspirin sensitivity is a marker toward possible tartrazine sensitivity, as *tartrazine allergy occurs in 13.2 percent of those with aspirin sensitivity.*

DANGER
Aspirin sensitivity may predict tartrazine allergies. Medications containing tartrazine should be relegated to second-line treatment in such patients. If chosen, small doses should be used initially and frequent follow-up ensured.

The identification of tartrazine allergies is important, since the patient may not be truly allergic to the underlying psychotropic compound. Such a patient may be changed to a different preparation or a different brand of the same psychotropic that does not include tartrazine, and may well be able to tolerate the psychotropic drug. Another strategy is to investigate whether other pill strengths of the same brand are manufactured without the dye. For example, a patient who is sensitive to the 150-mg strength pill that contains tartrazine, could, perhaps, take three 50-mg pills that do not contain the dye.

Reference

1   Bhatia MS. Allergy to tartrazine in psychotropic drugs. *J Clin Psychiatry* 2000;61:7.

Part V Competent Clinical Practice

Chapter 19

Misuse of medication - taking too much and taking too little

Despite our best efforts and conscientious practice, patients don't always take medications as prescribed. In order to properly assess and manage this problem, it is important to distinguish several key terms, and understand how they overlap or are distinct. While overutilization of medication is generally of more urgent concern to the clinician, underusage of medication can also occur and will be discussed later in the chapter.

Misuse of medication occurs in every clinical setting and in every practitioner's practice. No setting is immune. Particularly high-risk populations for medication misuse include:

- Predominantly adolescent populations, especially if adolescents are housed together
- Patients with personality disorders, particularly with sociopathic or borderline traits
- Forensic settings, such as prison or the penitentiary
- People who abuse alcohol, recreational drugs or other substances.

It is a common misconception that if the patient takes too much medication it is abuse, and the clinician has been deceived. This is not always the case, and knowing the various categories of overuse will help the clinician to understand when, and when not, to be concerned. Table 19.1 will serve as an outline for important terms and a framework for this chapter.

Misuse of medication is a general term describing the use of medication in an unauthorized or non-recommended manner. Misuse may be chronic or acute, accidental or intentional, and involve overusage or underusage. It may or may not include withdrawal or tolerance. It may be a part of "self-treatment" and a belief on the part of patients that they know what is "right" for them and what they "need," regardless of what the clinician prescribes. Patients' misuse of medications may occur in an effort to self-treat a psychiatric symptom or physical symptom. It may be a part of universal feelings about medications in general, be related to psychotropic medications only, or be limited to one particular medication. Misuse may be rationalized by patients ("if one pill is good, then four pills must be better"), or come from a belief about their physiological tolerance to medication ("I always need more medication than everyone else"). The broadest subtypes of misuse involve *overutilization* (using more medication than the clinician prescribes) and *underutilization* (using less medication than the clinician prescribes).

Overutilization may be accidental and unrealized by patients. On the other hand, it may be a conscious decision on their part to take excessive amounts of drug. This can lead to an excess of medication that may occur gradually over a period of time ("*chronic overdose*"), and sometimes leads to gradually increasing signs of medication intoxication. Overdose may also occur all at once in an intentional ingestion of a large amount of medications for various reasons (referred to, in this text, as an *acute overdose*).

Substance abuse is a maladaptive pattern of medication usage manifested by recurrent and significant adverse consequences related to the use of a substance or

---

Table 19.1 Misuse of medication

Overutilization of medication
1   Accidental overusage:
- From carelessness
- By persons who believe they are following directions
- "Chronic overdose"
2   Intentional overusage:
- Acute overdose
- Substance abuse
- Substance dependence (addiction)

Underutilization of medication
- Because of fear
- As a symptom of the illness being treated
- Because the patient can't afford the medication

Separate clinical issues that may overlap with misuse
- Physiological (physical) dependence
- Intoxication

medication. There may be physical debilitation, a decrease in school/work performance, neglect of family duties, legal problems, or other behavioral reactions accompanying substance abuse, but continued use of the medication occurs despite having persistent and recurrent social or interpersonal problems. *The term "substance abuse" does not automatically include physical tolerance, withdrawal, or a pattern of compulsive use; instead it includes only the harmful consequences of repeated usage.*[1]

Substance dependence (commonly referred to as "addiction") not only shows a pattern of repeated self-administration of a drug, but also results in physical tolerance, compulsive drug-taking behavior, and withdrawal when the medication is stopped. There may be a pattern of cognitive, behavioral and physiological reactions that result as the person continues to use increasing amounts of medication.[1]

Physical tolerance (the need for increased amounts of medication to achieve intoxication or the desired effect, or a diminished effect with continued use of the same amount of the substance) is common in substance dependence. Physical tolerance is, however, neither a necessary nor a sufficient condition to warrant the diagnosis of substance dependence (addiction). Similarly, *withdrawal*[1] (a maladaptive behavioral change with physiological and cognitive components, which occurs when blood or tissue concentrations of a substance decline in an individual who has maintained prolonged heavy use of the substance) also may or may not be present in a person with substance dependence. Persons with substance dependence often use the substance in larger amounts over a long period of time. They spend a great deal of time obtaining the substance, using it, or recovering from its effects. Often their daily activities revolve around obtaining, using or withdrawing from the use of the substance. They often have marked social, recreational, and occupational changes because of substance use. They may express a desire to decrease or regulate the amount that they use, and often have many unsuccessful attempts to decrease or stop using. Despite recognizing the pattern of usage in their overall life and the negative consequences thereof, they are unable or unwilling to discontinue use. *The crucial component of substance dependence is not overusage, but the inability to abstain from using despite having ample evidence that continued use is harmful.*

Physiological dependence (a physiological state that occurs when the individual has taken doses of medication for a long enough period of time that when the medication is stopped, symptoms of physiological withdrawal occur) is not automatically a sign of drug abuse, substance abuse, or inappropriate practice by the clinician or the patient. *Physiological dependence is a physical state based on usage of medication at a high enough dose for a long enough period of time.* It does not necessarily translate into substance abuse if it occurs from conscious rational decisions, made in partnership between the clinician and the patient, in order to treat certain psychiatric or medical problems. For example, a patient with chronic anxiety disorder treated over a long time with a benzodiazepine may become physically dependent on the medication (i.e. withdrawal will occur when the drug is stopped suddenly), but the patient does not necessarily abuse the medication.

Intoxication is a substance-specific syndrome that occurs shortly after ingestion of a substance, and may include symptoms of maladaptive behavioral and psychological changes, including impaired cognitive abilities, judgment, coordination, social or work functioning as well as perceptual changes and belligerence. The manifestations can vary greatly between individuals, and may depend on the substance ingested and the setting in which it occurs.[1] Intoxication can occur acutely or chronically.

How medication misuse presents

Evidence of medication misuse may present to the clinician from a variety of sources:

- By the patient volunteering a report
- On direct questioning by the clinician
- From investigating side effects and how the patient is dealing with them
- By an urgent telephone call from the patient saying, "I took too much"
- From emergency room staff or other medical clinic personnel treating your patient
- Via reports from a family member, caretaker or friend who is concerned about the patient's behavior
- After the clinician observes symptoms such as slurred speech, irregular gait, or sedation
- High serum blood levels of a medication on a laboratory report
- From a pharmacist's call requesting early renewal of a prescription by the patient.
- After the fact, when the overusage is no longer occurring

Whatever the reason, when a clinician becomes aware that the patient is taking too much medication, he or she must assess the cause, document the assessment, and take action.

Accidental and careless overutilization

Many confused, anxious, elderly, or visually impaired patients may accidentally take too much medication – occasionally or chronically. Patients with poor memory may not realize that they have already taken a dose, or may be oblivious to how much medication they have taken. Some patients will confuse various medications they are taking, overutilizing one medication and underutilizing another. Patients with visual problems may confuse one pill or pill bottle for another. Some patients feel that medications can be taken "whenever I need it," and do not keep track of how often they are dosing themselves. Patients who use medications along with alcohol or street drugs can become further confused and, when intoxicated, misuse their medications unintentionally.

If it is determined that the patient is accidentally but carelessly taking too much medication, resulting in chronic overdose:

- The clinician should verbally reinforce the specific instructions as to how much and how often the medication should be taken.
- Written instructions should be reissued and the patient educated about the risks of continued overutilization.
- The clinician may wish to use the help of family members – a spouse, parent, adult or child – to oversee the usage of medication. Elderly, confused patients, or minors who are overutilizing medication, may need supervision, with the responsibility of medication administration delegated to another person.
- The use of a "pill minder," in which pills can be filled into a partitioned container organized by days of the week and time, can often help forgetful patients to know whether or not they have taken their doses. These may also be useful for any patient who takes chronic medication, particularly with complicated regimens of medication.
- Patients with visual problems should have an optometric exam, use a magnifying glass and/or use color-coded bottles for their medications.

Accidental overdose when patients believe they are following instructions

Despite written instructions, repetition, and education, many patients still misunderstand instructions for dosing psychotropics. In some cases, patients may have left the clinician's office correctly understanding directions, but may be told by other family members or healthcare professionals that they should change their psychotropic dosage, and do so without contacting the prescriber. Occasionally, the patient is given the wrong pill from the pharmacy or the medication is mislabeled. The patient follows the instructions, not knowing they are incorrect.

In these circumstances, the clinician should re-emphasize the correct instructions or re-issue a correct, written schedule of dosing. If necessary, the patient or a family member should bring the pill bottle or read the label over the telephone. It may be necessary to call the pharmacy to verify that the correct medication, in the correct dosage, has been dispensed. If incorrect instructions are coming from the family or another healthcare provider, the clinician should contact that party to explain the rationale for the dosing schedule and ask that future dosing matters be left solely to the prescribing clinician, so as to eliminate confusion for the patient.

Intentional overdose

When the patient is not suicidal

When patients intentionally take a large dose of medication, their conscious (or unconscious) intent may not always be to harm themselves. Other reasons that patients may intentionally take a large amount of medication include:

1   To treat intolerable symptoms such as:
    - Insomnia
    - Excruciating anxiety
    - Emotional pain
    - Physical pain
    - Hallucinations.
2   To show anger or make a point ("I'll show you"). This may be part of an argument, and often occurs impulsively.
3   To attempt to make someone feel guilty ("You'll be sorry"). Although most often this is a family member, a boyfriend/girlfriend or a spouse, occasionally it may be the clinician!
4   To escape temporarily from what is perceived as an intolerable situation ("I just wanted to get away from it all and sleep").
5   For psychotic reasons. For example, patients may feel that by taking a large amount of medication they can escape delusional persecution, observation or taunting. They may also be responding to command hallucinations.

With suicidal intent

Suicide is a complex phenomenon with many facets, and the causes of suicide vary among cultures. Attempted or completed suicide through self-poisoning by ingestion of medications is a common methodology worldwide. By definition, when prescribing psychotropic medications to a patient the prescriber has enabled one of the risk factors for suicide (easy access to lethal toxins – prescription medications).[2] While it is beyond the scope of this book to explore all the causative, evaluative, and risk factors involved in suicide, this section explores the practical issues facing the practitioner when a current medication patient presents having possibly intentionally overdosed on medication.

On occasion, the patient appears in person directly after taking an intentional overdose. More commonly, the clinician receives an emergency telephone call after hours. The recommended evaluation procedure for the medicating clinician, whether on the telephone or in person, is to do a brief screening of the patient's condition, including any elements of physical danger, patient lucidity, and ability to communicate. Questions that should be asked at this time are:

- How much of your psychotropic medication did you take?
- When did you take the medication?
- Did you take any other prescription medicines with the psychotropic?

■ Did you take any alcohol or other street drugs with the medication?
■ Are you having trouble breathing?
■ What, if any symptoms, do you have now?
■ Are you feeling sleepy?
■ Have you vomited, or do you feel like vomiting?
■ Are you having trouble walking or performing other coordinated actions?
■ Are you feeling dizzy, lightheaded or faint?
■ Is anyone else present with you now?

If the patient is sufficiently alert and the clinician is not current with the patient's other possible medical conditions or medication regimens, the clinician should ask about the presence of any other medical problems and regularly taken non-psychotropic medications. Responses to the above questions in a lucid patient will dictate the clinician's immediate response. Any patient who cannot speak clearly and/or respond to initial questions presents a medical emergency. An urgent evaluation and/or transportation to an emergency room setting should be arranged for any patient who cannot respond clearly or sounds intoxicated.

Serious overdose

Because of potential serious medical sequelae, overdoses that include the following psychotropic medications should *always* have emergency medical clearance through face-to-face evaluation:

■ MAO inhibitors
■ Tricyclic antidepressants
■ Lithium
■ Bupropion.

Physical signs which, when present, should concern the clinician and necessitate a face-to-face evaluation, include:

■ Slurred speech
■ Fluctuating level of consciousness
■ Inability to remain awake
■ Mental confusion.

Other situations that mandate a medical evaluation include:

■ A mixed medication overdose with more than one prescription medication, or prescription medication plus an over-the-counter compound
■ Medication overdose mixed with alcohol, recreational drugs, or toxins
■ Any patient who cannot convince the clinician that the amount of medication ingested was small
■ When the patient is vague, manipulative, or gamey

- Any overdose with more than three times the daily dose of medication
- Any patient who is excessively worried and cannot be reassured. (For medicolegal reasons, it is generally safer to have such a patient evaluated than have the clinician assume full burden of responsibility, even if the risk is small.)

If a patient or a family member calls about an overdose, and the clinician cannot get a clear and convincing response that the overdose is minor, the patient should be sent to the emergency room or medical clinic for medical clearance. It is always better to be safe than sorry. With any serious overdose, in addition to arranging for the patient to go for medical evaluation, the clinician should assure that safe transportation is available. This can be another driver or a taxicab. If there is concern about the patient's ability to get to the hospital without further symptoms, call 911 for emergency ambulance transportation (999 in the UK).

Once the patient has been instructed to get to an emergency evaluation and transportation has been assured, the clinician should call the emergency room or clinic to provide historical data obtained from the patient or family, and any pertinent history from the patient's record. Once the patient has arrived and has been evaluated, the emergency staff should be asked to call the clinician with the results of their evaluation. The *time* of the first contact and when notification of the overdose was received must be recorded by the clinician, along with the results of his or her evaluation and recommendations made for treatment or evaluation, including emergency room referral, if made. Documentation of any follow-up care that is to be provided based on the emergency room's evaluation, should also be recorded.

Minor overdose

A healthy patient

- without the presence of a medical disorder
- in the absence of alcohol or illicit drugs
- in the absence of other medications
- who is not alone
- who did not ingest a high risk medication

can generally tolerate up to two to three times the usual daily dose of many newer medications without medical sequelae. Patients who meet the above criteria may have some increased side effects, but these are generally not life-threatening ones. SSRI antidepressants, other new generation antidepressants, typical and atypical antipsychotics, and benzodiazepines in minor amounts may cause sleepiness, gastrointestinal upset, or a confused feeling. As long as such patients are observed and are not alone, they generally do not need emergency care. If more than 6 hours have passed since the patient ingested the overdose and there are no side effects, it is unlikely that there will be any further effects.

Following such a minor overdose, if the clinician intends to continue the patient on the medicine prescribed, he or she should hold at least one dose, order the next scheduled dose at half the usual amount, and then resume regular dosing.

Using too little medication

While generally less urgently significant than taking too much medication, taking less medication than prescribed may lead to inadequate therapeutic effect, and partial or sporadic response. Reasons why patients take less medication than the clinician prescribes include:

■ Fear of excessive response ("it will control me," "change me," or "make me feel something I don't want to feel")
■ Fear of side effects
■ As a symptom of the illness being treated – patients with panic disorder or obsessive–compulsive disorder frequently catastrophize possible outcomes; they assume that medication response will be negative and seek to avoid problems by minimizing their medication dose
■ The patient feels "I'm medication sensitive"
■ The patient does not have enough money to pay for full therapeutic doses.

See Chapter 12 for a further discussion of underdosing in the geriatric patient.

Fraud and abuse with psychotropic medications

Any clinician who prescribes medications that have the potential for abuse is a potential target for patients who will fraudulently use and abuse medication. No practitioner is immune from this abuse potential. As has been described earlier, the vast majority of psychotropic medications are not abused or abusable. However, stimulants, sedative/hypnotics, benzodiazepines and anticholinergics are medications that some patients may obtain under false pretenses or use in inappropriate amounts. Although many people equate the fraudulent obtaining of prescriptions with personal drug abuse, this view is not always correct – there are exceptions. While the vast majority of patients seeking medication illegally are in fact abusing medications themselves, other reasons include:

■ Obtaining medication for sale on the street
■ Using the medications to moderate the effect of other recreational or prescribed drugs (for example, using benzodiazepines to "come down" from abuse of stimulants, or using anticholinergics to increase the "high" of narcotics)
■ Obtaining medications for others who may be abusing.

The most common methods of prescription fraud and abuse are shown in Table 19.2.

By following a few simple techniques and practices, clinicians can minimize the majority of these causes of fraudulent use of prescription medications. Any prescriber, however, no matter how diligent, will occasionally find that he or she has been fraudulently utilized.

Table 19.2 Methods of obtaining medication fraudulently
■ Altering a written prescription, particularly the number of pills dispensed
■ Falsely posing, by telephone, as a current patient in need of a refill to off-hours covering practitioners
■ Theft of blank prescriptions
■ Direct theft of medication
■ Falsely presenting symptoms that could be treated with abusable medications
■ Requesting excessive amounts of medication
■ Trading medications with others

Practitioner protections against abuse of prescription medications

To avoid prescription alteration

When stocking office supplies, alter-proof prescription pads should be ordered. While these are slightly more expensive than plain paper prescriptions, these alter-proof prescriptions will blur or smudge if there is an attempt to erase or rewrite the name of the medication or the number of pills prescribed. Any alteration is usually obvious to the pharmacist, who will often call the practitioner prior to dispensing. When writing the prescription the clinician should always clearly write the number of pills in words rather than in numbers. It is very difficult to alter the wording "dispense one hundred" whereas it is relatively easy to add a zero to "10" to make "100." It is also best to give a patient a prescription without cross-outs or alterations in the writing. If a mistake is made in writing a prescription, write it over.

Off-hours coverage issues

Most practitioners assume that the largest risk for medication abuse is altering prescriptions. While it does occur, an even more frequently practiced means of obtaining medications fraudulently occurs when somebody poses as an active patient of a clinician who is out of town or off-call. The drug-seeker will telephone requesting a renewal prescription for an abusable medication. Frequently stated reasons are that he or she has unexpectedly "run out," has had to cancel an appointment "just before" the clinician's absence, or has "lost" a prescription. If the off-hours call is for an abusable medication, this often presents a dilemma for the covering clinician. If the patient requests a large amount of medication, it is usually an ominous sign. The more clever abuser will call for smaller amounts of medications from a number of different clinicians covering the practices of multiple off-call providers. There are medication-abusing individuals who regularly and repeatedly spend weekends and holidays phoning numerous mental health practitioners fraudulently requesting "reasonable" amounts of controlled substance medications.

Remedying this situation requires the agreement of those practitioners who work together providing off-hours coverage. A ground rule for the group is that *any patient who calls off-hours for abusable medications must provide the covering prescriber with the telephone number of a pharmacy at which the regular prescriber has written a prescription that can be verified.* When the off-hours prescriber calls the pharmacy, it is an easy matter to verify if and when this patient has received previous prescriptions written by the clinician of record. If there is no record of this patient having received previous prescriptions, no medication is authorized. If the patient cannot give a pharmacy telephone number where previous prescriptions can be verified, the off-hours clinician simply refuses to prescribe any medication.

It is not uncommon for the abuser to offer a variety of excuses, such as: "I must have used a different pharmacy" or "the pharmacy I use is closed" or "I'm traveling and I need to have it filled here." In general, the off-hours clinician should ignore these excuses and simply refuse to provide medication until the primary clinician returns. On rare occasions, the covering clinician may be convinced to provide some amount of medication. If so, only enough pills should be provided to get the patient through until the regular clinician returns. Prescriptions for large amounts of abusable medications should not be written off-hours, regardless of the reasons presented. Drug-seekers can often protest strongly when refused medication, in an effort to badger the clinician. When routinely enforced, these procedures give the abuser the message that this prescriber is not vulnerable to prescription fraud. These procedures also have the benefit of reinforcing to the legitimate patient that waiting until the last minute to refill medications may be problematic.

Another common ploy of abusers is to request refills for several medications, one or more of which are non-abusable and one that may be abusable. If the clinician renews all the medications, the individual will then pick up only the abusable medication, feigning to the pharmacy that he or she lacks the money to pay for all the medications. Therefore, the above outlined guidelines should apply even if multiple medications are requested.

Since the vast number of psychotropic medications, particularly antidepressants, antipsychotics, and mood stabilizers, are generally not abused or abusable, a clinician covering for an off-duty provider can generally prescribe refills of these medications comfortably with at least enough medication until the return of the regular prescriber.

Theft of prescriptions

Simple preventative measures can easily address the issue of stolen blank prescriptions. Careful, locked storage of blank prescriptions is crucial. The clinician must take care not to leave prescription pads or blank prescriptions in easily accessible places. Common locations that are vulnerable to theft include:

- On a desk that may be available to the patient when the clinician leaves the room
- In an unlocked drawer

- In an unlocked car
- At home, in the practitioner's residence.

Despite reasonable precautions, it is still possible that prescriptions may be accidentally lost or stolen. Unfortunately there is relatively little recourse if this occurs, and missing prescriptions may fall into the hands of an abuser. When fraudulently filled out and presented for filling, a pharmacist is unlikely to recognize the problem and contact the prescriber.

The new patient who requests large amounts of abusable medicines

The clinician may be presented with a new patient requesting a large amount of an abusable medication. A typical scenario involves the patient who has recently relocated or is changing clinicians and now needs a "usual" dose of a benzodiazepine or stimulant. Some patients may ask specifically and exclusively for one particular abusable medication, refusing other non-abusable preparations. While some of these individuals are abusers, a certain number of them are legitimately seeking continuity of care. After a diagnostic evaluation, and if the request appears justified, the clinician may choose to prescribe a small amount of a controlled medication initially. It is incumbent upon the clinician at this first visit to obtain a release of information from the patient for the previously prescribing clinician. *The previous treater should be contacted before the next patient visit.* The previous prescriber can give relevant information – verifying the patient's legitimate medication profile and conscientious use of medications – or, on occasion, identify the patient as an abuser. If the patient cannot provide the name of a previous clinician or verifiable treatment information, the clinician should be quite cautious in prescribing abusable medications, and may refuse to do so at all. Regardless of the new patient's request, as with any treatment plan, it is not reasonable to prescribe large amounts of abusable medication with many refills, or to provide a long-term prescription without regular follow-up appointments to assess the patient's response and continued need.

The development of abuse

Some patients who begin using habit-forming medication during appropriate prescription may gradually slip into abuse. When this begins to occur, behaviors will emerge that suggest to the clinician that this problematic situation is developing. Common tip-offs include:

1 *Frequent early requests for renewal* of medication. This practice may initially occur with refill requests a few days early, but can worsen to the stage where requests come weeks or months early. The patient will have a rationale for needing an early renewal, such as the pills having been destroyed, lost, or damaged.
2 *Frequently missed appointments* with telephone contact (often after hours) requesting medication refills. Patients who are abusing medication may try to avoid face-to-face contact.
3 *Repeated requests for dose increases*, particularly beyond a safe dosage range.

4 *Requests for multiple abusable medications*, such as a tranquilizer plus a hypnotic, or a tranquilizer to counteract the effects of a stimulant.

If abuse is suspected

When the clinician begins to suspect abuse, direct and prompt action is necessary.
The initial clinical response is not always to refuse to prescribe or refill prescriptions. *The first step is the identification of the problem and the setting of firm
limits with the patient.* These may include clear timeframes at which renewals
will be authorized, and parameters as to when a lost or missing prescription will
be replaced. Some patients will accept these limits and guidelines without protest;
others may become overtly angry or act insulted.

While some clinicians will refuse, under any circumstances, to rewrite lost prescriptions for abusable medications, it is not unreasonable to rewrite a lost prescription for an abusable medication one time to an otherwise stable patient.
Further requests for replacement prescriptions, however, should be refused.

If a patient requests and/or insists on increasing doses of abusable medications,
the clinician needs clearly to outline the parameters of the treatment dosage. For
example, a scenario can occur when an anxious patient repeatedly complains of
feeling more anxious unless he or she takes a larger benzodiazepine dose. If the
patient's dose reaches the maximum level at which the clinician is comfortable,
other non-abusable medications with anti-anxiety effect (an SSRI, gabapentin, or
buspirone) can be added or substituted. The clinician should explore possible precipitants to the increased anxiety and offer counseling directly or through the psychotherapist working with the patient. If these remedies are ineffective,
sometimes the clinician's best response is to indicate that the patient may, unfortunately, continue to be mildly anxious at times, and that further escalation of
doses is not advised or permitted. Fortunately, the latter situation is not typical of
the majority of anxiety disorder patients, who will use medications responsibly. It
is generally the anxiety disorder patient with a history of substance abuse who
misuses benzodiazepines.

The pharmacist as ally

The pharmacist can be of great assistance in both identifying and dealing with
patients who abuse medications. It is not uncommon for a pharmacist to call the
prescriber to verify the accuracy of a prescription for a large number of habit-
forming pills. This is a reasonable precaution that the prescriber should welcome
and reinforce. Likewise, the pharmacist may question any apparently altered or
suspiciously-written prescription. The pharmacist is also in the best position to
recognize a patient using multiple prescribers for the same medication, or who is
prescribed multiple habit-forming medications. The call from the pharmacist
noting this concern may be the first indication to prescribers that they are
prescribing psychotropic medications while other providers are prescribing further
psychotropics, pain medication, or other habit-forming medications. A pharmacist
can also alert the clinician to requests for early refills or other suspicious behavior.

What to do when abuse occurs

When abuse occurs, the clinician should observe the following guidelines.

With the patient

- Educate the patient about the dangers of medication overuse and possible consequences.
- Set clear limits of dosage to be prescribed and frequency of any refills.
- Once possible abuse is identified, do not provide any further replacement prescriptions regardless of the reason. If a prescription is "lost," "stolen," or otherwise missing, the patient will have to go without medication until the next regularly scheduled renewal. It becomes the patient's responsibility to safeguard medications.
- If, despite education and clear limits, further excessive medication requests or abuse continues, stop prescribing that medication.
- If you have a release of information and intend to contact other providers about the abuse problem, remind the patient of this. If the patient "revokes" this release, use clinical judgment as to whether this revocation can be over-ridden. In general, mild to moderate drug overusage without emergency health or safety concerns does not justify overriding this revocation to release information. If there is an emergency or safety risk present with acute danger to the patient or other individuals, and you choose to override the lack of consent to release information, document the decisions and reasoning clearly. In the UK, the requirement for reporting suspected drug abuse is different from that in the USA (see the last section of this chapter).
- Decide if you are comfortable continuing to see the medication-abusing patient for any other services besides psychotropic prescription. If so, outline the parameters of this continued treatment.
- If you are not comfortable continuing any contact, send the patient a brief written letter documenting the abusive behavior and stating that, despite your efforts to educate the patient about the dangers, medication overuse has continued. State the dates and facts of overusage and/or renewals. Document the decision to terminate any treatment relationship and specify a date when this will occur.
- If, at the time of termination, the patient is at risk for serious withdrawal phenomena from the medication prescribed, offer to coordinate drug rehabilitation treatment or admission.

With the pharmacy

- You may receive and welcome information provided by the pharmacist about abuse of medications by a patient or information about prescriptions from other providers. *The information you may divulge to the pharmacist without a release of information, however, is limited.*

- A signed written release of information from the patient to speak with the pharmacist is unusual. The fact that you wrote a prescription for a patient does not constitute a release. When contacted by a pharmacist, the only information you may provide is your intent not to have your specific prescription or future prescriptions filled for this patient. If the pharmacist asks about a questionable prescription, you can also verify if you wrote a particular prescription or not.
- Although you may be tempted to do so, you are not permitted to discuss your knowledge of drug abuse, improper usage of medications, or other clinical information about a patient with the pharmacist without a release of information.

With other prescribers

- Preferably, the patient's release of information will have been obtained at the beginning of treatment so that contact with other prescribers/treaters is authorized. If not, this release of information must be obtained from the patient in order to contact other medical or mental health providers. If the patient is willing to permit it, you may then contact other health-care providers about medication overuse. If the patient is unwilling to consent, and no emergency situation exists, you may not violate confidentiality.
- If you are contacting other providers and have written consent, talk directly with any other prescribers of medication. Do not leave voice-mail messages, or speak through intermediaries or other staff members.
- If joint decisions are made regarding further prescriptive action, discuss and document the plan and who will notify the patient of the plan.
- One particularly effective strategy is to have the patient call other providers in your presence, from your office, informing the other providers of the abuse problem with a request that these providers stop prescribing abusable medications.

With the authorities

In the USA:

- Contacting the police or other law-enforcement authorities is only appropriate for clear criminal behavior such as theft
- Simple medication abuse is not justification for a police report.

In the UK, practitioners are expected to report, on a standard form, cases of drug misuse to their regional or national drug misuse center. All types of problem drug misuse, including opioid, benzodiazepine and CNS stimulant abuse, should be reported via the regional telephone numbers listed in Table 19.3.

Table 19.3 Reporting drug misuse in the UK*

England

Northwest

- Merseyside and Cheshire: telephone (0151) 231 4319; fax (0151) 231 4320
- North West: telephone (0161) 772 3782; fax (0161) 772 3445

Northern and Yorkshire: telephone (0113) 295 1337; fax (0113) 295 1310

South East (West) and Eastern: telephone (01865) 226734; fax (01865) 226652

South West: telephone (0117) 918 6880; fax (0117) 918 6883

Thames and South East (East): telephone (020) 7594 0811; fax (020) 7594 0866

Trent: telephone (0116) 225 6360; fax (0116) 225 6370

West Midlands: telephone (0121) 580 4331; fax (0121) 525 7980

Scotland

Telephone (0131) 551 8715; fax (0131) 551 1392

Wales

Telephone (029) 2082 6260; fax (029) 2082 5473

Northern Ireland

Administrative contact:

Health Promotion Branch

C4.22 Castle Buildings

Belfast BT4 3PP

Telephone (028) 9052 0532

*Adapted from *British National Formulary*, 43rd edn. British Medical Association, 2002, p. 9.

References

1   American Psychiatric Association. *Diagnostic and Statistical Manual of Mental Disorders*, 4th edn. American Psychiatric Association, 2000, pp. 192–204.

2   Tondo L and Baldessarini RJ. Suicide: an overview. *Psychiatry Clinical Management*, Vol. 3, Medical Education Collaborative, 2002. Available at http://www.medscape.com/medscape/psychiatry/clinicalmgmt/cm.v03

Chapter 20

"Difficult" medication patients, and how to treat them

If the principles in this book are followed, the majority of patients for whom clinicians prescribe psychotropic medications will be easily managed and successfully treated. There are, however, some patients who present special problems for a clinician in the medication prescriptive process. Often, the difficulty in treatment is a reflection of the patient's personality. When negative personality traits are strong, these may color the entire interaction with the prescriber. Clinicians may, at times, find themselves frustrated and wishing to avoid treating such patients. While these traits are annoying, knowledgeable clinicians can work within them. This chapter focuses on the most common "difficult patients" (see Table 20.1), and makes recommendations for clinical management.

Table 20.1 Some "difficult" medication patients

- The patient who abuses the telephone
- The overly anxious patient
- The patient preoccupied with side effects
- The minimal contact patient
- The non-compliant patient
- The patient who needs to be in charge
- The information overload patient
- The "naturalist"
- The borderline patient

Overriding principles of managing difficult patients

Some general principles that are useful in dealing with all "difficult" patients are listed in Table 20.2.

With time, each clinician develops his or her own personal style of dealing with patients. Special patients, however, may need a modification of the prescriber's style in order to achieve successful treatment. While it may take some amount of work and commitment on the part of the clinician, such minor modifications of interaction and approach will pay off with increased compliance and fewer points of friction. Some clinicians are reluctant to change their style, feeling they are "conceding" to the patient's personality. This is not true. As long as safety and clinical necessity are not compromised, the ability to modify style is a sign of the experienced and wise clinician.

At times, friction or irritation between clinician and patient may rise to the point that almost all interactions appear to be negative. Here, clinicians should realistically acknowledge to themselves that a particular patient is frustrating them, making them angry and/or leaving them feeling unable to help them as they would like. It is important for clinicians to distinguish those areas of interaction that must be insisted upon from those matters where they can accede to a patient's wishes. *Clinicians should choose their battles carefully. It is important to separate issues of clinical safety and necessity from issues of interactional style.*

If some small issues of style or "the usual way of doing things" that are not critical can be changed, it is much easier to insist on those points of safety and good clinical care on which there is no compromise. Clinicians who refuse to budge on even small issues may get grudging compliance temporarily, but this usually results in a major power struggle, or in a patient looking for care elsewhere.

Be positive where possible

One particularly useful technique in dealing with problem medication patients is to understand and verbally recognize those parts of the patient's personality style

Table 20.2 Principles of treating "difficult" medication patients

- Be prepared to modify your usual interactional style. To be successful with problem patients, you may need to take a slightly different approach.
- You do not have to change a patient's personality to work with him or her; you need only prescribe in a safe and effective manner. Indeed, it is unlikely that your interventions will change underlying, fundamental personality traits.
- If there is friction with a patient, carefully choose the issues on which you must stand firm, and those on which you can be flexible.
- Distinguish issues of safety and necessity from issues of personal style – yours and the patient's.
- When possible, find a way to give the patient acknowledgment and a measure of respect for their "difficult" behavior.
- When necessary, identify a patient's pattern of behavior gently, without criticism, and *after* acknowledging the "value" of their style.
- Keep your focus narrowed to the elements of the prescriptive process itself, and avoid the tendency to generalize critique and feedback.
- For particularly resistant patients, you do not need their agreement that your rules for treatment are correct. During the prescriptive interactions, you need only gently but firmly insist on compliance with your guidelines and expectations.
- Consider enlarging "the team" treating the patient.
- Engage the patient in trying to fix the "problem."
- Limit the number of "difficult" patients you see.

that, even though exaggerated, may provide positive benefit for the patient. To help bring these issues to light, clinicians can ask themselves:

- What does this style accomplish for the patient?
- Are there elements of how this patient is relating to me that can be interpreted as elements of positive, rational or helpful behavior?

Once understood, it becomes possible for the clinician to approach the patient with verbal interactions that are interpreted positively by the patient as being both understanding and respectful. Many of these patients have had chronically abrasive, troublesome and unsuccessful relationships with healthcare providers, and a clinician's display of understanding can diminish conflict and start the process of alliance with the patient that may have been difficult to achieve in the past. For example:

- A suspicious patient can be labeled as "careful"
- A patient who swamps the clinician with data and articles is "someone who wishes to be informed"
- A patient who avoids appointments is "busy and trying to be efficient"
- A substance-abusing patient is someone who "wants to feel good – as most of us do."

The team approach to problem patients

Difficult patients, even when skillfully managed by a primary clinician, often need the talents of multiple types of care providers. Coordinated assistance from several individuals or clinics not only provides multifaceted support and help, but also dilutes the difficult, sometimes abrasive, effects of these patients over several providers. If not already part of the patient's care, the clinician should consider using other medical specialists, a mental health counselor, a psychopharmacology provider, a social worker, a visiting nurse, a dietitian, or an occupational/vocational specialist. Conversely, but also true, these patients often do not do well seeing a different primary care provider with every visit (even though the providers themselves may see this as a benefit since each provider does not see the patient often). Trust needs to be built with one primary provider who coordinates care. If the patient has changing or multiple primary medical care providers, it is worth considering solidifying and coordinating the primary medical care with one central provider who, when needed, will use others with specific expertise as noted above.

The "team" should always include the patient when deciding how to manage problem behaviors.

TALKING TO PATIENTS

Particularly if progress is minimal and tensions are high, the clinician should not hesitate to engage the patient with interventions such as:

- *What do you think is wrong?*
- *What do you think would help?*
- *Here is the problem that I observe* [describe the behaviors]; *help me figure out a way that makes this situation better for you and provides the help you need, but also works for me (and my staff).*
- *I am willing to adjust how I work with you* [specify what you are doing or are willing to do]. *In what ways can you change to make our working together go more smoothly?*

PRIMARY CARE

If the problem patient is a person with multiple somatic complaints whose diagnosis remains elusive and/or does not improve with standard therapies, consider a mental health etiology. Many patients with large numbers of vague, changing somatic symptoms have an underlying mood or anxiety disorder. Begin inquiring into the patient's mood state with two useful screening questions:[1]

1 During the past month, have you often been feeling down, depressed or hopeless?

2 During the past month, have you often been bothered by little interest or pleasure in doing things?

Consider referral to, or collaboration with, a mental health specialist. Such patients often will not take a mental health referral smoothly and will show resistance, anger or a feeling of being misunderstood. Use the techniques outlined in Chapter 6 for making a mental health referral.

The patient who abuses the telephone

Abuse of the telephone is covered in Chapter 24, and will be reviewed only briefly here. Of critical importance is understanding the reason that the patient is abusing the phone. The clinician's approach will vary depending on the cause for phone over-utilization. Once a clear pattern of overuse is seen (this is often signaled by the clinician's frustration at receiving yet *another* phone call from this particular patient), the clinician should speak directly to the patient about the issue. Identify the pattern rather than waiting for patients to see "the error of their ways" – patients may not view their behavior in the way that the clinician does. Without direct action, the patient may continue to overutilize the clinician's time, increasing the clinician's frustration and perhaps leading to a future angry, explosive, or inappropriate interaction. The following guidelines should be observed:

- If the patient is calling about an issue that is not an emergency, identify this fact and that the matter can wait until the next scheduled visit
- Define what are appropriate issues for phone consultation, and what can be postponed until the next face-to-face consultation
- If necessary, set specific times for calls, and the length of time that you can spend on the telephone
- If repeated inappropriate telephone calls continue, label the call as inappropriate and minimize the length of the call
- If the patient continues to call inappropriately, it is reasonable to interrupt at the beginning of the call, and insist that the patient bring the subject matter to the next session, without continuing the conversation.

Specific *"Talking to patients"* interactions for telephone abusing patients are detailed in Chapter 24.

The overly anxious patient

Patients who have an anxiety-prone personality can show marked concern about the use of medication as one aspect of their treatment. The very notion that a clinician is recommending medication may make them more anxious. They may have multiple questions about suggested prescriptions. These persons are also anxious about many other issues in their life – job, children, parenting, finances, risk of accident, tragedy, or death. They often catastrophize and assume the worst outcome of a situation, even if its likelihood is rare. In applying this way of thinking to the use of medication, they expect problematic, uncomfortable, or disastrous response to medications.

Several strategies are useful in dealing with overly anxious patients. Whenever possible, medication should be *started only when* such *patients are ready*. Anxious patients may need to ponder the clinician's recommendation before they are willing to begin taking medication. Faced with mild to moderate symptoms, it may be totally appropriate to allow a patient to digest and consider the suggestion for medication before the prescription is actually written or filled. In the long run, even if the clinician would prefer that the medication be started sooner, it is often preferable to wait for a patient to become ready (albeit still hesitantly), than to insist on beginning a medication with an overly anxious patient who is not ready to accept the recommendation. If the patient is fundamentally not prepared to begin medication and the clinician insists, the person will usually find a reason for never starting or quickly stopping the medication. Initially, when beginning medication, *more frequent appointments* with these patients may provide the opportunity to ask questions and receive reassurance. When a change in medication is contemplated, it is often useful to *identify the need for this change as far in advance as possible* to give the patient time to adjust. It may take a very anxious person several visits to be ready to change medication or even change doses.

 TALKING TO PATIENTS

As a way of recognizing a patient for his or her anxiety, it can be useful to say: *"I can see that you are a person who wants to be very, very sure about the safety and effectiveness of anything you would take. This is a useful way of thinking, and I share your wish to ensure that any medicines you use are taken safely without serious adverse effects. Let's work together to make sure this happens."*

Even when clinicians feel they have provided sufficient education and reassurance to anxious patients, those with an overanxious personality style often require repeated reassurances. Such a patient may arrive at the next visit asking virtually the same questions that the clinician has previously answered. The person will again ask for reassurance that the medication is necessary, safe, and in the appropriate dose. While it can be tedious, particularly if repeated multiple times, this behavior is intrinsic to the patient's style. It cannot be ignored, or the patient will likely stop medication. Even if the clinician identifies this behavior pattern and describes it to the patient, the underlying personality style will seldom disappear.

For the exceptionally anxious patient who continues to call frequently between appointments for education, reassurance, and questions about the medication, a useful strategy is to ask the patient to call on a regularly structured schedule. By using a brief scheduled contact, the clinician decreases the patient's anxiety, keeps the patient on medication and avoids frequent annoying off-hours calls for reassurance. For example, the clinician could tell the patient to call every Thursday between 1 pm and 2 pm with any accumulated questions they have, but to hold routine questions at other times. Gradually, as the patient becomes more comfortable, the interval between telephone check-ins can be increased or the telephone calls perhaps discontinued.

The patient preoccupied with side effects and negative reactions

Patients with this behavior pattern will often have many of the same traits as the overly anxious personality style described above. Many of the principles of medication management of these two types of persons will also overlap. Patients solely preoccupied with negative side effects, however, are not, in general, overly anxious about other areas of their life. They may be particularly preoccupied with the effects of psychotropics on their mind or body. It should not be assumed that patients who ask many questions prior to taking medication will automatically become problem patients preoccupied with side effects. Some patients, once they have received answers to their initial questions and the necessary reassurances, will proceed comfortably with taking medication. Once medicated, they have few questions and do not develop the level of concern associated with the side-effect preoccupied patient. If, however, over several appointments it becomes clear that the patient has a long list of possible concerns about medication, and at each appointment presents the clinician with a long list of possible "side effects" that they attribute to this psychotropic, it may be necessary to take management steps.

First, it is important to listen carefully and *differentiate true or possible side effects from effects that are not likely to be related to the medication*. Early in the prescriptive process, this level of active listening reassures the patient that the clinician, too, will be diligent in looking for negative effects of the medication, and that the patient has an active partner in evaluating any discomfort experienced. It is seldom helpful to simply dismiss all the patient's concerns as "unrealistic" or "overreaction." The clinician should be clear and direct with such a patient as to which effects may, in fact, be side effects and which are probably unrelated.

It is not uncommon for these patients to bring a printed list of potential side effects that they have taken from a book or the Internet, or have heard from relatives or friends, without any sense of how likely it is that such effects will occur. When possible, in discussing the likelihood of possible side effects, actual percentages of incidence taken from source materials should be used (e.g. "This reaction does occur, but has been reported in 0.1 percent of people taking this drug. This means that for every 1000 patients, 999 will never have this problem.")

TALKING TO PATIENTS

One way of approaching a patient like this would be to say: *"Of the list you bring, these* are *potential side effects . . .* [specify]. *These* are not *likely side effects of this medication . . .* [specify]. *We will have ample warning if and when they are going to occur. Together we will be watching for these problems and certainly will consider stopping the medication if there any signs or symptoms that are dangerous. I know you are a very careful person; so am I. I doubt very much that these rare possibilities are going to be problems for you. If it were me, knowing what I know about the medication, and having the symptoms that you have, I would take the medication. I would not let these concerns prevent me from trying a medication that could be very helpful."*

Early in treatment, more frequent appointments with such patients will allay fears and deal with their concerns. Gradually, as they become more comfortable with the effects of the medication, intervals between appointments can be increased. It is also useful to have patients chart the occurrence and frequency of any negative effects that they perceive. This provides them with a sense of being actively involved in their own medication management. Such a chart or list additionally gives the clinician a rapid way to see if a particular side effect occurs frequently, or has any pattern of occurrence.

Patients who have continually persistent and changing complaints about their medication can also be approached in a manner similar to the process of dealing with the hypochondriacal patient. In this model, the clinician has regularly spaced appointments with the patient while using simple benign interventions without major changes in the medication regimen. This permits the patient to stay on medication, maintain a relationship with the clinician, and yet perceive that some active intervention "is being done." Small changes in timing or dosage, or the use of benign over-the-counter remedies, can be a temporizing measure. An occasional laboratory measurement to test for organ safety can also be reassuring to the patient. While these small changes or tests are performed, the central medication regime is neither discontinued, nor changed in a major way. The patient is allowed a longer time to identify the beneficial therapeutic effects of the psychotropic and to forge an increasingly strong alliance with the clinician.

When a patient has been identified in the clinician's mind as a "complainer," a "whiner," or a "worry wart" about negative medication effects, it may unfortunately be assumed that any new complaint about the medication is automatically a result of the patient's hypersensitive style. Even the most "side-effect preoccupied" patient may, at times, have genuine unwanted effects from the medications that are significant or troublesome. While it can be time-consuming, each claim of a new side effect must be evaluated on its own merit. At times, it may be necessary and very appropriate to change medications for these patients because of a problematic side effect.

The minimal contact patient

Patients with this style do not see the value of, or need for, follow-up medication appointments. Such patients will feel and, at times, verbalize: "You have seen me. I'm doing fine. I don't see why my prescription just can't be renewed without having to see you again." Although the underlying, driving force is their personality style, such patients will often cloak their resistance in the need to spend long hours at work, having multiple personal commitments, extensive travel, or a changing schedule, any of which will not permit making and keeping appointments. Even when scheduled, such patients may cancel a follow-up appointment and "forget" to reschedule it. When their prescription is nearly exhausted, they will often call the pharmacy for a refill and avoid talking to the clinician directly. If the clinician is willing to continue to renew prescriptions by telephone, the patient is likely to continue this pattern of behavior indefinitely.

Dealing with the minimal-contact patient involves recognition of this pattern and, at times, insistence on appropriate follow-up. As outlined in the earlier chapters of this book, the clinician must see a patient face-to-face periodically for safe, effective prescribing practice. Once stabilized, the patient should be seen at a minimum of every 3 months for at least the first year. It is totally appropriate for clinicians to require that they become acquainted with patients for whom they are prescribing, and these visits accomplish this task in addition to managing the prescription. When the minimal contact pattern is first discovered (often when the pharmacy calls for a refill at the request of a patient who has not made or kept follow-up appointments), the prescription should be filled for a small amount of pills and the pharmacy requested to have the patient contact the clinician prior to further refills. If the patient continues to request telephone refills, the clinician should deny the requests and require a face-to-face visit. Clinicians should not allow an inappropriate interval between visits if they feel a face-to-face appointment is necessary for safe management.

For the patient who consistently delays or fails to keep face-to-face appointments, the pattern should be identified, and the parameters of safe care laid out.

TALKING TO PATIENTS

"I know it may be inconvenient for you to come to the office for a visit. You have a very busy schedule and the last thing you need is another appointment. It is, however, essential for me to see you in person to prescribe safely and responsibly. I need to get to know you, assess your condition, order appropriate lab tests and monitor the safety of your prescription. Here is the frequency with which I can work with you . . ."

For appointment-resistant patients who are on long-term maintenance medication, it is possible to stretch out the intervals between their face-to-face visits to a frequency of every 4–6 months. Such longer intervals should only be permitted if:

- The clinician knows the patient, his or her clinical history, the diagnosis, and any complicating medical conditions
- The patient is on a stable, uncomplicated regimen of medication
- The patient does not have a rapidly changing or brittle *medical* condition
- The patient does not have a rapidly changing or brittle *psychological* condition
- The patient is responsible in taking medications
- The patient does not abuse alcohol or drugs.

The non-compliant patient

There are multiple ways in which a patient can be non-compliant, and multiple reasons why this occurs. Some patients do not follow through with appointments or do not take their medications on schedule; others do not follow through with requested serum blood levels, or run out of medications and fall into a symptomatic crisis. Several patient types described elsewhere in this book, such as the substance-abusing patient, the minimal contact patient and the confused patient, include non-compliance as part of the clinical picture.

Patients who are not compliant but do not fall into the above-mentioned categories often present to the clinician not for themselves, but because others have insisted upon treatment. These patients may be frankly involuntary, or simply not personally motivated. Some non-compliant patients feel they have no reason to improve and are reluctant to follow a medication regimen. It is these resistant individuals who do not fall into other categories that are discussed in this section.

Principles that cover the management of non-compliant patients include the following:

1 *Distinguish less than ideal treatment from unsafe treatment.* Although some patients may participate only partially in a medication regime, it does not automatically mean that they have markedly compromised their safety or health.
2 *Symptoms or discomfort may not constitute an unsafe situation.* Patients who stop medication prematurely or take medication irregularly may develop symptoms of the underlying illness for which they are being treated, or may develop a discontinuation syndrome. When symptoms emerge, patients may be a bother to their family, friends, neighbors, or co-workers. While this may be inconvenient and problematic for others, it does not necessarily constitute an unsafe situation or one in which the clinician must intervene, beyond encouragement, elucidation of the reasons for the behavior and continued recommendations for more consistency.

   Particularly when a patient is being treated at someone else's insistence, the clinician should make efforts to uncover reasons for taking a medication that would benefit the patient, regardless of the reasons why the family, the work supervisor, the courts, or other agencies have brought the patient to treatment. It is worthwhile trying to discover aspects of the patient's life that could be benefited by medication, even if such benefit is not the prime motivation for other people, nor the primary reason the patient is being seen. For example, a person may be court-ordered to treatment for psychosis, but be motivated to take medication because it allows him to keep a job that makes money for the car he wants to buy. A patient may come seeking medication for depression at the insistence of his spouse, but continue to take it because when not depressed, his sexual performance is better. A bipolar adolescent may not be motivated to take medication for her parents or teachers, but will do so because when medicated she does not "say weird things" that drive her friends away.

3 *Some treatment is often better than no treatment.* Some non-compliant patients fail to comply in ways that result in less than optimum treatment. While it is clear to many people around them that the ultimate outcome would likely be better if they were more compliant, patients still refuse to participate fully with medication recommendations, even with clinician encouragement. Rather than withdraw from prescribing or becoming angry with such patients, the treator should decide if some measure of compliance is better than none at all – which it often is. This does not mean that the treator would support non-compliance or would not be diligent in attempts to improve patient adherence; it simply means medication treatment need not be all or nothing.

4 *Some non-compliant patients will behave in ways that result in arrest, incarceration or other sanctions.* Even if such behaviors are a direct result of non-compliance with medication, it may ultimately be in such a patient's best interest to suffer the discomfort of incarceration or punishment in order to facilitate future compliance.

Parents dealing with adolescents and young adults who are disobedient, truant, or are involved in frankly illegal activities are often reluctant to involve the police or jail. Even when these behaviors are the result of a mental illness that could be treated with medication, the patient does not comply with medication recommendations and prescription. The clinician must often counsel the family that the use of the appropriate authorities may not only be necessary, but also advisable, to reinforce negatively the problematic behavior, including non-compliance.

5 *Non-response does not necessarily equate to non-compliance.* Having prescribed many medications to a patient with minimal or no success, some clinicians assume that because the patient has not responded, he or she must not be following the clinician's advice. While a majority of patients will respond, at least partially, to an aggressive psychopharmacological regimen targeted to an accurate diagnosis, some patients simply do not. Despite multiple medication trials, they are minimally better. This does not indicate that they are not complying with the prescriber's recommendations. Unfortunately, some mental health symptoms remain stubbornly non-responsive despite adequate and full patient adherence.

The patient who needs to be in charge

Many executives, supervisors, leaders in business or persons having a strong need for control may come to the prescriptive interview with difficulty because it signifies giving control or power to another person. They maintain a lifestyle of control – of themselves and of others. They want, and need, to be in charge, and feel unsettled when someone else is making decisions about them, and for them. Once begun on medication, these patients will often return in a follow-up session having altered the timing, dose, or start date of the medication. It will rapidly become clear to the clinician that such a patient needs to "run the show."

When such a pattern of control and subsequent unilateral decision-making becomes apparent to the clinician, several behavioral responses are useful.

First the clinician should take his or her ego out of the prescriptive process. The clinician need not always make all the decisions about the prescription but can allow the patient to be in charge, at least partially, of some portion of the medication process. With such a patient, it is particularly important that a rigid, set medication regimen is avoided. If the clinician requires a set schedule of medication, and insists upon it with such an individual, a power struggle will be inevitable. Because these patients need to be in charge and make decisions, they cannot, and will not, relinquish control totally to another person. While clinicians cannot abdicate responsibility for medication decisions and schedule, they can allow the patient some choices while retaining the larger decision-making position.

Once areas of limited choice within which the patient can make decisions have been identified, the clinician can outline broad limits of safe prescription while allowing the patient a limited choice that will permit him or her to feel more in control. There may be a dosage range within which the clinician will allow flexibility. The patient may be in charge of how many "as needed" (or "PRN") doses they need to take, within certain limits. The clinician can also permit patient input about when a regular dose is changed.

TALKING TO PATIENTS

Here is an approach to an "in-charge" patient when beginning a new medication. As can be seen in the following dialogue, the clinician makes references to the patient being in control and in charge: *"We are going to begin ...* [name of medication]. *Here are some general guidelines about when and how to take the medication, but I'd like you to be in charge of some elements of this. Let's start with 25 mg, and I'd like you to remain on that dose for several days. When you feel ready, and only when you feel ready, increase to 50 mg. Once you've adjusted to 50 mg you can, if you like, increase to 75 mg. My recommendation is that you do not go beyond 75 mg until our next visit. Obviously when you leave the office you'll be the one taking the pills, but I think you'd be taking an added risk of side effects if you increased the medicine dose too fast."*

[To a patient who, during a follow-up session, has returned having taken several extra doses more than was prescribed]: *"I know you're just trying to feel better as rapidly as you can, but I think you were actually fortunate that you didn't have any adverse effects of increasing the dose too fast. Had we talked, I might not have disagreed with your decision to increase your dose, but I think for future reference it would be best if we make this decision together."*

With sensitivity and tact, most of these individuals can be treated in a safe and effective manner. In the rare instance where such a person clearly and repeatedly takes medication in an unsafe manner or dose, the clinician may need to be more forceful, as shown in the following:

TALKING TO PATIENTS

"We have discussed the parameters of using your medication and I had hoped we could see eye-to-eye about this. You have continued to make decisions about how and when you are taking your medication without our making these decisions together. What you are doing is not medically safe. We will need to agree on a plan of how you will use the medication in order for me to continue working with you. I would like to hear your thoughts about how you are making the decisions about medication, so we can negotiate a schedule that will not compromise your health." After this discussion and your proposal for a schedule, write down what you agree upon, give a copy to the patient, and keep one in his or her chart. In the unusual circumstance when no agreement can be reached, or the patient makes an agreement but does not adhere to it, jeopardizing safety, the clinician will need to break off contact: *"I had hoped we could be a team in making decisions about your medication, but since you continue to violate our agreement, I think it best that you see another practitioner."*

The information overload patient

While many patients will, on occasion, bring articles about medication or mental health treatment to the clinician, there are some patients who take this to an extraordinary level. At virtually every appointment such patients arrive with a new article or set of data, asking "Is this appropriate for me?" or "Have you seen this?" Such patients are continually looking to refine their medication regimen or are hoping for an improved outcome. Their behavior can be independent of the adequacy of their medication response. Even when they are doing quite well, they seek "just a little bit more." These individuals may spend hours on the Internet, looking at journals or other sources for information about their illness and possible new treatments. For some patients it appears to be their hobby or avocation. Although most patients are genuinely trying to help themselves and to improve their treatment response, some are trying to show their intelligence or diligence, or match what they perceive as the practitioner's level of knowledge.

Requesting that patients cease bringing in articles or references is counterproductive and often misinterpreted. No matter how gently stated, the underlying message is that patients should not be involved in improving their level of care and this puts the clinician in a negative light. Therefore, the clinician should allow this behavior to continue without trying fundamentally to change such a patient's style. Although the prescriber should evaluate the pieces of information presented, there are keys to doing so in a time-efficient and useful way. The principles involved with this type of person include the following:

The clinician should ask the patient always to send or bring full copies of the articles or books to the office. If the patient brings only references, citations or website addresses for the clinician to follow up, he or she should ask the patient to make a hard copy and bring it at the next visit. Searching out such materials from the patient's suggestions can be quite time-consuming! Asking that the patient do the legwork also invites the patient to be selective in distinguishing material that is particularly relevant from "general information."

Sometimes an article is short and can be evaluated during a face-to-face session. At other times, it may be appropriate to peruse a lengthy article between appointments, which will allow the clinician to decide if more detailed reading is necessary. Usually this is not the case, and scanning of selected parts of the material is all that is needed to assess the material. It is not necessary to read in detail all the information that the patient has culled with hours of searching. The clinician can then correctly say at the next session that the material has been read, and make any appropriate comments regarding its applicability for this patient.

Many "information-seeking" patients find non-mainstream sources for their information. They may have connected to dubious Internet sites of biased, self-serving groups or organizations. The information may be primarily homeopathic in nature, or relate to "hormones," herbal remedies or medications available only in other countries. Some of the information may come from print advertisements or Internet sites that are trying to sell products for profit. Some sources advertise "comprehensive remedies" that will treat almost any condition. The clinician can then point out the obvious fact that, if such a "miracle cure" were genuinely as effective as claimed, it would very quickly become a common, mainstream standard of care.

At times, articles brought by a patient are genuinely useful and will inform even the knowledgeable clinician about a possible treatment that had not been considered. Despite any clinician's diligence to be updated and current with all medications, the number of sources of information on psychotropics available at this time is nearly overwhelming. Even the most well-read clinician can be challenged to stay current with all information available, and patient suggestions can be very helpful.

TALKING TO PATIENTS

One way of recognizing and "crediting" the patient for this behavior would be to say: *"I appreciate your interest in getting better. Most patients are not willing to go to the lengths that you are to investigate new possibilities. I'll take a look at this article and see if there is anything that applies to my treatment of you."* Clinicians need not feel compelled to prescribe a remedy or medication that they are unfamiliar with or doubt will be effective. It is quite acceptable to decline to act on a patient's request for an obscure, unusual treatment just because it is asked for (and possibly supported by "research" obtained by the patient). If the information is markedly complex, non-mainstream treatment, or inaccurate, the clinician could say: *"This is interesting, but I know of no research to support this treatment currently. You may be a little ahead of your time."*

The "naturalist"

For some persons, herbs, potions, hormones, and plant products are deemed to be "natural," and therefore better and safer than synthetic medications, which are considered "chemical." Often these individuals will first try the use of health food stores, herbalists, practitioners of Eastern medicine, over-the-counter medications, "home remedies," and vitamins to treat their symptoms. They may not arrive at a more traditional medical office until they have unsuccessfully tried many other alternatives. Even when they do come to the clinician's office, they are reluctant to accept a recommendation for prescription medicines, which they perceive to be artificial and potentially dangerous.

TALKING TO PATIENTS

In talking with a patient who has a strong preference for natural remedies, a clinician could use the following dialogue: *"You clearly want a treatment that is going to work in harmony with your body. I do, too. If there was a plant or herbal product that had sufficient research to support its use, I would suggest it. With your level of symptoms, however, I think that we should use a prescription medication which we know is pure, in a dose that is reproducible, and for which we have solid research evidence to support its results. I know that this is probably not your first choice, but there are some things we need to remember:*

- *A chemical is a chemical whether it's made by a plant or in a laboratory*
- *Many "natural" products have markedly varying amounts of active ingredient in each pill, and it is difficult to standardize the dose you are receiving*
- *Many things that come out of the ground I would not put in my mouth. Just because something grows, it does not mean it is healthy."*

If such a person has very mild symptoms or insists on a "natural" remedy, a clinician may choose to try one of the remedies listed in the text below. While research evidence for their effectiveness is limited and, at times, contradictory, some patients who are fixated on natural remedies will insist on a trial of any possible "natural" compounds before being willing even to try a prescription. Practitioners may, if they choose, initially use one of these "natural" medications in a mildly symptomatic patient, if for no other reason than to obtain a stronger alliance with the patient and demonstrate the willingness to work effectively together.

If the patient symptoms are moderate or severe, however, there is some medicolegal risk in pursuing an unproven natural remedy when other proven prescription medications exist. Therefore, with a more severe symptom picture, a clinician should be skeptical of using unproven "natural" alternatives.

CLINICAL TIP

For mildly depressed patients who insist on a natural remedy, the use of St. John's Wort[2–4] may provide some benefit, although research is contradictory. Use of omega-3 fatty acids (fish oil)[5–7] has also been shown to be of some benefit in patients with affective disorders. For individuals with bipolar disorder who insist on a "natural" remedy, consider the use of lithium carbonate. In prescribing it, stress the fact that lithium is a natural element that is mined from the earth, and not a synthetic chemical. (In contrast to St. John's Wort, for which the research is contradictory, lithium has a long and strong track record in treating bipolar disorder and can be used with confidence, even in a patient with significant symptoms.) Valerian root has been used with some success to diminish anxiety and promote sleep.[8–10] There are no known successful herbal remedies for psychosis.

The borderline patient

The person with borderline personality disorder (often referred to as "a borderline") is one of the most challenging types of patient with which to interact and treat with medication. The majority of these individuals are young women, with a prevalence as high as 2 percent of the population.[11] The disorder is marked by frequent crises, self-harmful, and markedly disruptive behavior ("acting out"). Such behavior is often repetitive, and these patients can rapidly become well known within a clinic, emergency department or group practice for difficult, problematic and, at times, seemingly outrageous behavior. Even when well managed, they engender strong reactions and responses from clinicians. Poorly managed, they can cause clinicians to experience intense anger, frustration and self-doubt.

The reader may notice that these patients are covered somewhat more in-depth than other "difficult" patients. Although not necessarily seen on a day-to-day basis, the intensity engendered by borderline patients, much of which emerges over medications and their prescription, merits a more thorough review. Clinicians currently treating one or more borderline patients will quickly recognize the issues presented here. When a clinician first becomes involved with such a patient (as is likely over time), the detailed information presented in this section will be welcome and deserving of review.

Medication prescription for borderline personality

Initially characterized in 1938 as a diagnosis that stood on the borderline between neurosis and psychosis, borderline personality disorder was later conceptualized to be a mild version of schizophrenia. This was reframed to the modern understanding of borderline personality disorder (BPD) by Kernberg in 1975.[12]

He characterized a person with BPD as a person who has problems maintaining consistent internal images and memories of people (poor "object relations") and displays primitive psychological defenses, including:

■ Splitting (a person is seen as all good or all bad)
■ Magical thinking
■ Projective identification (the projection of the person's own unpleasant characteristics onto others and trying to elicit in others feelings that the person him or herself is experiencing).

The DSM-IV-TR now lists nine characteristics of persons with BPD, of which five must be present to make the diagnosis.[13] These diagnostic criteria include:

1 Frantic efforts to avoid real or imagined abandonment
2 A pattern of unstable and intense interpersonal relationships characterized by alternation between extremes of idealization and devaluation
3 Identity disturbance with a marked and persistently unstable sense of self
4 Impulsivity in at least two areas, which can be self-damaging (such as spending, sexual behavior, substance abuse, reckless driving, or binge eating)
5 Recurrent suicidal behavior, gestures or threats, or self-mutilating behavior
6 Affective instability due to marked mood reactivity lasting several hours, and rarely more than several days
7 Chronic feelings of emptiness or boredom
8 Inappropriate and intense, poorly controlled anger, including frequent displays of temper or recurrent physical fights
9 Transient, stress-related paranoid ideation or dissociative symptoms.

Although the exact etiology of BPD is unclear, many patients diagnosed with this condition have strong histories of physical, sexual, or mental abuse during their upbringing, and have experienced parental neglect and/or inconsistent parenting.[14,15] There is some evidence from brain-imaging studies that persons with BPD inconsistently activate areas of their frontal cortex, which would normally be expected to inhibit or suppress negative emotions.[16]

Because of their primitive defenses, if a borderline patient perceives that the clinician has been non-understanding, it is as if there has been no previous contact with the clinician. The patient cannot see the currently perceived problem in the context of a greater pattern of positive and therapeutic interaction, and the clinician is often defined by how he or she last acted with the borderline person. If the medicating clinician is not providing primary psychotherapy, there may be frequent attempts to split the primary psychotherapist and the medicating clinician. The patient may report behaviors or negative interactions with the psychotherapist, inviting the medicating clinician to intervene or join in the patient's outrage. Also, the medication clinician should not be surprised to have the psychotherapist at times receive information about the medication clinician that is negative, degrading or distorted.

Because of the idealizing/devaluing ("black-and-white") thinking of persons with BPD, the medicating clinician can be initially idealized as the "best," "most understanding," or "most knowledgeable" practitioner with whom the patient has ever dealt, often accompanied by denigration and devaluation of previous medication clinicians. This belief and interaction may persist for weeks, months or even years, only to change suddenly and unexpectedly. Change can occur when the patient perceives the clinician to have been absent when needed, to have prescribed a medication that was not successful, or to have engaged in some other behavior that the patient perceives to represent lack of connection and understanding.

Because of strong affective fluctuations, particularly with anger and depression, the patient may repetitively request or demand a medication solution to his or her intense discomfort. Many borderline patients have a strong placebo response to medication. Therefore, there may be brief, overly positive responses to a medication intervention that are quickly lost. The patient may request further dosage increases in order to reclaim the initially perceived effect, at times requesting dosage levels beyond those normally given or safe. Persons with BPD have strong "oral" characteristics, and often will ingest medications, alcohol, drugs, or other substances in hopes of remediating their intense affect. Using the philosophy that if "one pill is good, then three or four must be better," they may accidentally overdose in an attempt to self-medicate their emotional state.

Because of their inability to self-soothe and manage crises, patients will often call the medicating clinician for help in calming themselves or for direct advice on how to manage interpersonal crises. These patients often feel "entitled," in that they can call the clinician whenever, and about whatever subject they please. Some borderline patients can significantly overutilize the phone with the medicating clinician, if firm boundaries are not set.

Suicidal threats are common with borderline individuals,[17,18] often in response to having perceived negative behavior on the part of someone important in their lives. At times, the source of their wrath or disappointment is the clinician and their suicidal threats can have a transparent, manipulative, or angry message. Despite the seeming obviousness of these angry messages, it is not wise to ignore suicidal threats in borderline patients, since serious suicide attempts and death by overdose are common. Even when suicide attempts are repeated or are perceived to be manipulative, borderline patients will need to be evaluated in an emergency department and/or be psychiatrically hospitalized short-term in the face of serious overdose or threat.

Behaviors of self-harm can include burning, cutting, scratching or self-mutilation in addition to frank overdose. It is estimated that 75 percent of borderline patients have had at least one deliberate episode of self-harm, and that up to 9 percent of these patients successfully commit suicide.[19]

Patients with BPD have significant problems maintaining clear boundaries with many people in their lives, and this may emerge in the medication prescription process. These patients can ask for exceptions to normal prescriptive practice, such as:

- Requesting unusual, large doses of medication
- Setting appointments outside of the regular treatment setting or after hours
- Personal friendship or support beyond that of the normal clinician–patient relationship.

Borderline patients often see themselves as special, and feel they deserve or need special treatment from the clinician. Their requests for special treatment can be repetitive and recurrent, but should, in general, be resisted. When granted unusual or special treatment, such patients often respond poorly, or ultimately take advantage of these special privileges. Any intimate or sexual contact is strictly prohibited, and even the appearance of impropriety or physical affection should be assiduously avoided. Borderline patients may change dramatically and suddenly. The idealized clinician who was the "best" may suddenly become "the worst," and accusations may be made about the clinician's behavior even when there is no solid reason.

Medication treatment principles with borderline patients

Borderline patients are particularly vexing, and can be problematic for even the most experienced medication clinician. The clinician should not hesitate to utilize consultation with other colleagues early in the course of treatment to discuss the management of a borderline patient. In general, because of the difficulty managing such patients, clinicians should avoid medicating large numbers of them simultaneously.

No medication should be provided in the absence of psychotherapy. If the medication clinician is not the primary psychotherapy clinician, it should be insisted that the patient be solidly involved in a psychotherapeutic relationship with another therapist prior to any medications being provided. In general, therapy for BPD is long term and difficult, with frequent crises. Individual therapy with a dialectical behavioral therapy or psychodynamic focus is crucial to long-term progress.[20]

Medications may have some symptomatic benefit, although they are not the primary treatment. Medications used in BPD do not treat the underlying, core personality itself. Target symptoms should be identified, and specific medications chosen to modulate these target symptoms. In general, the four most common target symptoms identified are:

1 Impulsive behavior
2 Affective dysregulation, particularly depression
3 Anger management
4 Short-term psychotic symptoms.

SSRI antidepressants have been the backbone of treatment for many persons with BPD.[21-24] They have usefulness in decreasing impulsive behavior and have some modest antidepressant activity. Even large doses, however, seldom preclude the intense dysphoric depressions that these individuals experience. There is some evidence that mood stabilizers[25–28] have been useful for affective disregulation and impulsiveness. Naltrexone can be used for dissociative states.[29]

Psychotic symptoms most likely evident in borderlines include hallucinations, distortion of body image, and ideas of reference. Transient psychotic symptoms are generally treated with low doses of antipsychotic medications. In general, atypical antipsychotics, such as olanzapine or risperidone, are safer than traditional antipsychotics, with fewer extrapyramidal side effects, lowered incidence of tardive dyskenesia, and increased safety in overdose. Olanzapine[30] and risperidone[31] have also been shown to be useful with symptoms of aggression and depression in the patient with BPD. Doses should be small and the medication continued for relatively short periods of time – usually several days to several weeks. Most borderline patients do not require chronic antipsychotic medication unless there is clear re-emergence of symptoms quickly after the medication is withdrawn.

When first evaluating a patient with a borderline personality disorder, it is important to attempt to *establish a strong initial medication contact with the patient*. The clinician should emphasize the necessity of psychotherapy as being the central treatment issue, with medications being a supplemental aid. The prescriber will need to be specific about any guidelines for appointment frequency, directions for medication usage and "lost" prescriptions. It is essential to obtain a clear agreement from the patient as to safe and controlled use of medications. The risk from overdose should be described in detail.

Despite a strong initial contact, many borderlines will inappropriately use medications – overutilizing them chronically, episodically, or erratically. In the context of a deep depression or intense anger, such patients may transiently take large amounts of medications to compensate for their lack of the internal, psychological ability to soothe themselves.

In general, medications that are dangerous in overdose, are habit-forming, or have narrow therapeutic indices should be avoided with borderline patients. These include tricyclic antidepressants, MAOIs, lithium carbonate, and benzodiazepines. Beyond their habit-forming potential, benzodiazepines have the added property of disinhibition, which may exacerbate impulsiveness – one of the central features of BPD.

A calm, even-handed demeanor is essential in dealing with borderline patients, who can be affectively excitable, demanding, irritable, and manipulative. It is important to maintain adherence to good prescribing principles and medication safety, despite repeated requests, insinuations, manipulation, or threats. Calm but firm reiteration of how much medication will be prescribed, for what period of time and for what indications may be periodically necessary. When a clinician is in doubt (as is common with these patients), firmness, consistency, and predictability are more useful than "giving in" to inappropriate requests, even when minor. The overvaluation and/or devaluation of the clinician should not be taken personally, nor be allowed to alter good prescribing practice.

When primary psychotherapy is provided by another individual, it is important to maintain *frequent communication with the psychotherapist* to minimize splitting. Regardless of any information provided by the patient about the behavior of the psychotherapist, no action should be taken until that therapist has been contacted and the reality of the situation discerned. If the medication clinician acts on a negative report, the issues may actually be the patient's misinterpretation and be partially (or totally) untrue. Other issues that should be discussed with the primary clinician include which person is going to be available for telephone contact and when, and which treatment issues will be handled by each clinician. Since borderline patients are particularly sensitive to absence, issues of coverage and availability during vacations should also be clearly outlined between clinicians, and then with the patient.

Since there is strong comorbidity of borderline personality disorder with substance abuse, eating disorders and medication abuse, the medicating clinician should be alert to signs and symptoms of these problems.

Consultation and disengagement

All difficult patients can upset, anger, frustrate, and disorganize clinical staff. When such patients' behavior is intense and repetitive, clinicians may lose perspective on their role, their interventions and their goals. At any time, but particularly if the above interventions are not working, a consultation may be utilized. This may be with a colleague in the same discipline, or with a mental health specialist. A telephone call specifically for advice, a brief meeting or a meal with the expressed purpose of discussing a problem case will often yield more results than a "curbstone consult" in the hall or the parking lot.

Despite clinicians' best efforts, consultation, skill, and tact, some patients will not match well with some providers. There are situations when a clinician will feel unable to work productively with a patient who is unwilling or unable to participate in working together as a team. While not generally the first, second, or third alternative, there *are* times when a practitioner must explore whether another clinician could work more effectively with a patient. When a clinician begins to question his or her ability to prescribe effectively and safely, despite efforts to modify the situation, he or she should raise the issue with the patient directly *as a possibility* before actually implementing a termination.

TALKING TO PATIENTS
"Miss Carpenter, I have begun to wonder whether I am the best clinician to treat you. We have had some differences of opinion about your care and we have attempted to come up with a plan to work together. From my view, this is not working. How are you feeling about working with me? Unless things change, I will need to withdraw from prescribing for you. This is what I need from you in order to continue working with you." Be specific and list the behaviors that need to occur, change or stop.

If the patient cannot or will not comply, the patient should be sent written notice of the clinician's intent to stop providing care/medication as of a specific date, with advice to find another caregiver.

The patient is not always the problem

If a clinician finds that gradually (or suddenly) there are many "difficult" patients to be dealt with in the practice, clinician-centered difficulties, not the patients, may be the primary problem. Overwork, a large caseload, an excessive number of gravely ill, complicated patients, lack of sleep, inadequate personal time, failure to take vacations, as well as personal and family stresses, can all lead to clinician burnout. Initially, one sign of this problem can be frequent irritation with patients, intolerance for small patient idiosyncrasies, or finding multiple patient management issues burdensome. This can be accompanied by other warning signs, including:

- Regularly being unable to stop thinking about "problem" patients
- Allowing feelings about "difficult" patient interactions to intrude on family or social relationships
- Inability to sleep well or relax when not at work
- An uncharacteristic emotional outburst at a patient
- Excessive irritability with office staff or colleagues.

The presence of any of these signs should raise the warning flag that some alteration of workload, caseload mix, or amount of non-work personal time is necessary. Although sometimes painful to accept, the difficulty at the office may be most clearly seen in the mirror.

References

1 Whooley MA and Simon GE. Managing depression in medical outpatients. *JAMA* 2000;343:1942–1950.
2 Phillip M *et al.* Hypericum extract versus imipramine or placebo in patients with moderate depression: randomized multicentre study of treatment for eight weeks. *BMJ* 1999;319:1534–1538.
3 Shelton RC *et al.* Effectiveness of St. John's wort in major depression: a randomized controlled trial. *JAMA* 2001;285:1978–1986.
4 Laakman G *et al.* St. John's wort in mild to moderate depression: the relevance of hyperforin for the clinical efficacy. *Pharmacopsychiatry* 1998;31(suppl. 1): 54–59.
5 Hibbeln JR. Fish consumption and major depression. *Lancet* 1998;351:1213.
6 Tanskanen A *et al.* Fish consumption and depressive symptoms in the general population in Finland. *Psychiatr Serv* 2001;52:529–531.
7 Stoll AL *et al.* Omega-3 fatty acids in bipolar disorder. A preliminary double-blind, placebo-controlled trial. *Arch Gen Psychiatry* 1999;56:407–412.
8 Wagner J *et al.* Beyond benzodiazepines: alternative pharmacologic agents for the treatment of insomnia. *Ann Pharmacother* 1998;32:680–691.
9 Heiligenstein E and Guenther G. Over-the-counter psychotropics: a review of melatonin, St. John's wort, valerian, and kava-kava. *J Am Coll Health* 1998;32:680–691.

10 Santos MS *et al.* Synaptosomal GABA release is influenced by valerian root extract involvement of the GABA carrier. *Arch Int Pharmacodynamics* 1994;327:220–231.

11 Clarkin JF *et al.* Proptotypic typology and the borderline personality disorder. *J Abnorm Psychol* 1983;92(3):263–275.

12 Kernberg PF. *Borderline Conditions and Pathological Narcissm.* Jason Aronson, 1975.

13 *Diagnostic and Statistical Manual*, 4th edn. American Psychiatric Association Press, 2000.

14 Zanarini MC and Frankenburg F. Pathways to the development of borderline personality disorder. *J Pers Disord*, 1997;11(1):93–104.

15 Zanarini MC. Childhood experiences associated with the development of borderline personality disorder. *Psychiatric Clin North Am* 2000;23(1):89–10.

16 Davidson RJ *et al.* Dysfunction in the neural circuitry of emotion regulation – a possible prelude to violence. *Science*, 2000;289(5479):591–594.

17 Soloff PH *et al.* Self-mutilation and suicidal behavior in borderline personality disorder. *J Pers Disord* 1994;8(4):257–267.

18 Gardner DL and Cowdry RW. Suicidal and parasuicidal behavior in borderline personality disorder. *Psychiatric Clin North Am* 1985;8(2):389–403.

19 Lineham MM *et al.* Naturalistic follow-up of a behavioral treatment for chronically parasuicidal borderline patients. [Published *erratum* appears in *Arch Gen Psychiatry* 1994;51(5):422]. *Arch Gen Psychiatry* 1993;50(12):971–974.

20 Koerner K and Linehan MM. Research on dialectical behavior therapy for patients with borderline personality disorder. *Psychiatric Clin North Am* 2000;23(1):151–167.

21 Coccara EF *et al.* Fluoxetine treatment of impulsive aggression in DSM-III-R personality disorder patients. *J Clin Psychopharmacol* 1990;10:373–375.

22 Cornelius JR *et al.* A preliminary trial of fluoxetine in refractory borderline patients. *J Clin Psychopharmacol* 1991;1:116–120.

23 Kavoussi RJ *et al.* An open trial of sertraline in personality disorder patients with impulsive aggression. *J Clin Psychiatry* 1994;55:137–141.

24 Salzman C. Effect of fluoxetine on anger in borderline personality disorder. [Abstract] *Neuropsychopharmacology* 1994;10(suppl.):826.

25 Cowdry RW and Gardner DL. Pharmacotherapy of borderline personality disorder. Alprazolam, carbamazepine, trifluoperazine, and tranylcypromine. *Arch Gen Psychiatry* 1988;45:111–119.

26 Gardner DL and Cowdry RW. Positive effects of carbamazepine on behavioral dyscontrol in borderline personality disorder. *Am J Psychiatry* 1986;143:519–522.

27 Hollander E *et al.* A preliminary double-blind, placebo controlled trial of divalproex sodium in borderline personality disorder. *J Clin Psychiatry* 2001;62:199–203.

28 Frankenburg FR and Zanarini MC. Divalproex sodium treatment of somen with borderline personality disorder. *J Clin Psychiatry* 2002;63:442–446.

29 Finley E. Personality Disorder: Borderline. On: http://www.emedicine.com/ped/topic270.htm

30   Zanarini MC and Frankenburg FR. Olanzapine treatment of female borderline personality disorder patients: a double-blind, placebo-controlled pilot study. *J Clin Psychiatry* 2001;62:849–854.

31   Rocca P *et al*. Treatment of borderline personality disorder with risperidone. *J Clin Psychiatry* 2002;63:241–244.

Chapter 21

Prescription writing and record keeping

This chapter will focus on the written elements of the prescriptive process, including the elements of a well-written prescription and the records necessary to document prescriptive practice.

The written prescription

A patient comes to a prescriber for the prescriber's knowledge, judgment, evaluation, and thinking. The end product of these endeavors is usually a written prescription. The essential elements, without which a prescription cannot be valid, are listed in Table 21.1. Additional elements that may or may not be included in a prescription are in Table 21.2.

A model prescription is shown in Figure 21.1.

Stylistic elements and recommendations

Attention to several other items will help make prescriptions consistent, and less open to misinterpretation. The clinician should therefore observe the following guidelines:

■ *Use legible handwriting.* If handwriting is not easily readable, consider printing prescriptions. It is extraordinarily easy for a pharmacist to confuse "Lamictal" for "Lamasil, Ludiomil, and Lomotil" or "Fluoxetine" for "Fluvoxamine." *If writing is not clear, mistakes will be made* by the pharmacist or the patient.

■ *Use the metric system* for the amounts of medication, wherever possible.

■ *Avoid abbreviations of medications* (e.g. "Lith" for lithium, "MOM" for milk of magnesia).

Table 21.1 The essential elements of a prescription

■ *Patient name.* Include the patient's full first name. Do not use initials or nicknames.

■ *Date the prescription is written.* Although the vast majority of prescriptions are dated on the day the prescription is written, it is legal to write a prescription for a future date. While it should not be standard practice, this could occur, for example, with a patient who is taking a stimulant. Since stimulant medications can be only dispensed in the USA for a month at a time, a practitioner might, when prescribing for a long-term, stable patient at a 90-day medication management visit, write two future prescriptions dated for subsequent months so that the patient need not return to the office. In general, however, most prescriptions are dated on the day they are written.

■ *The medication to be dispensed.* Use the generic or brand name, as appropriate.

■ The *strength* (usually in number of mg or μg) and *dosage* form of the medication (pills, capsules, liquid, suppositories, or other format).

■ The *number of units to be dispensed* preceded by "Dispense" or "Disp #." Spell out the number of units in words rather than using numbers (e.g. "one hundred tablets" instead of "100 tablets").

■ The number of *refills* allowed, if any.

■ *Specific directions for use,* including how many units are to be taken, how often they are to be taken, and by what route (oral, intravenous, rectal, etc.). If the medication is to be given as needed (PRN), specify how often the dose is to be taken and for what purpose. Preface the exact directions with "*sig*" (Latin for sign or mark – literally, how the prescriber wants the vial marked for patient usage).

■ Some American states may legislate other items to be included in the written prescription. Contact the licensing board relative to your specialty for this information.

Table 21.2 Optional elements on a prescription

■ Patient age

■ Patient address

■ Generic substitution allowed. Some prescriptions contain a check-off box to permit generic substitutions. If generic substitution is to be specifically *disallowed*, write "DAW," or "dispense as written," on the prescription

Sample Prescription

Christopher M. Doran, MD

Name: _____Mary Jones_____   Date: <u>06/15/03</u>

Lithium carbonate
300 mg
Disp # Ninety
Sig: Three capsules by mouth at
bedtime

Label ☒   _____(signature)_____ MD

Refill   None   Times

Figure 21.1 Sample prescription

- *Avoid the use of abbreviations in giving directions* (for example, spell out "four times a day" rather than writing "qid," which can be easily confused with "qd" – once a day).
- Always use a zero before strengths of less than 1 mg (for example, use 0.5 mg not .5 mg).
- Avoid using a terminal or trailing zero after a decimal (for example, use 0.1 mg, not 0.10 mg).

Record keeping

Written records of the prescriptive process are crucial to treatment documentation. Whether the interaction process occurs in an outpatient office, a clinic, or a hospital, written records should be consistently made of every patient contact no matter how brief. Specifically, there should be written documentation of every:

- Face-to-face appointment
- Telephone contact
- E-mail contact
- Message left on an answering machine for the patient about a clinical matter
- Original prescription or prescription refill.

Elements of a clinician's prescriptive note

The elements of an initial prescriptive evaluation are covered in Chapter 3, including the elements necessary to the written record, and will not be repeated

Table 21.3 Elements of a prescriptive note
■ Date of the contact
■ Patient data, including target symptoms and significant changes in the clinical state. This should include changes in psychological condition, medical condition or medication use
■ Pertinent negatives if important questions are asked and responded to negatively (e.g. patient denies presence of suicidal ideation)
■ Side effects present or denied
■ Laboratory results, including any psychotropic blood levels
■ Clinician assessment of the current condition. Is the patient improving, unchanged, or regressing? Is the medication effective in the overall treatment? If not sufficiently effective, what changes are needed?
■ Plan and recommendations
■ Specify:
■ Any change in medication regimen. If the patient is to maintain the current regimen, specify this in writing
■ Any warnings or recommendations
■ Any prescriptions written
■ Any laboratory tests needed or consultations requested
■ Date of the next evaluation for medications

here. The elements of a note documenting a follow-up session consultation or any other contact that results in a revision of the medication regimen are included in Table 21.3.

A signature is necessary on institutional records, unless the note is solely in an outpatient clinician's private files.

Taking and preparing notes

There are many equally useful methods of recording patient clinical notes. What is crucial, however, is that the clinician:

■ Has a system of taking, filing, and storing notes that is used consistently
■ Notes every clinical encounter at the time of the contact, or directly thereafter, and does not wait until a later date or time. If delayed, notes will inevitably be vague, inaccurate or forgotten.

Within these broad parameters, which clinicians can adapt to their personal style, notes can be documented in various ways:

■ Handwritten
■ Typed
■ Dictated and transcribed by others
■ Spoken into a computer and transcribed automatically.

As voice-recognition computer software improves in speed, accuracy, and ease of use, it is likely that the last method will become universal and most written medical records will ultimately be documented in this way.

Some clinicians take written notes during their face-to-face meeting with the patient. Others prefer more eye contact and a greater sense of connection to the patient, and wait until the end of the visit to compose and document their clinical thoughts. Some practitioners feel that it is useful to dictate the patient's note in the patient's presence so he or she knows exactly what is being documented about the visit. Others are more comfortable waiting until after the session to dictate or write, particularly if sensitive material is to be documented or precise wording is necessary. Although it is desirable that all dictation be reviewed for accuracy and completeness, not all practitioners routinely review their dictated notes until the next time the chart is opened. If any dictated note documents a sensitive issue, is involved in a negative patient outcome, or is to be sent to others outside of the treatment setting, each dictation should be promptly reviewed for accuracy.

CLINICAL TIP

No matter how experienced or confident a clinician may be, *he or she must not attempt to write a document about one subject while discussing another*. This applies to writing prescriptions, medical record notes, laboratory test requests, or any other written document while talking to patients, office staff, or using the telephone. In particular, if the clinician feels rushed, it can be tempting to try to do two tasks at once. This practice will inevitably result in errors on the written document and/or poor verbal communication. For example, even experienced clinicians cannot satisfactorily write prescriptions while discussing side effects, order a lab test while giving the patient medication directions, or make a clinical record note while making a referral to a colleague on the telephone.

It can, however, be valuable to clinician and patient alike for the clinician to say out loud what he or she is writing. For example, it is reinforcing to speak what is written on a prescription as it is being done. *"Mrs Harrison, I am writing this prescription for [name of medication]. I am giving you 60 pills with two refills. You are to take two of these by mouth every night at bedtime."* This practice may improve the accuracy of both the written and the verbal communications.

Some clinicians may delay writing notes that document negative outcomes, particularly serious ones in which the records could ultimately be scrutinized. The rationale can be to await complete information to compose a note as accurately and thoroughly as possible. While this practice is not totally without merit, it is generally preferred to document notes on negative outcomes soon after the event. It is important to document clinical decision-making at the time, with as much data as is then known. Information that is pending or missing should be noted, then followed up later with an additional note. If new or additional data affect the treatment plan, clinical thinking or assessment, the clinical reasoning should be explained simply. It is perfectly reasonable for the clinician to refine his or her thinking or change an assessment based on new data. *Under no circumstances should a previously written note be altered, rewritten, deleted, or otherwise changed* in an effort to make it "look better" or make the decision-making appear more sound. Changed or altered records or notes, written after the fact, can raise medicolegal suspicion, particularly if there are negative outcomes.

Systems for note taking

Several systematized methods of writing progress notes have been devised and widely promulgated. Although the acronyms vary, the elements are similar. Each system includes information to be gathered, the clinician's assessment or impression of the data, the recommendations, and the plan. Some of the common acronyms are:

■   SOAP (subjective data, objective data, assessment, and plan)
■   DAP (data, assessment, and plan)
■   DAR (data, assessment, and recommendations).

An inexperienced clinician would do well to adopt and practice one of the systematized formats to ensure that all necessary elements are included.

Style items in a medication note

Medication notes should be targeted and concise, as very long notes are often not read. As to content and wording, a useful guideline is that the clinician *should not include words or items in a note that he or she would not want read aloud to the patient or to a colleague.* Slang, derogatory, or disparaging terms should be avoided, as should assessments that cannot be documented by observation and fact

Regardless of the format used, clinical notes are best recorded on standard-sized paper ($8\frac{1}{2} \times 11$" in the United States, A4 in the UK), which is easily copyable. Clinicians who prescribe medications will often have need to copy their records for other clinicians or for insurance companies, or as documentation of the session. If the size of the paper is other than standard, it is often cumbersome to copy. *Spiral notebooks* or other bound volumes, which cannot easily be copied, should be avoided, and notes must always be written in ink pen, not in pencil.

Separate medication lists

In addition to whatever clinical notes of patient contact are maintained, it is useful for the prescriber to maintain a current, easily modifiable list of all medications so that the entire regimen prescribed for each patient is easily viewed at one time. Additionally, such a medication list permits the clinician rapidly to see when medications were started, when they were stopped, and previous medications tried.

In modern psychopharmacology, when patients are often prescribed multiple medications, it is not only convenient, but also safe practice to list all medications on one document. If clinicians document medication data solely in the body of a written paragraph, or in the "Plan" section of a progress note, it is difficult to follow which medications have been used, their start and stop dates, and when combinations of medications may have been tried. While maintaining a separate medication list in an outpatient chart requires additional writing on the part of the clinician, it results in superior organization and safety. An example of such a medication sheet, which shows dates, names, doses, and includes a space for serum blood level results, is shown in Table 21.4. By circling dates when a medication is stopped, it is clear which medications have been tried, when, and for how long they were used.

Ongoing laboratory monitoring

Although not all psychotropics require periodic laboratory tests, some medications require serum blood levels of the psychotropic itself (see Chapter 22) or periodic assessment of liver function, blood count, or other parameters, as has also been described previously in this text. During follow-up appointments and throughout the length of prescription, the clinician will need to devise a system to know when repeat tests need to be ordered and to manage reports of lab tests in the client's chart. There is a variety of ways to do this, but if some methodology is not followed, clinicians will have difficulty in remembering to order necessary

Table 21.4 Sample medication list

Medication log of *(name of patient)*_____

Date	Name of medication	Dose/freq	Disp #	Refills	Comments/blood level/lab tests

Circle on stop dates   Medical conditions   Other medications   Allergies/sensitivities tests at appropriate times and in consistently organizing their laboratory records. This becomes particularly problematic when a patient is on multiple medications and is seen over a long period of time.

Clinicians practicing in inpatient or clinic settings may have a standard chart format with dividers, one of which is usually reserved for laboratory results. In an outpatient setting, where such a system is not required, clinicians should organize their office records so that *lab test results and reports of any physical examinations/consultations are kept separately in chronological order* in one section of the patient's chart. This provides a consistent place at which to review past medical results, view any trends, see when exams or tests were performed, and collate any physical exam and laboratory information where needed – e.g. when preparing a report of the patient's care for a third party.

Although the clinician will want to mention appropriate physical exams and lab results in a progress note, in general it is not wise to insert these actual reports haphazardly or "as they arrive" into the patient's progress notes. While this may seem intuitive or an easy way to file, chronological filing within the progress notes can lead to confusion and an increasing likelihood that important results may be overlooked, especially when the patient's file becomes large.

Some clinicians will prefer to record serum blood levels and/or other lab test results on the patient's medication list as mentioned in the previous section of this chapter. Others may prefer to devise separate forms specifically for monitoring laboratory values, with prompts for the clinician in ordering subsequent tests. An example of such a system is shown in Table 21.5.

When using this format, the clinician will necessarily be succinct and likely use abbreviations to save documentation time. Only significant findings need be documented, as long as a copy of the full lab report is contained elsewhere in the chart.

The form shown in Table 21.5 could be filled out as in Table 21.6, which is an example of a patient initially started on lithium, who later had the dose increased to treat breakthrough symptoms.

Table 21.5 Sample laboratory test results form

Laboratory Monitoring for (*patient's name*)_____

Date	Test	Significant positive or negative results	Information conveyed to patient	Changes in treatment plan or medication	Date of next test

Table 21.6 Sample laboratory test results form (filled in)

Laboratory Monitoring for (*patient's name*)_____

Date	Test	Significant positive or negative results	Information conveyed to patient	Changes in treatment plan or medication	Date of next test
9/4/03	Chemistry profile CBC TSH	WNL WNL 1.05	✓ ✓ ✓	Start lithium	1–2 weeks
09/14/03	Lithium level (on 900 mg)	0.47 meq/l	✓	Increase dose to 1200 mg	2 weeks
10/01/03	Lithium level (on 1200 mg)	0.70 meq/l	✓	Maintain dose	6 weeks
11/15/03	Lithium	0.68 meq/l	✓	Maintain dose	3 months
2/18/04	Lithium TSH	0.52 meq/l 2.1	✓	Increase dose to 1500 mg	1–2 weeks
3/1/04	Lithium (on 1500 mg)	0.91 meq/l	✓	Maintain dose	3 months
6/7/04	Lithium	0.85 meq/l	✓	Maintain dose	6 months
12/02/04	Lithium Chemistry profile TSH CBC	0.86 meq/l WNL 2.0 WNL	✓	Maintain dose	6 months

WNL = Within normal limits.

Confidentiality and security of records

All medical records require attention to confidentiality and safe storage. Because of the special nature of mental health records, including those of medication prescription, even more attention is required in ensuring that written records and conversations about patient treatment are kept confidential.

Any written records that include documentation of mental health prescriptions should always be kept safe and locked. Whether active or in storage, such records are typically kept in locked file cabinets, locked offices, or locked storage rooms. A breach of confidentiality can occur when records are carried away or left in unusual places where they can be read by others. Some common locations where records are accidentally left and their confidentiality endangered include:

- Left open on a desk when the clinician leaves the room
- In patient exam rooms

- In a hospital room
- In a patient waiting room
- In cars
- In a personal residence
- In public areas such as a staff cafeteria or meeting rooms.

It is only clinicians themselves or certain select clinical/clerical staff who should have access to records, especially in clinic settings. It is important to ensure that records are not observed by non-authorized individuals, including custodial staff, repairmen, package delivery persons, or other patients.

Discussing clinical matters

Oral communication is another way by which confidentiality of clinical and medication information can be easily and inadvertently violated. In general, verbal communication about patients should be only undertaken within an office or over the telephone in private. Common situations that can lead to violation of confidentiality include:

- Discussing one patient's status while a second patient is in the office
- Discussing a patient's case in a room with an open door
- Talking with clinic staff outside of an office, in a hallway, or another public area of a clinic
- Talking about patients in a clinic waiting area
- Discussing clinical material in an elevator
- Discussing patient information at a hospital nursing station
- Discussing a patient's condition "on rounds"
- Discussing patient histories at a meeting or conference
- Discussing patient information over lunch or dinner
- Discussing patient information on a cell phone when others are present.

Chapter 22

Serum blood levels of psychotropics

A prime example of the mixture of art and science in mental health medication is the use of serum blood levels of psychotropic medications. The introduction and successful use of serum blood levels (sometimes referred to as Therapeutic Drug Monitoring, or TDM) has scientifically "legitimized" psychiatry to both clinicians and patients. It supports the notion that mental health prescriptions are scientific and in line with other specialties of medicine. Utilizing the results of blood levels, however, still requires the art of flexibility and judgment, rather than rote treatment decision-making based on numbers.

When blood levels help

Serum blood levels may have several clinical applications:[1]

- To increase efficacy by using the optimum amount of medication
- To increase safety by decreasing side effects and minimizing the likelihood of toxicity
- To monitor compliance
- To protect against medicolegal actions.

Those types of medications where blood levels can be of significance include:

- Medications that have a *narrow therapeutic index* (a small difference between a therapeutic level and a level resulting in toxicity/side effects), such as TCAs or lithium
- Medications where there is a *proven, useful therapeutic range* that can be correlated to clinical response, such as nortriptyline or clozapine
- Medications that have a *wide variability* in *absorption, metabolism or excretion* between individuals (e.g. TCAs).

Specifically, the medications in which serum blood levels have been useful are listed in Table 22.1.

The therapeutic range for each of these medications is listed in Table 22.2. These data are also included in Appendices 2, 4 and 5.

Small changes in blood level are generally not of clinical significance, and it usually serves no purpose to adjust medications to change blood levels by less than 5–10 percent.

Instructions to patients

Fortunately, regardless of what medication is being monitored through blood levels, instructions to the patient are virtually identical. Clinicians measure *trough blood levels*, typically timed 12 hours after the last medication dose. Since the timing is critical to obtaining levels that are accurate, for most patients this requires drawing the blood level in the morning (12 hours after an evening dose). The timeframe is approximate, and a level drawn within 10–14 hours from the last dose is generally accurate. There is no intrinsic reason why a patient could not have a blood level drawn in the early evening (12 hours after a morning dose), but most outpatient laboratories are not open to draw the level.

Most psychotropics will generate a steady-state blood level within four half-lives. Therefore, in order accurately to measure the amount of medication at steady-state it is necessary for the patient to be on a consistent dose of medication for at least 4 days prior to the blood level. Inconsistent dosing before a blood level can have a variable effect on the result. If the only dose missed was on day one or day two, some reasonable estimate of the blood level may still be

---

Table 22.1 Psychotropic medications for which serum blood levels are helpful

- Lithium
- Carbamazepine
- Valproic acid
- Clozapine
- Nortriptyline
- Imipramine
- Desipramine
- Amitriptyline
- Clomipramine

Table 22.2 Therapeutic serum blood levels of commonly used psychotropic medications*

Medication	Therapeutic range (meq)	Toxic levels (where established)
Lithium[1]	0.6–1.2/l	>1.5 mmol/l
Carbamazepine[1]	4–12 µg/ml	>12 µg/ml
Valproic acid[1]	50–100 µg/ml	
Clozapine[2]	> 350 mg/ml	
Nortriptyline[3]	50–150 mg/ml	
Imipramine[4,5] (Parent compound plus metabolite)	200–250 mg/ml	>450 mg/ml
Desipramine[4]	110–180 mg/ml	
Amitriptyline[4]	150–250 mg/ml	

[1] Bezchlibnyk-Butler K and Jeffries JJ. *Psychotropic Drugs*, 9th edn. Hogrefe & Huber, 1999, pp. 111–124.
[2] Kronig MH *et al*. Plasma clozapine levels and clinical response for treatment refractory schizophrenic patients. *Am J Psychiatry* 1995;152:179–182.
[3] Perry PJ *et al*. The relationship between antidepressant response and tricyclic antidepressant plasma concentrations. *Clin Pharmacokinet* 1987;13:381–392.
[4] Hales RE. *Textbook of Psychiatry*, 3rd edn. American Psychiatric Association Press, 1999, p. 294.
[5] Kaplan HI and Sadock BJ. *Comprehensive Textbook of Psychiatry*, 6th edn. Lippincott, Williams & Wilkins, 1995, p. 1164.

obtained. However, if the missed dose occurs on day four, just before the blood level, the value obtained can be affected by as much as 25–50 percent.

Written instructions are helpful for most patients to ensure that they follow the methodology necessary to obtain accurate values. A typical instruction sheet for serum blood level testing is shown in Table 22.3.

Although it may vary by locale and laboratory used, lithium levels, valproic acid levels, and serum carbamazepine levels are generally returned within 12–36 hours. Stat levels may be obtained more quickly in situations of crisis or serious toxicity. Serum tricyclic antidepressant levels and clozapine levels take 48–96 hours to return to the clinician, since these tests are often not performed locally and need to be sent to a specialty lab.

On occasion, patients will call urgently from the lab saying that they are there to have their blood level drawn, but now realize that they took their morning dose an hour or two before. Such patients should be advised NOT to have the blood level drawn that day, to continue taking their regular dose and to return on another day. Drawing a level 1–2 hours after the last oral dose registers a meaningless number that cannot be reliably extrapolated to yield valuable information.

Table 22.3 Instructions for blood level testing

1 Draw your first level on [date]_____. Blood levels require 4 days on the same dose of medication in order to be accurate. If your dose of medicine has been changed recently, maintain a consistent dose for at least 4 days before testing. Do not miss any doses in the 4 days before the test.
2 Have the level drawn approximately *12 HOURS AFTER YOUR EVENING DOSE* (a range of 10–14 hours is allowed, but not shorter or longer).
3 If you usually take a dose of medicine in the morning, *WAIT UNTIL AFTER THE BLOOD IS DRAWN TO TAKE YOUR MORNING DOSE ON THE DAY OF THE TEST*. If you forget and take your morning dose that day, the test will not be accurate. *Have the blood level drawn another day.*
4 You may eat a normal breakfast on the day of a blood level test. It is *not* necessary to fast for this test. You may also take any other prescribed medication (that is not being measured in the blood level) on the morning of the test.

Frequency of blood levels

How often a blood level is drawn depends on a number of factors, including the particular medication monitored, the medical health or fragility of the patient, and the patient's level of improvement (or lack thereof). *Lithium levels* are ordered both more frequently and more regularly over the long term than are levels of other psychotropics. The serum level of lithium can be significantly affected by various prescription and non-prescription medications (such as NSAIDs and diuretics), changes in salt and fluid balance, and gastrointestinal illness, particularly diarrhea. Therefore, lithium levels are typically measured in the outpatient clinic within a week after starting lithium and every 1–2 weeks thereafter until the medication is stabilized. Once stabilized, lithium levels should be drawn every 3 months for the first year. Thereafter, levels can be drawn every 3–6 months. A serum creatinine, BUN, CBC and TSH should be monitored every 6–12 months for changes in kidney function, blood count and lowered thyroid function.

Serum carbamazepine, valproic acid or clozapine levels should be drawn 5–7 days after an initial target dose is reached, and every 1–4 weeks thereafter until an appropriate blood level is stabilized. If the patient is doing well clinically, blood levels may then be monitored every 2–4 months during the first year. Clinicians have variable ways of dealing with blood levels for patients remaining on these medications over the long term. Some clinicians choose to check blood levels at regular intervals even if the patient is doing well, whereas other clinicians will not draw routine blood levels unless there is some clinical indication to do so. Even if clinicians choose not to check routine blood values when a patient is doing well, it is appropriate to check a panel of liver function tests and a CBC to monitor for hepatic or hematological side effects at least once a year.

For *tricyclic antidepressants*, an initial level is generally drawn 5–7 days after an initial target dosage of medication has been reached. Follow-up blood levels may be drawn every 1–3 weeks thereafter, depending on patient response and the presence or absence of side effects. Once stabilized, tricyclic levels need not be drawn on a regular basis provided the patient remains clinically stable and symptoms are in remission.

Some of the exceptions to these general time guidelines for serum blood monitoring are listed in Table 22.4.

A *clinical relapse* or the emergence of *new or troublesome psychiatric symptoms* is a clear indication to check the blood level of any psychotropic medication currently prescribed to the patient. Blood levels may have changed, and a simple adjustment of dosage may be all that is necessary to re-establish remission.

The *addition or removal of a medication* that might affect the serum level of a psychotropic is also a good reason to check a blood level. Many of these occur because of P-450 interactions (see Chapter 17). Common psychotropic medications with such potential interactions include adding an SSRI to a TCA (which can raise the blood level of the TCA), adding valproic acid to lamotrigine (which can raise the level of lamotrigine), or adding an SSRI to carbamazepine (which can raise the level of carbamazepine).

A third reason for rechecking a blood level is the *emergence of new side effects*. Subtle or significant changes in blood levels over time may result in side effects that were not present when the patient initiated the medication. A check of a blood level and comparison with baseline blood levels on which the patient had no side effects may alert the clinician to lower the dosage and possibly eliminate the side effect.

Occasionally, it is necessary for a clinician to monitor *medication compliance*. A blood level will give valuable information as to whether the patient is taking the medication at all. From the numerical value and comparison to previous levels, it can usually be determined if the patient is following the full regimen.

It is prudent to check a serum blood level of a measurable psychotropic at the time of a *psychiatric or medical hospitalization*. Regardless of the reason for hospitalization, by definition there has been a major change in health status, and it is useful at these times to know the baseline level of the psychotropic. A psychiatric hospitalization indicates that a psychiatric crisis has occurred. Decisions about medications may need to be made, and blood levels can be helpful with this determination. A very low or zero blood level may also indicate that poor compliance can have contributed to the crisis. If the hospitalization is medical, there may be a significant medical illness or the possibility of surgery. In either case, knowing the current blood level of the psychotropic is helpful to the medical/surgical team.

Table 22.4 Reasons to obtain more frequent serum psychotropic levels

- Clinical relapse
- Addition/removal of an interacting medication
- Emergence of new side effects
- When the patient is hospitalized or institutionalized
- Suspected non-compliance

There can be some changes in absorption or pharmacokinetics with certain *generic medication* compared to the branded version. When a patient changes from brand name to generic or *vice versa* and the patient's clinical state changes proximate to that time, a check of blood level is indicated (see Chapter 23).

Using clinical judgment

The presence of numerical blood levels should not override the clinician's judgment and clinical observation. It is a simple but unfortunate error to assume that all patients will do best when a blood level is within the published therapeutic range. Ultimately, the most important parameters to monitor are the patient's functioning and emotional state, and the presence of side effects, if any. If the clinician finds that either a higher or lower blood level provides solid, consistent clinical control of symptoms, the clinician may choose to maintain the patient on this dose of medication. It is important, however, when using a dose that gives higher or lower than "normal" published levels, that the clinician document the rationale for this exception. Notably lithium, valproic acid, and carbamazepine can provide adequate clinical response even if a patient's blood level is technically "low." There are numerous examples of patients who show satisfactory mood stabilization on sub-therapeutic blood levels, and in fact get significant side effects when their blood levels are brought into the therapeutic range.

Where blood levels do not help

There are many psychotropic medications for which blood levels are either unavailable or yield no significant clinical information. A list of such medications appears in Table 22.5.

For these drugs, clinically it would be helpful to have valid therapeutic dose ranges or some other biological measure of the amount of medication absorbed for a given oral dose. While the technology for *qualitatively* measuring the presence of these medications in the blood stream exists, clinically helpful *quantitative* results are not possible. Technological problems for accurate lab values may not exist, or the results may not be reproducible. Even more commonly, medication levels may be measured but there is no significant correlation between the numerical medication levels and clinical response. This is especially true for SSRI

Table 22.5 **Psychotropic medications for which serum blood levels are of no value**

- All SSRI antidepressants
- Bupropion, nefazodone, mirtazepine, venlafaxine
- Traditional and atypical antipsychotics
- Benzodiazepines
- Buspirone
- Anticholinergic medications
- Cholinesterase inhibitors
- Any medication used for alcohol abuse

antidepressants and traditional antipsychotics, where patient A may respond very well to significantly low blood levels and patient B may require exceptionally high blood levels. In typical practice, a clinician would have no reason to draw a blood level of the medicines listed in Table 22.5 except to assess compliance.

Necessary documentation

Blood levels are only useful when seen and evaluated by the clinician. The clinician needs to indicate that the results of a blood level have been noted, which is usually done by initialing the report. It is useful to comment on the results of the blood level in the progress note for that day or the appointment note for that session. It is also crucial to document what action was taken based on the blood level received, particularly if the blood level was outside the therapeutic range:

- Was the clinician satisfied with the blood level?
- If not, are there to be any changes in dosage?
- When is the next blood level to be drawn?

Serum blood level results outside of the therapeutic norm that are not noted and/or acted upon can present a medicolegal risk. In the event of an untoward response, the presence of a blood level that was not noted, not acted upon and not documented may prove to be the legal undoing of the clinician. Similarly, a timely blood level noted by the clinician may be a strong legal defense against a poor outcome of medication.

Reference

1   Jamicak PG *et al. Principles and Practice of Psychopharmacotherapy.* Baltimore, Williams & Wilkins, 1997, p. 77.

Chapter 23

Generic medications

Brand-name medications are protected by a patent, issued to the pharmaceutical company that develops the medication, to compensate the firm for the time, money and testing invested in bringing the medication to market. When the patent expires 17 years after being issued, other companies may manufacture the same medication. Formulations of the same product are marketed and sold under its generic (chemical) name, which usually leads to lower prices (see Table 23.1). Relatively few of the newest mental health medications are available as generics today, but over the next 5–10 years the patents of many branded products will expire and generic preparations may then be manufactured.

The generic share of the prescription market increased from 18.6 percent in 1984 to 41.6 percent in 1996.[1] Research shows that during the first year in competition with a generic, brand name medications lose an average of 44 percent of their share to generic drugs. Retail prices of generics cost an average of 25 percent less than the original brand name.[1]

The fate of a medication when its patent expires depends on the extent of usage of the medication and what, if any, alternatives exist. When a medication is little used and/or there are better alternatives, generic formulations seldom emerge. The medication can still be prescribed through its branded name, and the price for this branded preparation usually remains relatively high. For a medication that is commonly used and/or there are few superior alternatives, one or more generic preparations will emerge. The medication can then be prescribed as

Table 23.1 Generic medications

These are

- Chemically identical to the branded medication in regard to their active ingredients
- May have different bioavailability
- May contain different dyes, fillers or coatings
- Are usually plain in color and packaging
- Are usually less expensive than branded medications, but not always

a less expensive generic. It may continue to be prescribed through the higher-priced branded name as well.

When generic preparations are available, pharmaco-economics drive pharmaceutical manufacturers to try one of several strategies to ensure continued prescription of a branded version of the medication. A different preparation that still contains the same active ingredient (e.g. a unique combination of more than one product or a new delivery system) may be marketed. In the USA, if the Food and Drug Administration (FDA) deems the medication to be sufficiently different, unique and effective, a new patent is issued. An example of this is valproic acid sodium, which was available as a useful generic medication, but gave some patients significant side effects. It was reformulated with a special coating to ensure more gradual absorption of the drug, thus having fewer side effects than the generic version. This newly formulated version of valproex sodium was marketed in the USA under the brand name Depakote with significant success.

Other companies have developed and marketed stereo-isomers (mirror images) of the initial product. If such an isomer is valuable, more targeted, has fewer side effects than a mixture of isomers, or has some other advantage, a new patent may be issued for the preparation. An example of this is S-citalopram (marketed in the USA as Lexapro), which is a product containing just one stereo isomer of citalopram rather than the mixture of stereo-isomers of citalopram contained in Celexa. Whether this new preparation will have significantly increased effectiveness and/or a lower side-effect profile will emerge as the drug comes into common clinical usage.

Another manufacturing option is to repackage a medication under a new name for a new indication. Examples of this include fluoxetine (Prozac) remarketed as Serafem for premenstrual dysphoric disorder, and bupropion (Wellbutrin) remarketed as Zyban for smoking cessation.

Table 23.2 lists commonly used mental health medications that have a generic preparation.

In general, the FDA maintains that generic drugs are safe and effective. Clinically, this is also the experience of most practitioners. When generics are substituted for branded products, the majority of patients who have previously responded will continue to experience positive therapeutic benefit. The one and only reason to switch to a generic preparation is cost. Some patients have a strong preference for branded *vs* generic preparations. When this is so, there is little reason not to prescribe the branded preparation, if the patient is willing to pay the difference.

Table 23.2 Commonly used mental health medications that have a generic preparation
■ TCAs, all
■ MAOIs, all
■ Lithium carbonate
■ Carbamazepine (Tegretol)
■ Traditional antipsychotics, all
■ Benzodiazepines, all
■ Antihistamines, virtually all
■ Beta blockers, virtually all
■ Valproic acid (Depakote, Depakote ER)
■ Benztropine (Cogentin)
■ Disulfiram (Antabuse)
■ Bupropion (Wellbutrin)
■ Fluoxetine (Prozac)
■ Clozapine (Clozaril)

To allow or specify a generic product, write the chemical name of the medication on the prescription. Some prescriptions have a check-off box that can be marked to allow generic substitutions for a branded product.

If the clinician does not wish to allow generic substitutions for a brand-name product, the prescription should include the phrase "Dispense As Written" or "DAW" on the prescription to instruct the pharmacist that a generic drug may not be substituted.

Generic substitution problems

Although most people tolerate generic preparations well, and receive comparable therapeutic effect, when problems do occur with generic substitutions, it is generally because of the reasons listed in Table 23.3.

An issue of concern with a generic versus a branded product is bioequivalence. Two medications are considered bioequivalent if they have the same biological effect in the body at equivalent doses. This is usually determined by equal bioavailability – i.e. equal doses of both preparations become equally available to the target tissue in the body. For oral medications, this means that they will be equivalently absorbed from the gut, carried through the bloodstream to the target tissue in similar concentrations, and metabolized equally. Preparations that are

Table 23.3 Potential generic problems
■ Non-bioequivalence of generic medication may lead to differing blood levels for a specific patient and, therefore, a changed clinical state
■ Patient sensitivity to inactive ingredients (e.g. dyes, fillers) in the generic preparation
■ Manufacturing/processing problems with the generic (uncommon)

absorbed more quickly or slowly, transported at significantly different rates, or broken down and excreted at different rates may not be bioequivalent. Differences in any of these steps could result in varying amounts of drug at the tissue site, markedly different peak concentrations of drug, differing clinical response, as well as fewer side effects.

In order for a generic drug to be considered legally bioequivalent to the branded product, the confidence intervals for absorption and maximum drug concentration must fall entirely between 80 and 125 percent of the reference (branded) drug. This range is quite wide, and in actuality a narrower range is usually preferred. A difference of 8–10 percent, while technically falling within the range, is still unlikely to pass FDA approval. Average differences of 3–4 percent in absorption and maximum drug concentration are more typical for the majority of approved generic medicines on the market.

Because each person has variables in his or her gastrointestinal capacity for drug absorption, protein binding in the blood, and metabolic capacity, there may occur significant differences in bioavailability and bioequivalence even when the drugs have been deemed "bioequivalent." This can occur because the capsule/pill coating, filler or pill size is different for the branded and generic products, leading to changed absorption rates or peak drug concentrations. When the amount of drug differs at the site of action, "too little" or "too much" drug effect may occur, and new side effects may emerge.

Occasionally a patient has an allergy or adverse effect to an inactive component of the generic, such as a dye, filler or capsule coating.

In the past, on rare occasions, the manufacturing process of a generic drug may have been poorly controlled, resulting in marked variability in the amount of active medication in each pill or, even more rarely, contamination.

Generic change without the clinician's knowledge

Patients may be switched to a generic preparation when the primary clinician is unaware of the change. Such unexpected transitions can occur in the situations listed in Table 23.4.

If a patient begins to experience a change in clinical state, the practitioner should investigate, as one possible reason for the clinical change, whether a new generic drug preparation was given to the patient.

Table 23.4 Changes to a generic

These could occur when there is:
- A move to a new geographic location
- Admission or discharge from hospital
- Entrance into, or exit from, a nursing care facility or hospice
- A change to a new pharmacy or insurance plan

Tips for generic use

When a generic preparation is available and the clinician chooses to prescribe it, some practitioners prefer to start with the generic and titrate blood levels and/or clinical response with the generic medication alone. Other clinicians prefer to start with the branded preparation, stabilize the clinical condition and blood level, then switch to a generic at a later date. Either method is valid and clinically responsible.

When prescribing a generic medication, it is useful to suggest that patients continue to receive the same brand of generic preparation to minimize any likelihood of differing capsules and fillers that could affect absorption. This may be accomplished by suggesting that they always use the same pharmacy to obtain their generic medication. Have patients ask the pharmacist to supply the generic from the same manufacturer, and report to the clinician if their pills "look different."

If and when a clinician switches a patient from a branded product to a generic, most patients will do well clinically with no significant difference in their clinical state. It is, however, wise to suggest that the patient report any changes in therapeutic effect, or new or increased side effects.

Serum blood levels and generic substitution

When serum blood levels of a medication are available and accurate (see Chapter 22), they can be used to investigate the cause of altered clinical state or change in side effects when a generic switch is undertaken. The result of a generic serum blood level can be easily compared to a level drawn when taking a branded preparation. A blood level change of greater than 5–10 percent could signify that the amount of drug in the serum is different with the generic preparation, even if the oral dose is the same. While the clinician may not know whether this represents a change in absorption, metabolism or excretion, the oral dose can be relatively easily adjusted to re-establish the previously useful blood serum level. Differences of less than 5 percent in blood level are generally not clinically significant for mental health effects.

If no clinically valid serum blood level test exists and a clinical change occurs when a generic alternative is substituted, the clinician may try to guess whether a larger or smaller oral dose is necessary to re-establish clinical equilibrium. If this procedure is not successful and the patient remains symptomatic, an empirical trial of returning to the branded product may be helpful.

Mandated generics

Some institutions, insurance plans or managed care entities will mandate that the clinician prescribe generic preparations when available. This is usually a cost-saving measure that may, or may not, create a problem for an individual patient. In general, a patient's simple desire to have a branded product is an insufficient reason for the clinician to insist that the patient receive the branded product. It is usually not useful, or successful, to insist on branded products for all patients and all medications as a general principle. There may, however, be reasons when a clinician will choose to address the use of generics and insist on a branded product for a particular patient. Usually, this is best done after having tried the patient on a generic version and having documented a poorer response from the generic product. Clinicians should choose their battles carefully for those patients for whom they feel that clinically, it is indicated to insist on a brand-name product. Information should be documented and reasons outlined when calling the person authorizing such decisions. If there is a particular patient for whom the clinician wishes to have a branded product, a carefully reasoned proposal will usually receive approval.

Reference

1   The generic-ization of drugs: will patients benefit?, *Psychopharmacology Update* 2001;12(8):1,4–5.

Chapter 24

The telephone and e-mail – mainstays and millstones

The telephone is the most frequently used method of communication between clinician and patient. Its clinical and administrative uses are almost taken for granted. Telephone contact often provides the first impression that a patient receives of the clinician and his or her office. Used wisely and appropriately during medication management, the telephone can speed up assessments of medication changes, provide the therapist with rapid feedback, and perhaps save the patient an unnecessary trip to the office.

Electronic mail has rapidly become a fixture of world-wide communication that will likely become an ever larger part of the way patients and prescribers interface. It has unique advantages, but puts the clinician one more step removed from cues regarding the patient's condition and behavior.

Both methodologies can facilitate a prescriber's practice life or become intrusive and a chore. This chapter describes the intelligent use of both telephone and e-mail, and identifies their potential pitfalls.

The telephone can be used to manage efficiently many clinical needs, including questions about response, side effects, dosage and interaction with other medications. The patient may be asked to call the clinician on a particular day to give feedback on the effectiveness of a new medication or dosage change. Further clinical refinement of dosage can be accomplished in a brief telephone call, thus saving both clinician and patient significant time and energy. When a patient calls with a question about a drug interaction or side effect, the clinician can quickly intervene, saving the patient discomfort and perhaps avoiding premature discontinuation of medication.

At the same time, when used inappropriately or overutilized the telephone can be both the bane of the practitioner's existence and medicolegal quicksand. This chapter describes the appropriate use of the telephone and how to manage patients who use it inappropriately.

Being available by telephone

Telephone service is a lifeline to the clinician from the patient. There is an old adage: "If patients know they can call, they won't; if they feel they cannot call, they will." In the practice of medication prescription, this is extraordinarily true. Patients feel reassured when they know they can reach the clinician. If patients know that urgent questions will be responded to quickly and consistently, they can often tolerate minor side effects and need not bother the clinician with trivial issues. When patients feel the prescriber is unavailable, does not return calls, or cannot be reached, their anxiety increases and they often magnify minor complaints into "crises." By making themselves available to patients by telephone, clinicians can effectively manage time and gain a reputation as a practitioner with whom patients have a solid alliance.

Appropriate use of the telephone by clinicians

- The clinician should always return all telephone calls from a patient personally or through office staff – if possible promptly, but always by the end of the business day.
- If unable to speak with the patient directly, the clinician should leave a message indicating when a return call was made, and if and when another contact will be attempted. If the message machine is confidential, brief replies to questions can be left. *Clinical information must not be left on a message machine or voice mail unless it is known that confidentiality will be maintained.*
- Having pre-arranged blocks of time available for telephone contact with patients is useful, but not always possible. If such times are publicized, the clinician must be sure to be available during those specified times.
- The patient can expect medication management 24 hours a day, 7 days a week. When the clinician is not personally available, competent coverage needs to be arranged.
- If an emergency exists and it cannot be evaluated satisfactorily over the telephone, an appointment should be made for a face-to-face evaluation and/or the patient sent to an Emergency Department.
- *All telephone contacts should be documented*, including clinical content, medication recommendations or dosage change. Such documentation should include the date and time of the call, the reason the patient called and any response given.

■ *Medication for new patients must not be prescribed over the telephone without a face-to-face evaluation.* In general, major medication regimen changes should not be made over the telephone.

If office staff answer the telephone for the clinician, it is important to ensure that they:

■ Are trained in professional, courteous, and prompt response
■ Are trained in triage to recognize urgent matters
■ Can quickly reach the clinician personally, if necessary
■ Maintain appropriate patient confidentiality
■ Keep a log of the time and content of all calls
■ Have been appropriately trained and credentialed, if they are to provide clinical information/guidance to patients or authorize prescription refills. Purely clerical staff should not be allowed to provide clinical recommendations without documented approval/input from the clinician.

Telephone appointments

On occasion, it may be reasonable to have a "telephone appointment" with the patient. While this should not be routine, it can, at times, be both expedient and clinically appropriate. Conditions that might justify a telephone appointment include inclement weather, infirmity of the patient, patient travel difficulties, a suddenly emergent clinical matter, or another need to have patient contact when a face-to-face evaluation is not possible.

A telephone follow-up appointment can be conducted using a similar structure to a face-to-face appointment (see Chapter 6). Although the clinician is deprived of facial gestures, body movements or other signs that might help in assessing the patient, safe evaluation and treatment can be accomplished. Particularly for a patient who has a stable medication regimen, it is possible to cover the items of a usual follow-up appointment and to provide a renewal prescription. Documentation of a telephone visit should be similar to that for the typical face-to-face evaluation, and should include all the elements normally contained in a written note for such a visit. The vast majority of patients will not abuse the offer of a telephone appointment, and will be grateful for the opportunity when the situation warrants.

A regular pattern of prescribing over the telephone, or repeated telephone appointments, does not generally constitute safe, medically sound practice. If the clinician is thinking about giving medical/medication advice or prescribing over the telephone, the following questions should be considered:

1 Is this an established patient?
2 Do you know this patient well enough to treat over the telephone?
3 When was the last face-to-face visit?
4 How does this telephone treatment fit into the overall treatment of this patient?

5 How often is phone treatment occurring?
6 If a prescription is authorized,
   ■ Is it for a limited time?
   ■ Is it for the least amount of medication?
   ■ When will the next face-to-face visit occur?
7 Is the telephone appointment a pattern for *this patient*?
8 Is the telephone appointment a pattern for *me*?

If the patient has moved away and requests telephone follow-up, further questions should be considered:

1 Can I provide safe, high quality evaluation and treatment without personal interaction?
2 Can I evaluate the patient's changing status over time?
3 What measures are in place for emergency care in the new locale?
4 Would a clinician in the new locale better serve the patient's condition?

When a patient has made a decision to relocate permanently, it is almost invariably preferable to transfer care to a local practitioner, if medication needs will continue.

Inappropriate use of the telephone

There are temptations, both to the patient and clinician, to overutilize the phone. Each of these considerations will be addressed separately.

Patient's overusage

Patients may misuse the phone in various ways, including:

■ With inappropriate frequency
■ For inappropriate reasons
■ At inappropriate times.

Causes for patient overutilization of the telephone include:

■ Anxiety
■ Mania
■ Personality disorder, particularly borderline personality
■ It's "easier" to reach the mental health prescriber than other, more appropriate primary care medical clinicians
■ Lack of funds to pay for appointments
■ The patient feels it is inconvenient to come to the office
■ The patient feels a follow-up appointment is not necessary
■ The patient feels embarrassed to come to a mental health office.

Depending on the reason overutilization occurs, each situation requires an individualized response from the clinician.

Anxious patients may telephone the clinician to interpret possible side effects or solely for reassurance in taking their prescribed medication. Mentally scattered or extremely nervous patients who have little support in their lives may call the prescriber frequently with medication questions. They will reach for what they perceive as their "life preserver," the clinician, when they feel overwhelmed with anxiety. Despite this anxiety, it is not therapeutic for them relentlessly to seek reassurance through repeated telephone calls.

Manic patients can overutilize the telephone with many individuals including family, friends, neighbors, acquaintances or even strangers. A prescriber may be caught in a manic pattern of verbosity and hyperlogia. At times, manic patients can call frequently, unaware that their repeated calls are inappropriate.

Some patients with personality disorders, particularly *borderline personality disorders*, feel "entitled" and special. They feel they can expect immediate access to the prescriber at whatever time and about whatever issue comes to their minds. Repeated or inappropriate access to the prescriber is just one part of what they perceive as their special rights.

Some patients' use of the phone is inappropriate not because of frequency, but because of the nature of the call. These patients may call a medication prescriber about issues that can and should be dealt with elsewhere. When the patient has a regular psychotherapist, psychotherapy issues, marital issues, parenting issues, or other issues relative to the patient's life should be referred to the psychotherapist. The medication prescriber is not the most direct (or most appropriate) resource. If, however, the prescriber is seen as an interested, available, and knowledgeable resource, the patient may choose to bypass the regular therapist and call the prescriber. Gently redirecting the patient to the regular therapist is the appropriate intervention.

Patients may call the prescriber for medically unrelated issues. Patients may wish to use the mental health prescriber as a general practitioner, calling about headaches, blood pressure, rashes, pain, cough, antibiotics, or other medical issues. If the prescriber has a minimal telephone barrier, patients may perceive that he or she is easier to reach than a primary care provider and may call the mental health prescriber rather than attempting to deal with what they perceive as a difficult maze of resistance to reach a family practitioner in a large family practice office, or a specialist in another field. It is not uncommon for a patient to request a renewal for a non-mental health prescription just because "I can never reach Dr X" or because "my nurse practitioner is out of town." Rather than attempting to reach the appropriate clinician's back-up or coverage person, such patients will call the mental health prescriber.

Anxious or desperate individuals who are not current patients may telephone requesting medications for anxiety, sleep, depression, or other mental health symptoms without an in-person evaluation. Although a practitioner may empathize with the patient's plight, *prescription without face-to-face evaluation is inappropriate and dangerous*. These requests should be denied, and such patients referred to an Emergency Department or a more available colleague.

There are occasions when a previous patient, well known to the clinician but who has not been seen in months or years, calls in a crisis. It may be reasonable to re-institute a temporary, small amount of medication until the patient can be seen in person. At the time of this telephone contact, the clinician should ask about intervening medical issues that may have changed before automatically re-starting a previously utilized medication:

- Have there been any medical changes?
- Are there new or ongoing medications or allergies?
- Is there ongoing suicidal ideation or substance abuse?

Face-to-face follow-up should be arranged as soon as possible.

In other situations, patients who have neglected to arrange a follow-up visit will telephone requesting prescription renewals. This is usually done when a patient's medications are nearly depleted. Initially, when this happens, the clinician may appropriately ensure continuity of medication by providing a short-term prescription to cover the patient until the face-to-face evaluation is performed. Although this may be reasonable for an occasional lapse, if the situation becomes repetitive, the clinician will need to define the rules of safe prescription. When the patient continually fails to make or keep appointments, and repeatedly asks for telephone renewals, the clinician should give a clear verbal message that further renewals will not be provided over the telephone without face-to-face evaluation. This should be documented in the patient's record (see Chapter 20 for further information).

Some patients may also abuse the telephone by deliberately calling the clinician after regular business hours. They call off-hours, reaching coverage personnel, in hopes of gaining further medication renewals without the need for face-to-face evaluation. This behavior must be addressed by a coordinated effort between the primary clinician and coverage clinicians. Standard practice for weekend or holiday coverage personnel should be to provide only enough medication to last the patient until the primary clinician becomes available. On the next regular work day, the primary clinician can then appropriately assess the situation for further prescription.

When a patient calls too much

Some general principles are helpful for managing inappropriate telephone usage in a medication practice.

First, the clinician should ensure that there is an established pattern of inappropriate telephone usage before setting rules. One unnecessary call does not automatically mean a patient is being inappropriate. Particularly early in treatment, a patient may not know what is, and what is not, an appropriate call. Education about the use of the telephone will lay the groundwork for a workable agreement between patient and clinician.

If inappropriate phone calls become a pattern, the clinician must deal promptly and directly with the patient about this behavior.

TALKING TO PATIENTS

"We need to talk about your telephone calls to me and your treatment plan."

The discussion should be specific regarding the issues of frequency of calls, nature of calls, timing of calls, or any other telephone issue that is problematic. The clinician should be firm, but not display anger. A specific outline of therapeutic use of the telephone should be detailed, including specifics about *when* the clinician can be called, *how often*, and *about what issues*. It is important that the clinician also adheres to the newly established parameters. If for some reason the clinician deviates from the outlined plan for a telephone-abusing patient, this instance must be identified as a deviation and why it is being done. It is quite reasonable to tell the patient to bring certain issues to the next face-to-face appointment, and that these issues do not require an extra-session telephone call.

Clinicians should not cut off all telephone contact with an active patient, even though with some particularly troublesome patients they may wish to do so. While medications are being prescribed, the patient must continue to have emergency access to the clinician. It may be necessary, however, for the prescriber to define what constitutes an "emergency." Once outlined, the plan should be documented in the written notes and a copy given to the patient.

TALKING TO PATIENTS

If telephone calls continue to be abused after initial parameters are set and reinforced, the clinician can state: *"We have talked about your use of the telephone, and you have continued to use it in ways that I do not feel are helpful. This is the last time I will discuss the matter. If you do not use the phone appropriately, in the ways I have outlined in our plan, you are putting your relationship with me in jeopardy and we may need to stop your treatment."* Then, reiterate the parameters.

When repeated last-minute telephone requests for medication renewal have been identified as problematic, further telephone requests for medication renewal should be refused, even if the patient may run short of medication or experience some rebound side effects from having a medication-free interval.

When the clinician identifies a particular telephone call as inappropriate from a patient who has done it before, the clinician should interrupt the call and identify it as a non-urgent one. Identification of the call as an inappropriate one is the only necessary response; such an interruption is quite professional and necessary. Usually this intervention will alter the behavior of even intractable patients. However, if a patient continues to use the telephone inappropriately and ignores guidelines, the therapist may need to terminate the relationship. The patient should be given written notice that his/her treatment, therapy and/or medication relationship with the clinician has ended, along with a date after which the clinician will provide no further prescriptions. It is appropriate to provide several weeks of medication to allow the patient time to find another prescriber. The patient will have the responsibility of finding a new prescriber.

Clinician's overusage of the phone

When a clinician finds that he or she is scheduling frequent telephone appointments without face-to-face evaluations, it is a warning sign that the clinician may be overutilizing the telephone. The busy clinician may see telephone therapy as a way of fitting large numbers of patients into a small space of time. While useful as a temporary measure, it should not become standard practice. Clinician overutilization of the telephone is often accompanied by offering excessive numbers of medication refills over an extended period without re-evaluation.

E-mail and the medication prescriber

E-mail has become a common form of personal and business communication. Some patients may find e-mail a useful way to communicate from their workplace, since they are already at computer terminals much of the workday. In confined areas where telephone conversations may be overheard, patients may be more comfortable utilizing e-mail. Patients traveling overseas may find e-mail the most convenient way to communicate with the clinician over long distances.

Regardless of the clinician's degree of computer sophistication, some decisions about the use of e-mail will need to be made. If the clinician does not wish to use e-mail as a potential medium for communication with patients, the e-mail address should not be made available. Even so, resourceful patients may find the address through Internet search engines. If the clinician does not wish to communicate via e-mail, he or she must directly indicate this to the patient, and not respond to e-mail message requests.

In general, unsecured e-mail presents more risks than benefits for the prescribing clinician in keeping patient matters confidential. If a secure line is available, however, there may be reasons to use this modality. If a clinician chooses to use e-mail, it should be disclosed whether or not the line is secure and/or that communications via e-mail may not be confidential. With increasing frequency, secure e-mail lines are being provided to medical clinicians and this confidentiality issue may gradually wane. Currently, however, most e-mail, like many other areas of the Internet, is not confidential, and it is important that the patient be informed that others may gain access to the content of messages sent to the clinician.

E-mail communications made by patients should be printed in hard copy rather than stored electronically where they may be easily erased or destroyed. These hard copies should be treated as patient notes and stored in the patient's file. Any responses that the clinician provides through the e-mail should also be printed out and kept in the patient's file with other written documentation.

If e-mail is utilized, the clinician will need to decide how often and when to read and respond to messages. Most busy clinicians do not have time during the day to respond to e-mail requests as quickly as they might to telephone requests.

Many clinicians find that picking up e-mail at the end of the day or at home may serve to lengthen the workday.

As with telephone calls, some patients may prefer e-mail prescription renewal requests to face-to-face interactions and follow-up. If such requests become a pattern, it is recommended that the clinician not respond to them, since e-mail is one more step removed from the patient than the telephone. Without voice and other behavioral signs and signals, it is even more difficult accurately to assess the patient's current state.

Some unscrupulous clinicians have offered to prescribe medications for patients over the Internet without any face-to-face evaluation. Usually this is an attempt to establish a high-volume prescription-writing business with profit as a motive. This practice is unacceptable and is poor medical practice. A prescription written for medication constitutes a therapeutic relationship, and all legal liabilities that accompany this relationship are in force. The clinician who prescribes without any face-to-face contact with the patient runs the risk of serious legal liabilities.

Chapter 25

The pharmacist, the pharmaceutical industry and the clinician

Interacting with the pharmacist

When utilized appropriately, the pharmacist can be a significant resource in the practice of psychopharmacology. An experienced pharmacist can often answer queries about drug interactions, dosage forms or strengths, and identify possible medication substitutions. Today's pharmacies are busy places, but most pharmacists are eager to be of help to practitioners.

When pharmacists telephone the clinician, it is often because they have some concerns about a prescription. It may be as simple as being unable to read the clinician's handwriting and needing clarification, or an important element of the prescription may have been inadvertently omitted. Which drug was required? How many pills were prescribed? What is the dosing schedule?

The pharmacist may also have clinical concerns about what has been written. A dose may be higher than usual, or the number of pills to be dispensed may be of concern. At times the pharmacist may see an aberration, crossed-out writing or some other indication that raises suspicion, and call to document the authenticity of the prescription. Some of these issues may be largely resolved in the near future as we move toward the era of computer-generated prescriptions sent directly from the clinician's office to the pharmacy across the street or across the country.

Many pharmacies at this time have computer-generated programs that produce complete patient medication profiles, and interaction and safety information about the medication prescribed. This information can be given to the patient as a print-out, and contains warnings, precautions, possible side effects, and interactions with other medications. Such programs also contain a list of patient drug allergies and a chronological medication prescription history from all prescribers. Some programs automatically highlight possible drug interactions. When the program identifies a possible interaction, the pharmacist's call can provide useful information to the prescriber, who may have been unaware that the patient is using a medication from another prescriber. It is important to know, for example, if a patient who is starting lithium is already taking large doses of a prescription non-steroidal anti-inflammatory medicine that could, in some instances, raise the patient's lithium level by 50–100 percent. An episode of toxicity can then be avoided by starting the lithium at lower than normal doses.

Pharmacist's calls based on computer programs and the notifications they generate do not, however, create a mandate for the clinician, nor automatically require a change of prescription. Such programs may highlight very rare interactions that, while possible, are quite unlikely for a particular patient. Sometimes only one case of an interaction may have been suspected, but never proven. At other times the potential interaction highlighted is common, but the clinician, in concert with the patient, has decided to accept any possible interactional risk for reasons of clinical necessity. If there is good justification for the medication regimen prescribed, and the clinician is aware of the possible interactions with other medications, he or she may reassure the pharmacist to proceed with filling the prescription. When proceeding with a combination of medications that may carry some additional risk, the clinician should document the clinical rationale for proceeding with this recommendation.

Preauthorization – a fact of American practice

In the USA, where many patients receive medication coverage as an insurance benefit, the pharmacist will call if the medication prescribed is not on the approved list covered by the patient's insurance. The pharmacy will require "preauthorization" of a medication from the insurance plan before the insurance company will pay for the medication. Sometimes the pharmacist will ask if the clinician wishes to prescribe another medication that is covered by the insurance, almost as if the medications are interchangeable. The medications are on the approved list will vary from insurance plan to insurance plan, and may change over time. Such approval has more to do with corporate decisions based on cost, and does not necessarily reflect the clinical value, safety or utility of medications not covered. If the clinician has good reasons for prescribing the original medication, he or she may not want to change medications just because it is not on the patient's formulary. If this is the case, it is necessary for the clinician to call the insurance company to receive "preapproval." If other medications on the approved list have been previously prescribed and have failed, or if there is a good clinical reason for using a specific medication without substitution, it will usually be approved if the clinician takes the time to justify the clinical necessity.

The pharmaceutical industry

The presence of the pharmaceutical industry is a visible and growing factor in clinical practice. A delicate balance exists between the practitioner and pharmaceutical manufacturers with regard to the prescription of medications. Pharmaceutical firms are large, multinational companies with enormous budgets. These manufacturers must have the alliance of practitioners to prescribe their products, since there is no direct way to distribute their medications except through licensed, trained professionals. In turn, practitioners depend on the pharmaceutical industry to develop new medications and test them for safety. Industry-sponsored research has become a large segment of the medication data on which clinical decisions are made.

Since the field of mental health has been "discovered," increasing expenditures of pharmaceutical dollars are devoted to research into mental health medications. Mental illnesses that improve with the use of medication may require medication recurrently or, at times, on a lifelong basis. With this incentive, it can be expected that, over the next 10–20 years, research into psychotropics will continue to be one of the dominant forces in pharmacological research. Unfortunately, individual practitioners are likely to have little influence on the focus of research, how it is funded, or the ultimate cost of medications to the patients.

Pharmaceutical representatives

The relationship between clinicians and the pharmaceutical industry is primarily structured through interaction with pharmaceutical representatives. These representatives will be eager to meet with practitioners as often as possible. Pharmaceutical representatives are, first and foremost, employees of the pharmaceutical company and promoters of their products. Additionally, however, they are educators in the use of their products and facilitators of clinical practice. The services they offer are listed in Table 25.1.

Table 25.1 Services provided by pharmaceutical representatives

- Printed literature about their products and about mental illnesses in general
- Educational material, diagnostic and treatment aids, including a wide variety of paper, audio, and video products for the clinician, the patient and families
- Access to professional educational opportunities taught by experts in the field and sponsored by the pharmaceutical company
- Availability of research studies on questions about the use of their products in various clinical illnesses
- Free medication samples for professional distribution
- Access to indigent care programs to provide low- or no-cost medications to needy patients
- Product-labeled office items such as pens, clocks, and calendars

---

The practitioner's interface – opportunities and risks

The practitioner's level of connection with one or more pharmaceutical companies is an issue that has stimulated much controversy and many differences in practice. Some clinicians will refuse to have any contact with pharmaceutical representatives, feeling that it is unnecessary, or may bias their prescriptive decisions. Others will see representatives on a regular basis, obtaining samples and attending sponsored educational conferences. Clinicians will need to decide what level of comfort they have with pharmaceutical industry interaction. Some guidelines about interaction with pharmaceutical companies are provided in the American Medical Association policy (see Appendix 7).

On 1 July 2002, the Pharmaceutical Research and Manufacturers of America (PhRMA), a voluntary trade association of pharmaceutical companies, adopted a "Code of Interactions with Healthcare Providers." Although it does not represent all companies, the group's adoption of a set of standardized principles may minimize excessive and inappropriate inducements to prescribing professionals. The text of this Code is contained in Appendix 8. It may also be viewed along with clarifying questions and answers on the Internet at http://www.phrma.org/.

Regardless of what level of contact is maintained, some potential pitfalls for the clinician should be highlighted:

- It may be easy to be drawn into ethically questionable practices with pharmaceutical companies. Even well-intended clinical decisions can be affected by inducements, dinners, travel, products, or gifts. Involvement in non-educational entertainment inducements is of particular concern. Attending a theater, sporting event or trip sponsored by a pharmaceutical company with no educational agenda is ethically questionable. At the same time, avoidance of industry-sponsored educational programs may unnecessarily limit the clinician's exposure to useful clinical information. When attending such a program, it is important during the presentation to identify a speaker who is truly objective and is presenting unbiased material. Some presenters may be employed by the pharmaceutical company, or be speaking primarily to promote a particular product. Clinicians will need to listen carefully and judge for themselves if the presentation is objective or unnecessarily slanted.

- The availability of product samples can be a convenient and money-saving way for patients to begin an initial trial of a new medication. Making decisions about which product to prescribe solely on the convenience of having samples available, however, is not sound clinical practice.

- If the clinician places product-labeled materials in the office where they can be seen or used by patients, it may convey an unintended message. When a patient sees a labeled pen, clock, calendar, or other item in the practitioner's office, it tacitly puts the clinician's stamp of approval on this particular brand or product, which the clinician may not wish to do.

Indigent care medication programs

Many pharmaceutical companies provide indigent care programs for low-income patients. These can be quite helpful for a patient who benefits significantly from a particular medication, but cannot afford it. Although there is paperwork involved for the clinician, the patient can be maintained on medication at no cost, at least on a short-term basis. Although each company's procedure may vary slightly, once the clinician fills out the appropriate request a medication supply is shipped to the prescriber, who then distributes it to the patient.

A list of indigent care medication programs by manufacturer, with contact addresses and telephone numbers, can be seen on the Internet at http://www.phrma.org/pap.

Media advertising and mental health medications

Over the last several years, television, radio and print media have begun to accept direct-to-consumer medication advertisements from pharmaceutical companies. While initially limited to allergy products, gastrointestinal remedies and cholesterol-lowering medications, the practice now has spread to a wide variety of drugs, including mental health medications. More recently, companies have broken the longstanding prohibition of advertising scheduled, potentially habit-forming medicines, by running print advertisements about the use of stimulants for ADHD or hypnotics for sleep. Even though these are couched in a "for your information" format and suggest that patients seek advice from their doctor, such advertisements for possibly habit-forming medications create even more controversy about the overall wisdom of media advertising for medications.

Professionals have varying responses to such advertisements, and there are both benefits and drawbacks for mental health. When such advertising applies to mental health medication, the positives are that it can legitimize mental health problems and de-stigmatize seeking help for emotional problems. Some patients who would not otherwise do so will seek treatment solely because they have seen symptoms mentioned on television that correspond to what they have been feeling. Given that we, as professionals, continue to treat only a fraction of those people who suffer with most mental health conditions, advertising has some value for societal mental health management.

Negatives to this advertising include trivializing prescriptions and the prescription process itself. Patients who expect a prescription for medicine A that they have seen on TV may be less favorably disposed to medicine B, even if the prescriber thinks it is more appropriate. Additionally, the cost of such media advertising ultimately contributes to the high overall cost of pharmaceuticals for patients.

Chapter 26

Preparing an office for mental health prescribing

A clinician may open an office for prescribing mental health medication within an organization, clinic, or hospital, in a government-sponsored setting, or as an independent practitioner. Depending on the clinician's discipline and training, it may be as an independent practitioner with independent prescribing authority or as a collaborative practitioner requiring consultation or collaboration with another professional.

Depending on the setting, basic necessities and paperwork may be set up and provided by an institution. When opening an independent practice, however, clinicians will need to arrange for each item themselves. This chapter will provide a checklist of important issues to be addressed by the provider of mental health prescriptions who is not also setting up a general medical practice.

Mandatory issues

Clinicians must:

1 *Consult state or national law* regarding the limits of their practice and prescriptive authority.
2 *Maintain a copy of their prescriptive authority agreement* and any legal limitations on their prescriptive authority *at the office site*.
3 If practicing within a group, devise and sign a contract with any other group members and specify any contractual arrangements. This agreement should be in writing, and a copy maintained at the practice.
4 *Obtain malpractice insurance for prescription*. This should include limits of a minimum of $1 million per occurrence and $3 million per event. Ensure that

premises liability insurance is included, for any accidental occurrences that occur in the office (such as the patient who trips, falls and suffers an injury). *Under no circumstances should the clinician begin writing prescriptions until malpractice insurance coverage has been obtained in writing.*

5 In America, *obtain a Bureau of Narcotics and Dangerous Drugs (BNDD) certificate number* for prescription of scheduled medications. Although it is possible to prescribe without such a number, a practitioner without this certificate will not be able to write for benzodiazepines, sedative/hypnotics, or stimulants, resulting in a limited practice. In America, an application may be obtained by calling the Bureau at (202) 307-7255. In some states, a state license may also be required. In the UK, issues of prescribing scheduled medications are handled at the Home Office, Drug Branch, Queen Anne's Gate, London SW1H 9AT, telephone (020) 7273-3806.

6 If required by their licensure, *choose a consultant*. Although it may vary by state law, a consultant for a nurse practitioner can be any physician. When possible, a psychiatrist with psychopharmacological expertise is a desirable choice as consultant. Depending on location and availability, a family practitioner, internist, pediatrician or other medical specialist may also serve as a consultant. Such physicians, in general, do not have advanced psychopharmacology expertise. While they are within the limits of the law, such consultants may not be able to provide in-depth consultation about psychotropics. The clinician should keep a copy of the consultative agreement on the office premises.

7 *Lease or sublease office space.* It is not advisable to work out of a personal residence. Although in times past this has been popular for certain mental health practitioners, mixing personal life with professional life is not, in general, good safe practice. Of considerable importance is an office that maintains *adequate soundproofing*. Patients generally feel much more comfortable if they know their verbalizations cannot be heard in the waiting room or in another office. To maintain adequate confidentiality, special soundproofing may be needed in ceilings and walls. Use of a radio, fan, or "white noise" machine in the waiting room also reduces sound from the office to the waiting room.

8 *Establish coverage with other licensed practitioners 24-hours a day, 7-days a week*, as medication prescription requires availability by a qualified practitioner around the clock for emergencies. Practitioners may be of the same discipline or other disciplines with prescriptive authority. This is considerably different from standard psychotherapy practice, in which some practitioners may not require (or provide) such emergency availability. A patient who experiences a medication emergency and cannot reach a qualified practitioner may have grounds for medicolegal action.

9 *Establish a telephone service*, including a means of off-hours and weekend notification such as an answering service, pager, answering machine, or other method. The prescription of medications does require the availability of rapid access to the clinician or to covering personnel off-hours. The system should be tested periodically to make sure it operates consistently and smoothly.

10 *Arrange to have laboratory tests ordered through their consultant* or another provider/clinic if their licensure does not allow for independent ordering of laboratory tests.

11 *Obtain pads of prescriptions.* Personalized prescriptions written on alter-proof paper are preferred. Many medical supply houses such as Colwell (800-6371140) or Histacount (800-645-5220) in the USA provide these at reasonable prices. Some clinicians prefer to have their address, BNDD number (required to prescribe potentially habit-forming medications), state license number or other information on the prescriptions, while others do not. Non-personalized prescriptions with no identifying information are legal, but are perhaps more open to fraud. Some states require specialized embossed prescription blanks.

12 *Obtain reference books* such as the *Physician's Desk Reference (PDR)*,[1] *The Maudsley Prescribing Guidelines*,[2] *The USP D1*,[3] *Drug Facts and Comparisons*[4] and this text! Obtain the latest version of the *Diagnostic and Statistical Manual (DSM)*,[5] with a list of mental health diagnoses and their code numbers (American Psychiatric Association, 1400 K Street, NW, Washington, DC 20005).

13 *Devise paperwork* for medication prescription, which should include:
   ■ A consent to treatment form
   ■ A consent to share clinical information with a consultant or colleague
   ■ A patient registration form (this may be devised by the clinician or preprinted)
   ■ A sheet describing fees, including missed appointment charges
   ■ Written instructions for commonly prescribed medications, which should include side effects, interactions and warnings (these may be preprinted from a manufacturer or self-composed)
   ■ Laboratory test request forms – obtain a list of codes for commonly used tests from the laboratory
   ■ Patient instruction sheets for having laboratory tests drawn
   ■ Checklists of various symptoms for commonly diagnosed conditions (such as depression, bipolar disorder, obsessive–compulsive disorder, panic disorder, etc.) to serve as an outline for initial evaluations
   ■ Medication record forms to document medications prescribed (these may be preprinted or self-devised; see Chapter 5 for an example)
   ■ Initial evaluation and progress note forms, unless the plan is to use plain notepaper.
   ■ Appointment cards with the address and telephone number of the office
   ■ Letterhead stationery for reports and other correspondence.

14 *Devise a system for organizing and storing medical records* that maintains privacy, safety, and confidentiality of records, and consider how the capacity can be expanded as further patients are seen.

15 Obtain folders, charts, file cabinets, paper, notebooks, a clock, calendar, and appointment book.

16 For safe storage of medication samples, *obtain locked cabinets* or identify a locked storage room.

Optional measures

Optional measures that may be helpful but are not essential include the following:

1 *Interview and hire clerical help* to perform reception work, telephone answering, typing, billing, accounting, and/or insurance preparation.
2 *Obtain an automated blood pressure cuff* for convenient monitoring of blood pressure or a standard cuff and stethoscope.
3 *Obtain pharmaceutical samples* from drug company representatives, if these will be used. Local representatives' names and telephone numbers can generally be obtained through a pharmaceutical company's central phone number. These are listed by company at the front of the *Physician's Desk Reference*.
4 *Obtain a computer* with Internet access and printer for word processing and online information gathering.
5 *Obtain a fax machine* to receive faxed lab work, medical records, consents for treatment and other data from practitioners and insurance companies.
6 *Begin subscriptions to psychopharmacology journals* or journals relative to your specialty (see Chapter 27).
7 If planning to medicate children, set up a play area and obtain toys, age-appropriate dolls, and other suitable materials.

Before beginning the prescription process, the clinician should have a clear understanding as to the limits of his or her own ability. Together with the consultant, the clinician should identify and document which patients, if any, will be restricted by a collaborative agreement. For example, without consultation and oversight the inexperienced practitioner might be limited from prescribing to:

- The acutely, seriously active suicidal patient
- The acutely psychotic patient
- The patient with acting out borderline personality
- The patient in acute alcohol withdrawal
- The complicated medical patient with multiple physical illnesses and multiple non-psychiatric medications.

Periodic re-evaluation of image

As with any business or organization, a healthcare provider's presentation to a patient reflects positively or negatively on the quality of care to be delivered. This is particularly true for the psychotropic medication prescriber. For all the reasons listed in the first two chapters of this book, mental health medications and the persons who prescribe them are not automatically or universally accepted without doubt, apprehension, and skepticism. A professional, organized office and care delivery system can start the prescriptive process off on the right foot. The appropriate atmosphere gives a sense that quality, safe, professional decisions are made in this practitioner's setting. When the office and environs are disorganized, cluttered or non-professional, it may predispose the patient to wonder if the quality of care is likewise.

Even when the parameters detailed in this chapter are followed, time passes and circumstances change. Buildings age, offices can become shabby and furnishings outdated, and professional forms can become obsolete or inaccurate. Service provision by office staff may not meet the standards originally set. *It is extraordinarily valuable periodically to view the office, staff, and service provided through the eyes of a potential patient.* What will they see? Who will they encounter? What is the level of interaction with the clinician or any staff, by telephone or in person? Do all these elements meet the desired professional image? Are education materials (print, videotape, audio tape, CD-ROM) current and accurate? Are available medication samples within printed expiration dates?

First impressions count and can color the way in which patients view the clinician's treatment. It is important to make sure the initial impression given is the one intended.

References

1   *Physician's Desk Reference*. Medical Economics Inc., published annually.
2   *The Maudsley Prescribing Guidelines*. Martin Dunitz, published annually.
3   *The USP D1*. Micromedex, published annually.
4   *Drug Facts and Comparisons*. Walters and Kluwer, published annually.
5   Diagnostic and Statistical Manual, American Psychiatric Association, published periodically.

Chapter 27

Keeping current

Principles of medication usage change slowly. Many of the principles in this book will be little different 10 or 20 years from now. Books, such as this one, which provide principles of treatment, will still be valuable for many years in the future. Drug facts, medications and uses for medications change rapidly, however. Medication details in books are, as often as not, out of date before they are printed, whereas medication information in journal articles, presented in conferences and on the Internet all can be updated quickly and continuously.

Prescribers of psychotropic medications should consider themselves on a life-long learning curve. With the advent of new medications, new treatments, and new uses for various medications, clinicians will need to educate themselves continually in order to remain expert.

To maintain this level of currency, the practitioner should read psychopharmacology journals whenever possible. Although there are many useful journals, some particularly useful journals with direct clinical applicability include:

■ *Essential Psychopharmacology* (The Hatherleigh Company Ltd, 1114 First Avenue, Suite 500, New York, NY)
■ *Biological Therapies in Psychiatry* (Gelenberg Consulting & Publishing LLC, PO Box 42650, Tucson, AZ 85733-2650. Internet http:/www.btpnews.com)
■ In the UK, *The Maudsley Prescribing Guidelines*[1] provide yearly updated medication recommendations by disease entity and contain a wealth of information. American prescribers should strongly consider obtaining a copy

of this book since the vast majority of information is applicable to American practice, and there are few comprehensive yearly updated psychotropic medication guides in the USA

■ *Curbside Consultant* from the Massachusetts General Hospital Department of Psychiatry Bulfinch 436, 55 Fruit St, Boston, MA 02114, or e-mail curbside@partners.org

■ *Currents* (7000 Carmichael Avenue, Bethesda, MD 20817 301-320-6915)

■ *Clinical Handbook of Psychotropic Drugs* (edited by Bezchlibnyk-Butler and Jeffries, Hogrefe and Huber Publishers) is in book format but is updated quarterly to remain current with new information

■ The *Journal of the American Psychiatric Association* also provides good research information and review articles. In general, nurse practitioners who prescribe will find specific psychopharmacology journals or psychiatric journals more detailed and comprehensive than nursing journals for prescribing information.

Every effort should be made to attend conferences hosted by local universities, medical and nursing schools, non-profit organizations, and pharmaceutical companies. Depending on the practitioner's interest, availability and location, such conferences can be evenings, half-day, all-day, or for a week at a time. The opportunity to directly hear and question leaders in the field is invaluable in maintaining up-to-date information.

The Internet and clinicians

The advent of computer linking via the Internet has led to an avalanche of available data for practitioners. There are a vast number of sites that provide useful information to the clinician about various medications, side effects, drug interactions, medication statistics and treatments for an array of mental health conditions.

While a complete listing of all sites on the Internet associated with mental health could alone fill a 500-page book,[2,3] a selected, categorized listing of Internet sites that provide useful mental health, pharmacology and psychopharmacology information is as follows:

Information on psychiatric/mental health disorders

■ National Institute of Mental Health (NIMH): Public Resources
http://www.nimh.nih.gov/publicat/index.cfm

■ Journal of Affective Disorders, at
http://www.elsevier.nl:80/inca/publications/store/5/0/6/0/7/7

■ Journal of Anxiety Disorders, at
http://www.elsevier.nl:80/inca/publications/store/8/0/1

■ Journal of Clinical Psychiatry, at
http://www.psychiatrist.com

■ Mental Health Links, at
http://www.mentalhealth.org/links/KENLINKS.htm

- MentalHealthSource.com Directory, at
  http://www.mhsource.com/hy/links.html
- Psychiatric Disorder Info Center, at
  http://www.neuroland.com/psychiat.htm
- NYU Department of Psychiatry – Psychiatry Information for the General
  Public, at
  http://www.med.nyu.edu/Psych/public.html
- DSM-IV Complete Criteria for Mental Disorders, at
  http://www.chesco.com/~snowbaby/DSM-IV.html
- American Academy of Child and Adolescent Psychiatry (AACAP): Teenage
  Mental Illness Glossary, at
  http://www.aacap.org/Web/aacap/about/glossary/index.htm

Detailed articles for the prescribing professional

- Medscape: Psychiatry News, at
  http://www.medscape.com/Home/Topics/psychiatry/directories/
  dir-PSY.News.html
- American Journal of Psychiatry, at
  http://ajp.psychiatryonline.org
- Archives of General Psychiatry, at
  http://archpsych.ama-assn.org
- Psychiatry Online, at
  http://www.priory.com.psych.htm

Conferences on continuing medical/nursing education

- CMECourses.com, at
  http://www.cmesearch.com/search.asp?special
- Professional Events Calendar by Month for Mental Health
  http://www.mentalhealth.org/calendar/searchcal.cfm
- PCMEWeb, at
  http://www.cmeweb.com/#pdr
- Current CME Reviews: Psychiatry, at
  http://www.cme-reviews.com
- Medical Conferences & Meetings: Psychiatry, at
  http://www.medicalconferences.com/scripts/search_new.pl
- MediConf Online: Psychiatry Forthcoming Meetings, at
  http://www.medicon.com/online.html

Search engines that are specific to mental health

- Search Engine at NIMH, at
  http://www.nimh.nih.gov/search/search_form.cfm
- Health Sciences Library Psychiatric Resources Arranged by Topic, at
  http://www.hsls.pitt.edu/intres/mental/psyreso.html

■ MEDLINE Plus: Health Information: Mental Health and Behavior Topics, at http://www.psych.org/clin_res/prac_guide.html

Sites devoted to mental health in primary care

■ Behavior and Mental Disorder: Reviews for Primary Care Providers, at http://library.mcphu.edu/resources/reviews/psych.htm
■ Journal of the American Medical Association, at http://jama.ama-assn.org
■ International Clinical Psychopharmacology, at http://www.intclinpsychopharm.com
■ Journal of Clinical Psychopharmacology, at http://www.psychopharmacology.com
■ University of Iowa Family Practice Handbook, at http://www.vh.org/Providers/ClinRef/FPHandbook/15.html
■ Using DSM-IV Primary Care Version: A Guide to Psychiatric Diagnosis in Primary Care, at http://www.aafp.org/aft/981015ap/pingitor.html

Specific psychopharmacology sites

■ Harvard Mental Health Letter, at http://www.health.harvard.edu/newsletters/mtltext.html
■ Harvard Review of Psychiatry, at http://www3.oup.co.uk/harrev/contents
■ Antipsychotic Drugs, at http://www.gvsu.edu/adrianb/HS311Web/antipsy.htm
■ Neuroleptics, at http://www.neuroland.com/psy/neuroleptics.htm
■ Newer Generation Antipsychotic Drugs, at http://www.nlpra.org.hk/1stSymposium.NGAD.html
■ Medication Profiles: Benzodiazepines, at http://anxieties.com/8Meds/BZs.htm
■ Psychopharmacology Links, at http://www.links.co.nz/culture/drugs/psycho.htm
■ Psychopharmacology Tips, at http://uhs.bsd.uchicago.edu/~bhsiung/tips/intro.html
■ Psychopharmacology, at http://link.springer.de/link/service/journals/00213/index.htm
■ Pharmacology, at http://www.walkers.org/noframes/stabilizers.htm

Health sites for the general public that may have mental health sections

■ American Academy of Family Physicians Health Information Page, at http://familydoctor.org

- American Medical Association (AMA): Health Insight, at
  http://www.ama-assn.org/consumer.htm
- Columbia University College of Physicians and Surgeons Complete Home Medical Guide, at
  http://cpmcnet.columbia.edu/texts/guide
- Combined Health Information Database (CHID), at
  http://chid.nih.gov
- InteliHealth: Home to Johns Hopkins Health Information, at
  http://www.intelihealth.com/IH/ihtIH?t=408&st=408&r=WSIHW000
- Mayo Health: Home to the Mayo Clinic Health Information, at
  http://www.mayohealth.org/index.htm
- MEDLINEplus, at
  http://www.nlm.nih.gov/medlineplus
- Virtual Hospital: University of Iowa Health Care, at
  http://www.vh.org

The Internet and patients

Beyond the information provided to clinicians, the Internet is a rich source of information for patients – if they are educated in using it wisely. Many patients, unfortunately, do not adequately differentiate accurate, factual sites from sites with a bias or slant that may make the information therein suspect. When it comes to medications, patients may assume that anything "in print" and published on the Internet will be valid, and will apply to them. Therefore, guidelines are necessary to help patients use this treasure trove of information effectively and selectively.

A handout to patients left in the waiting room, such as the following, can be helpful.

TALKING TO PATIENTS
The Internet and your treatment
There are ever-increasing numbers of sites on the Internet that purport to give information about mental health problems, general health issues, medications, and possible side effects. In general, I am supportive of your having information about your treatment and any medications that you may be taking. Some of these sites are quite helpful and informative, while other sites contain merely opinions without adequate factual backup, biased information disguised as "fact" and, occasionally, information that is simply inaccurate. Even solid, authoritative sites may present data or mention side effects that are highly unlikely, or will not apply to you.

Here are some tips on assessing the possible usefulness of Internet sites:

- Your "search engine" results do not guarantee quality.
- Just because information is "in print" on a website says

nothing about its accuracy, or relevance to you, even if it is, colorful and eye-appealing.

■ Even sites allegedly "sponsored" by official-sounding organizations may not be unbiased.

■ Who sponsors the site? More reliable sites are sponsored by those with credible medical credentials, including medical and nursing associations, hospitals, medical centers, and accredited schools of medicine and nursing.

■ Is the information factual or opinion?

■ Does the site have a vested interest? Does it attempt to get you to buy any product or service? This is usually a sign of possible bias.

■ How up to date is the information? Has it been updated recently? The date of the most recent revision should be clearly evident on the site. Sites that are the most accurate and medically valid are updated regularly, but recent updates do not necessarily guarantee quality content.

■ What is the privacy policy? How does the site treat any personal information given?

Even if you see something on one of these sites, I would suggest not making any changes in your regimen or the medicines that I prescribe for you without discussing the issue with me first.

Practice guidelines

As the science of psychopharmacology and mental health treatment has become more evidence-based and scientific, numerous practice guidelines have been developed for the treatment of various illnesses. These practice guidelines include decision trees for the treatment of mental health conditions and/or specific psychopharmacology decision trees for the use of medications or combinations of medications in the treatment of specific illnesses. Some guidelines are rapidly becoming standards against which competent practice is measured.

These practice guidelines can provide a number of advantages. They are useful to novice prescribers or practitioners who prescribe infrequently, in providing a framework for thorough and consistent treatment of mental illnesses. More experienced practitioners may find such practice guidelines periodically helpful to review their own competence and practice patterns. In treatment-resistant patients, a review of practice guidelines may unearth a treatment possibility that the clinician had not considered. As the clinician gains more experience, he or she may not need to use the guideline as a regular tool, but may do so only intermittently or in particularly difficult cases.

The American Psychiatric Association, various state agencies, and numerous managed care organizations have devised many such guidelines after multidisciplinary input. Copies of practice and medication guidelines for many mental health conditions may be obtained via the Internet at:

- American Psychiatric Association (APA) Practice Guidelines, at
  http://www.psych.org/clin_res/prac_guide.html
- Clinical Practice Guidelines in Psychiatry, at
  http://www.guideline.gov/body-home
- Expert Consensus Guidelines, at
  http://www.psychguides.com/index.html
- National Guideline Clearinghouse, at
  www.guideline.gov/body_home
- Texas Medication Algorithm Project, at
  www.mhmr.state.tx.ws/centraloffice/medicaldirector/tmaptoc.html
- Harvard Psychopharmacology Algorithm Project, at
  www.mhc.com/algorithms/

Summary

If you have followed and applied the principles in this book you will be a competent and knowledgeable practitioner of psychopharmacology. Your wisdom and expertise will help countless patients ease the burden of mental health problems and provide increased satisfaction in their lives. If you have read this book at the beginning of your career, and make an effort to incorporate these principles as part of your standard practice habits, you will soon be seen as a knowledgeable and compassionate practitioner by both patients and fellow clinicians.

References

1   *The Maudsley Prescribing Guidelines*, 6th edn. Martin Dunitz, 2001, p. 195.
2   Slavney PR (consulting ed.) *Psychiatry 2000: An Internet Resource Guide.* eMedguides.com, 2000.
3   Stamps RF and Barah PM. *The Therapists Internet Handbook*. Norton Publishing, 2001.

Appendix 1

Mental status testing

The *de facto* standard for a brief mental status exam, often used by primary care professionals and mental health clinicians alike when a rapid, repeatable assessment of mental status is necessary, is the Mini Mental Status Exam or MMSE.

Mini-mental status examination

See Exam A: Mini-Mental State Examination (MMSE) – opposite

Instructions for administration of mini-mental status examination

Orientation

1 Ask for the date. Then ask specifically for parts omitted, e.g. "Can you also tell me what season it is?" 1 point for each correct.
2 Ask in turn "Can you tell me the name of this hospital?" (town, country, etc.). 1 point for each correct.

Registration

Ask the patient if you may test his memory. Then say the names of three unrelated objects, clearly and slowly (about 1 second for each). After you have said all three, ask him to repeat them. This first repetition determines the score (0–3), but keep saying them until he can repeat all three, up to six trials. If he does not eventually learn all three, recall cannot be meaningfully tested.

Attention and calculation

Ask the patient to begin with 100 and count backward by 7. Stop after five subtractions (93, 86, 79, 72, 65). Score the total number of correct answers.

EXAM A: MINI-MENTAL STATE EXAMINATION (MMSE)

Maximum Score	Score	
		Orientation
5	( )	What is the (year) (season) (date) (day) (month)?
5	( )	Where are we: (state) (country) (town) (hospital) (floor)?
		Registration
3	( )	Name 3 objects: 1 second to say each. Then ask the patient all 3 after you have said them. Give 1 point for each correct answer. Then repeat them until he learns all 3. Count trials and record. Trials:
		Attention and calculation
5	( )	Serial 7's. 1 point for each correct answer. Stop after 5 answers. Alternatively, spell "world" backward.
		Recall
3	( )	Ask for the 3 objects repeated above. Give 1 point for each correct answer.
		Language
9	( )	Name a pencil and watch (2 points). Repeat the following "No ifs, ands, or buts" (1 point). Follow a 3-stage command: "Take a paper in your right hand, fold it in half, and put it on the floor" (3 points). Read and obey the following: Close your eyes (1 point). Write a sentence (1 point). Copy design (1 point).

_____ Total Score

Assess level of consciousness along a continuum: ☐ Alert ☐ Drowsy ☐ Stupor ☐ Coma

Source: Folstein MF *et al.* Mini-Mental State: a practical method for grading the state of patients for the clinician. *J Psychiatric Res* 1975;12:189–198.

If the patient cannot or will not perform this task, ask him to spell the word "world" backward. The score is the number of letters in correct order, e.g. dlrow = 5, dlorw = 3.

Recall

Ask the patient if he can recall the three words you previously asked him to remember. Score 0–3.

Language

Naming: Show the patient a wristwatch and ask him what it is. Repeat for pencil. Score 0–2.

Repetition: Ask the patient to repeat the sentence "No ifs, ands or buts" after you. Allow only one trial. Score 0 or 1.

Three-stage command: Give the patient a piece of plain blank paper and repeat the command. Score 1 point for each part correctly executed.

Reading: On a blank piece of paper, print the sentence "Close your eyes" in letters large enough for the patient to see clearly. Ask him to read it and do what it says. Score 1 point only if he actually closes his eyes.

Writing: Give the patient a blank piece of paper and ask him to write a sentence. Do not dictate a sentence; it is to be written spontaneously. It must contain a subject and verb and be sensible. Correct grammar and punctuation are not necessary.

Copying: On a clean piece of paper, draw intersecting pentagons, each side about 1", and ask him to copy it exactly as it is. All ten angles must be present and two must intersect to score 1 point. Tremor and rotation are ignored.

Estimate the patient's level of sensorium along a continuum, from alert on the left to coma on the right.

More detailed evaluation

When a more detailed evaluation of a patient's mental status is necessary, it is often useful to document a more thorough examination, which will be outlined here. It contains some elements used in the MMSE with elaboration and the addition of other measurements. Even the basics of this mental status exam can be completed in 5–8 minutes once the technique is mastered. Optional elements listed at the end may be added for further detail. Principles of performing this mental status exam are as follows:

- A significant portion of the exam involves educated observation of the patient's appearance, behavior, speech, and mood, and can be done during the course of history taking or in the course of performing the specific mental status tests below.
- Each of the questions should be asked in a routinized way that the clinician states consistently each time the questions are asked. Examples of how to word these questions are listed with each item below.
- When recording the responses to the mental status examination, make brief notes, which may be elaborated upon at a later time for purposes of the

patient's chart. A report generated by this mental status exam should 'paint a picture' of the clinician's observations and experience of this patient, such that a reader of the evaluation can visualize, as clearly as possible, how the patient presented and interacted. Examples of these reports are included at the end of this Appendix.

Appearance and behavior

Look for:

- Dress, grooming
- Gait, motor activity
- Relatedness to the interviewer
- Eye contact, expression
- Somnolence, fluctuating attention
- Hyperventilation, nervous gestures
- Autonomic reactions (sweating, flushing)
- Personality traits (effort level/apathy, response to difficulties, attempts to please or resist).

Speech

Look for:

- Pace (slowed or rapid, pressured)
- Volume
- Grammar (for education)
- Dysarthria (slurring)
- Amount of verbalization
- Organization (circumstantial or tangential, overinclusiveness)
- Neologisms (new, nonsensical words)
- Clanging (rhyming associations)
- Blocking (abrupt stoppage of thought or speech).

Affect

Look for:

- Appropriate reactions to content
- Flattened, monotone
- Exaggerated reactions
- Labile (changing affect).

Mood

Look for:

- Sadness
- Elation, grandiosity
- Anxiety
- Anger, rage
- Fear
- Suspiciousness.

Verbal introduction to memory tests

- "Now I'm going to ask you some questions that will help me evaluate your memory and concentration. Some will be easy and others may be difficult, I want you to do your best."
- Give the patient a motive to try hard on the testing (e.g. "This will help me to determine if you can handle your money matters or manage your own medications, etc . . .").

Concentration and memory

Three objects

- "Now I'm going to give you three things to remember, and I'll ask you to repeat them in a few minutes" (use three unrelated objects, with at least two elements in each object – e.g. a blue fountain pen, a pair of used roller skates, and the address 37 South Broadway)
- "Can you repeat them for me now, just to make sure you have them?" (Immediate recall)
- 5 minutes later – "What were those three things I asked you to remember?" (Recall)

In the interim, you can go on to other questions assessing orientation, memory and calculations. Don't forget to ask for recall of the three objects before you complete the exam.

Orientation

- "What is the date today?" (date, month, year)
- "What is the day of the week?"
- If necessary, "What is the season?"
- "Where are we right now?"
- "What is your full name and birth date?"

Concentration and memory

Serial 1s, 3s and/or 7s (choose one test or all)

- "Now I am going to have you do some counting. Start at 100 (50 or 30) and count backwards by 7s (3s or 1s). I want you to subtract 7 from 100 and keep subtracting 7 (3 or 1) from the total." (If the patient looks for reassurance after one or more answers, "I won't tell you if you are right or wrong, just keep going.")
- Note the responses, time, consistency, response to errors, perseveration
- Presidents (USA):
  "Who is the president of the United States right now?"
  "Name the presidents before him in order, as far as you can go" (George W. Bush, Clinton, George Bush, Reagan, Carter, Ford, Nixon, Johnson, Kennedy, Eisenhower, Truman, Roosevelt)
- Prime Ministers (UK):
  "Who is the prime minister now?"
  "Name the prime ministers in order as far as you can go." (Blair, Major, Thatcher, Callaghan, Wilson, Heath, Wilson, Douglas-Home, Macmillan, Eden, Churchill)

Calculations

- "Let's say you were going to the store and wanted to buy . . . (e.g. a can of beans) . . . and it costs . . . (e.g. 57 cents) . . . If you gave the clerk a dollar, how much change would you get?" (43 cents)
- "If you wanted to buy (four) cans of (e.g. soup) and they cost (e.g. 28 cents) each, how much would you have to pay?" ($1.12)

Other helpful tests

- "Spell the word *world* backwards."
- "Repeat the phrase, 'no ifs, ands or buts'."
- "Trail test" of numbers and letters. Write a random array of numbers from 1 to 10 and letters from A to H at various places on a sheet of paper. Ask the patient to connect the numbers in order from 1 to 10 with a pencil. Then connect the letters in order from A to H in order with another pencil line.
- Fill in a clock face. Ask the person to draw the way a clock face looks. Ask them to draw the hands of the clock so it shows the time 10 minutes after 7 o'clock.
- Name common objects in the room (pen, pad, computer, picture).
- Follow a two- or three-step command (e.g. place your left hand on your right ear, then cross your legs).
- Write a sentence (e.g. I expect I will be feeling much better within a few weeks).

Psychosis

Look for:

- Darting glances
- Responding to internal stimuli
- Illusions
- Delusional thought content.

Ask:

- Do you see or hear things that other people don't see or hear?
- Do you hear voices when no one is around?
- Do you get "big ideas" that you, or other people, think are "too much" or not accomplishable? (Grandiosity)
- Do you ever feel people are watching or following you, or trying to conspire to cause you harm? (Paranoia)

Other information

Assess presence or absence of:

- Suicidal ideation
- Homicidal ideation.

(As outlined in Chapter 3.)

Optional elements

Judgment:

- "What would you do if you were in a movie theater and suddenly smelled smoke?" (Walk to the exit; alert the manager)
- "What would you do if you were walking along the street and came upon a letter on the ground with an address and stamp on it?" (Put it in a mailbox)

Abstraction:

1 "How are the following pairs of objects alike?"
   - An apple and an orange (fruits)
   - A bathtub and the Atlantic Ocean (they both hold water)
   - A table and a chair (pieces of furniture)
   - A fly and a tree (living things)
2 "Listen to these sayings, and tell me what is the most general meaning they have to most people" (Proverbs – ability to abstract)

- Don't count your chickens before they hatch. (Don't expect something to come true before it actually happens.)
- Even monkeys fall out of trees. (Even experts can make mistakes or fail.)
- People who live in glass houses shouldn't throw stones. (If you have faults, you shouldn't criticize others.)

Intellectual functioning (USA)

- "How far is it from New York to Los Angeles?" (about 3000 miles)
- "Name the five largest cities in the United States." (New York, Los Angeles, Chicago, Houston, Philadelphia)
- "Who is the governor (mayor) of . . .? (the state or city you are in)

Intellectual functioning (UK)

- "How far is it from London to Birmingham?" (about 150 km)
- "What are the five largest cities in Britain?" (London, Manchester, Birmingham, Liverpool, Leeds)

It should be mentioned that neither the mini-mental status exam nor those items mentioned in this Appendix will consistently identify the subtle, minor memory/mental status changes in the well-compensated individual. A person who is not having significant behavioral abnormalities and who functions adequately in a work or school environment, but complains of poor memory or decreased concentration, may give "normal" responses to the tests mentioned here. When present, subtle memory, concentration and retention problems may only be revealed through a formal battery of neuropsychological tests administered by a psychologist trained in neuropsychological evaluation.

Examples of possible mental status exam reports

A person with minimal impairment and "normal" mental status

Mrs Smith is a 47-year-old African American female who looks her stated age. She was seen for a diagnostic evaluation on 12 April. She is dressed casually in a skirt and a light sweater appropriate to the fall season. She sits quietly in her chair during the interview and maintains good eye contact with the interviewer. She relates in a pleasant, cooperative manner to the interviewer, and answers all questions asked, in a matter-of-fact tone. She is alert and oriented to person, place and time. Her speech is logical and coherent without sign of thought disorder or disorganization. The pace of her speech is normal in rate and rhythm. Her affect is normal in range and appropriate to content. Her mood is neutral, without significant signs of elation, depression or anxiety. She denies any suicidal or homicidal ideation. There is no evidence of hallucinations or delusions. She does appear moderately anxious when she begins talking about her daughter, who is failing in school and has been a behavior problem at home.

A depressed man

Mr Jones is a 64-year-old Caucasian male who was evaluated for pharmacotherapy on 8 November 2002. He looks older than his stated age, walks slowly with labored steps coming into the office, and appears to be in a modest amount of physical pain. He has a worried, apprehensive look on his face, and sits slumping in his chair. He can maintain eye contact with the interviewer, but often looks down at the floor or at his lap. He is alert and oriented to person, place, and time; however, he shows psychomotor slowing in his speech and body movements. He wrings his hands at times and grips the arms of the chair tightly. His affect is moderately constricted and his mood is moderately depressed. He is tearful several times during the interview when talking about the death of his wife. At these times, it takes him several minutes to compose himself to go on with the rest of the interview. He says that he has had thoughts of killing himself by shooting, but does not own a firearm. He denies any homicidal ideation. He is able to recall three of three objects immediately after being given them, and two of three objects at 5 minutes. He does serial 7s with three errors out of 15 subtractions done in a 2-minute span. He knows the current president of the USA and is able to name three presidents in order before Bush. He is able to make change correctly from $1 and is able to spell the word *world* backwards without error, although he struggles to remember each letter. He denies any auditory or visual hallucinations, or paranoid ideation.

A psychotic young man

Mr Abernathy is a 21-year-old man of Jamaican extraction who was seen for a medication examination on Thursday, 10 June 2002. He was dressed in tattered pants, worn shoes and a dirty T-shirt. His hair was tousled, and he had several days' growth of beard. His eyes were widened. He was markedly agitated, and had difficulty sitting in the chair to complete the evaluation. He showed frequent agitated movements and darting glances around the room, looking suspiciously off in corners. He talked primarily in a monotone, except when he glanced around the room, when he appeared anxious and agitated. He maintained a perplexed facial expression and displayed thought blocking. When asked about this, he initially denied it was of any significance. When asked a second time, he said that "I thought I saw something that scared me," but would not elaborate. He was oriented to person and place, but thought it was July instead of June. On specific questioning, he admitted to hearing voices, which he thought were those of his father, telling him that he was "no good" and a "failure." He appeared to be responding to internal stimuli, although he denied this. He stated that he had tried to kill himself two weeks ago by "eating himself to death," but said he had no plans to try to kill himself at this time. He denied any homicidal thoughts or behavior. He believed that several people in his apartment building had been watching him closely "to see if I was working for the government, but I'm not." Further, formal mental status testing was attempted, but the patient became increasingly agitated. He expressed concern that perhaps the interviewer was also trying to find out if he was "working for the government," and he refused to answer any further questions.

Appendices 2–5

Appendices 2–5 present the same data organized in different ways for easy reference.

Appendix 2 lists commonly prescribed psychotropics by *medication function with subgroups of chemical class listed alphabetically by generic name*.

Appendix 3 lists common psychotropic medicines *alphabetically by generic name*.

Appendix 4 lists common psychotropics *available in the USA listed alphabetically by* brand *name*.

Appendix 5 lists common psychotropics *available in the UK listed alphabetically by* brand *name*.

Each list includes starting doses and standard therapeutic dosage ranges.

Abbreviations:

STD	Standard release preparation
-SR	Sustained release preparation
-XR	Extended release preparation
NA	Not available
ng/ml	nanograms per milliliter
μg/ml	micrograms per milliliter
meq/l	milliequivalents per liter
QD	once a day
BID	twice daily
TID	three times daily
QID	four times daily

Collated from:

1 *British National Formulary*, Vol. 43. March 2002.
2 DeBattista C and Schatzberg AF. Current psychotropic dosing and monitoring. *Primary Psychiatry* 2001;8(3):59–77.
3 *Maudsley Prescribing Guidelines*. Martin Dunitz, 2001.
4 Pharmaceutical company product package inserts.
5 Schatzberg AF and DeBattista C. *The Black Book of Psychotropic Dosing and Monitoring*. MBL Communications Inc., 2002.

Appendix 2

Common psychotropic medications by class

These drug categories list those compounds commonly used in mental health treatment or in amelioration of mental health medication side effects. They are not exhaustive of every medication in each category.

Chemical (generic) name	USA brand name(s)	UK brand name(s)	Starting dose (mg) except as specified	Standard therapeutic dose (mg)	Useful blood levels
Antidepressants					
Non-SSRI new generation					
Bupropion	Wellbutrin, Wellbutrin-SR, Zyban	Zyban	100 QD (STD) 150 mg QD (-SR)	200–450 (STD) 150–400 (-SR)	No
Mirtazepine	Remeron	Zispin	15	15–45	No
Nefazodone	Serzone	Dutonin	100 QD–100 BID	200–600	No
Reboxetine	NA	Edronax	4 BID	8–12	No
Venlafaxine	Effexor-XR, Effexor	Efexor-XR, Efexor	37.5 BID (STD) 37.5–75 (-XR)	75–375 (STD) 75–225 (-XR)	No
SSRIs					
Citalopram	Celexa	Cipramil	20	20–60	No
Escitalopram	Lexapro	NA	10	10–20	No
Fluoxamine	previously Luvox, generic	Faverin, generic	50	50–300	No
Fluoxetine	Prozac, Serafem, generic	Prozac, generic	20	20–80	No
Paroxetine	Paxil, Paxil CR	Seroxat	20	10–60	No
Sertraline	Zoloft	Lustral	50	50–200	No
Tricyclic					
Amitriptyline	Elavil, generic	Lentizol, Triptafen, generic	25–50	50–300	120–250 ng/ml
Amitriptyline + chlordiazepoxide	Limbitrol	NA	1 tab TID	1 tab–2 tabs TID	No
Amitriptyline + perphenazine	Etrafon, Etrafon Forte	NA	2–25 tab TID	2–25 tab BID–QID	No
Amoxapine	(previously Asendin), generic	Asendis	50 BID	50–600	No

Chemical (generic) name	USA brand name(s)	UK brand name(s)	Starting dose (mg) except as specified	Standard therapeutic dose (mg)	Useful blood levels
Clomipramine	(previously Anafranil), generic	Anafranil, Anafranil SR, generic	25–100	25–250	100–250 ng/ml
Desipramine	Norpramin, generic	Pertofrane	25 TID	100–300	115–180 ng/ml
Dothiepin/Dosulpein	NA	Prothiaden, generic	75	150–225	No
Doxepin	Sinequan, generic	Sinequan	25 TID	75–300	200–250 ng/ml Blood level of parent compound plus metabolite
Imipramine	Tofranil, generic	Tofranil, generic	25 TID	75–300	200–250 ng/ml Blood level of parent compound plus metabolite
Lofepramine	NA	Gamanil, generic	70	40–210	No
Nortriptyline	(previously Pamelor), Aventyl, generic	Allegron, Motipress, Motival	50–100	75–150	50–150 ng/ml
Protriptyline	Vivactil	Concordin, generic	15	15–60	70–250 ng/ml
Trimipramine	Surmontil	Surmontil	75	50–300	No
Heterocyclics					
Maprotiline	(previously Ludiomil), generic	Ludiomil	25 TID	75–225	No
Mianserin	NA	generic	30–40	30–90	
Trazodone	(previously Desyrel)	Molipaxin, generic	50–100	150–600	No
MAO inhibitors					
Isocarboxazid	NA	generic	10	20–60	No
Meclobemide	NA	Manerix	100–300	300–600	No
Phenelzine	Nardil	Nardil	15	15–90	No
Tranylcypromine	Parnate	Parnate	10	30–60	No

Mood-stabilizing medication

Carbamazepine	Tegretol, generic	Tegretol, Teril, Timonil, generic	100–400	400–1600	4–12 µg/ml
Gabapentin	Neurontin	Neurontin	300	1800–3600	No
Lamotrigine	Lamictal	Lamictal	25	100–400	No
Lithium carbonate	Eskalith, Eskalith CR, Lithobid, generic	Liskonum, Camcolit	300–600	600–1800	0.6–1.2 meq/l
Oxcarbazepine	Trileptal	Trileptal	300 BID	600–2400	No
Topiramate	Topamax	Topamax	25	200–400	No
Valproic acid	Depakote, Depakote-ER, Depakene, generic	Epilim, Convulex, Depakote, generic	250 TID	750–4200	50–100 µg/ml
Verapamil	Verelan, Calan, Isoptin, generic	Cordilox, Securon, Univer, Verapress, Vertab, generic	40 TID	80–120 TID	No

Anti-anxiety/hypnotics
Benzodiazepines

Alprazolam	Xanax, generic	Xanax, generic	0.25 TID	0.25–10	No
Chlorazepate	Tranxene	Tranxene	7.5	7.5–60	No
Chlordiazepoxide	Librium, generic	Tropium, Librium, generic	10 TID	15–100	No
Clobazam	NA	Clobazam	20	20–60	No
Clonazepam	Klonopin, generic	Rivotril	1	1.5–20	No
Diazepam	Valium, generic	Valium, Rimapam, Tensium	2 TID	4–40	No
Estazolam	Prosom	NA	0.5	0.5–2	No
Flunitrazepam	NA	Rohypnol	0.5–1	0.5–2	No
Flurazepam	Flurazepam (previously Dalmane)	Flurazepam	15	15–30	No
Loprazolam	NA	(previously Dormonoct)	1	1.5–2	No
Lorazepam	Ativan, generic	Ativan, generic	1–2	1–10	No
Lormetazepam	NA	generic	0.5	0.5–1.5	No
Nitrazepam	NA	Somnite, Mogadon	5	5–10	No
Oxazepam	(previously Serax), generic	generic	10	30–120	No
Temazepam	Restoril	generic	15	7.5–30	No

Chemical (generic) name	USA brand name(s)	UK brand name(s)	Starting dose (mg) except as specified	Standard therapeutic dose (mg)	Useful blood levels
Triazolam	Halcion	N/A	0.125	0.125–0.5	No
Non-benzodiazepine anti-anxiety medication					
Buspirone	Buspar, generic	Buspar, generic	5–10 TID	30–60	No
Sedative hypnotics					
Chloral Hydrate	generic	Chloral Elixir, Welldorm	500	500–2000	No
Clomethiazole	NA	Heminevrin	1 capsule	1–2 capsules	No
Zaleplon	Sonata	Sonata	5	5–20	No
Zolpidem	Ambien	Stilnoct	5	5–10	No
Zopiclone	N/A	Zimovane	3.75	3.75–7.5	No
Antipsychotics					
Traditional					
Benperidol	NA	Anquil, generic	0.25–1.5	0.25–1.5	No
Chlorpromazine	Thorazine, generic	Largactil, generic	25 TID	30–800	No
Flupentixol	NA	Depixol	3–9 BID	6–18	No
Fluphenazine	generic, (previously Prolixin)	Moditen, Modecate	2.5–10	1–40	No
Haloperidol	Haldol, generic	Haldol, Dozic, Serenace, generic	1–3 BID	1–100	No
Levopromazine	NA	Nozinan	25–50	100–200	No
Loxapine	Loxitane	Loxapac	10–25 BID	20–250	No
Mesoridazine	Serentil	NA	50 TID	100–400	No
Molindone	Moban	NA	50 TID	15–225	No
Oxypertine	NA	generic	80–120	80–300	No
Pericyazine	NA	Neulactil	25 TID	75–300	No
Perphenazine	Trilafon, Etrafon, generic	Fentazin	4 TID	12–64	No
Pimozide	Orap	Orap	2	2–20	No

Drug					
Promazine	NA	generic	25–30 QID	400–800	No
Sulpiride	NA	Dolmatil, Clopixol, Sulpital, Sulpor, generic	200–400	400–2400	No
Thioridazine	generic (previously Mellaril)	Mellaril, generic	50–300	20–600	No
Thiothixene	Navane	NA	2 TID	6–60	No
Trifluoperazine	Stelazine, generic	Stelazine, generic	5 BID	2–40	No
Zuclopenthixol	NA	Clopixol	20–30	20–150	No
Atypical					
Amisulpride	NA	Solian	50–100	50–1200	No
Aripiprazole	Abilify	NA	10–15	10–30	No
Clozapine	Clozaril, generic	Clozaril	12.5 BID	12.5–900	> 350 mg/ml
Olanzapine	Zyprexa	Zyprexa	2.5–10	2.5–20	No
Quetiapine	Seroquel	Seroquel	25	50–750	No
Risperidone	Risperdal	Risperdal	0.5	0.5–16	No
Ziprasidone	Geodon	NA	20–40	40–160	No
Zotepine	NA	Zoleptil	25 TID	50–300	No
Miscellaneous					
Anticholinergics					
Benztropine	Cogentin, generic	Cogentin (generic as benztropin or Benzatropin	0.5–1	1–8	No
Biperidon	Akineton	Akineton	1 BID	2–8	No
Procyclidine	NA	Arpicolin, Kemadrin, generic	2.5 TID	7.5–20	No
Trihexyphenidyl	Artane, generic	Broflex, generic	1	2–15	No
Antihistamines					
Cyproheptadine	Periactin, generic	Periactin	4 TID	4–32	No
Diphenhydramine	Benadryl, generic	generic	25 BID	50–400	No
Hydroxyzine	Atarax, Vistaril, generic	Atarax, Cerax	25	50–100	No
Beta blockers					
Atenolol	Tenormin	Tenormin	50	50–100	No
Pindolol	generic	Viskin, Viskaldix	5 BID	15–45	No

Chemical (generic) name	USA brand name(s)	UK brand name(s)	Starting dose (mg) except as specified	Standard therapeutic dose (mg)	Useful blood levels
Propanolol	Inderal	Inderal, generic, Inderetic, Inderex	10–20 BID–TID	20–320	No
Stimulants					
Detroamphetamine and Amphetamine	Adderall, Concordia	NA	2.5–5 BID	5–60	No
Dexamphetamine	Dexedrine	Dexedrine	10	10–60	No
Dextroamphetamine	Dextrostat	NA	10	10–60	No
Methamphetamine	Desoxyn	NA	5 BID	5–25	No
Methylphenidate	Ritalin, Ritalin SR, Concerta, Concerta extended release, Metadate, Metadate ER, Methylin, Methylin ER, generic	Ritalin, Equasym	5–10 BID	10–60	No
Modafanil	Provigil	Provigil	100–200	200–400	No
Pemoline	Cylert	NA	37.5	37.5–112.5	No
Cholinestrase inhibitors					
Donepezil	Aricept	Aricept	5	5–10	No
Galantamine	Reminyl	Reminyl	4 BID	16–32	No
Rivastigmine	Exelon	Exelon	1.5 BID	6–12	No
Tacrine	Cognex	NA	10 QID	40–160	No
Drugs used in alcohol abuse/dependence					
Acamprosate	NA	Campral EC	666 BID	2000	No
Disulfiram	Antabuse, generic	Antabuse	250	125–500	No
Naltrexone	Depade	Nalorex	25	50	No

Anti-obesity agents

Drug					
Orlistat	Xenical	Xenical	120 TID	120 TID	No
Appetite suppressants					
Phentermine	Ionamin, Apidex	NA	37.5	18.75–37.5	No
Siburamine	Meridia	Reductil	10	5–15	No
Other medications mentioned in this book					
Diphenoxylate and Atropine	generic	Lomotil	1 tab QID	2 tabs Q 6 hours	No
Docusate	Colace, Peri-Colace, generic	Dioctyl, Docusol	50	50–200	No
Ispaghula husk	NA	Fybogel, Isogel, Ispagel, Konsyl, Regulan	1 packet BID	1 packet QD–TID	No
Levothyroxine	Levoxyl, Levothroid, Synthroid, Unithroid	Levothyroxine, Liothyronine, Terroxin	12.5–50 µg	12.5–500 µg	No
Loperamid	Immodium	Immodium, generic	4	6–16	No
L-Tryptophan	NA	Optimax	1 TID	6	No
Meprobamate	Miltown, Equagesic, generic	Equagesic, generic	400 TID	1200–1600	No
Psyllium husk	Metmucil, generic		1 tsp in water	1 tsp in water	No
Senna	Senekot	Manevac, Senekot, generic	15	15–30	No
Sildenafil	Viagra		50	25–100	No

Appendix 3

Common psychotropic medications listed alphabetically by generic name

These drug categories list those compounds commonly used in mental health treatment or in amelioration of mental health medication side effects. They are not exhaustive of every medication in each category.

Chemical (generic) name	USA brand name(s)	UK brand name(s)	Class of medication
Acamprosate	NA	Campral EC	Medication for alcohol abuse
Alprazolam	Xanax, generic	Xanax, generic	Benzodiazepines
Amisulpride	NA	Solian	Atypical Antipsychotic
Amitriptyline	Elavil, generic	Lentizol, Triptafen, generic	Tricyclic Antidepressant
Amitriptyline + chlordiazepoxide	Limbitrol	NA	Tricyclic Antidepressant
Amitriptyline + perphenazine	Etrafon, Etrafon Forte	NA	Tricyclic Antidepressant
Amoxapine	(previously Asendin), generic	Asendis	Tricyclic Antidepressant
Aripiprazole	Abilify	NA	Atypical Antipsychotic
Atenolol	Tenormin	Tenormin	Beta Blocker
Benperidol	NA	Anquil, generic	Traditional Antipsychotic
Benztropine	Cogentin, generic	Cogentin (generic as benztropin or Benzatropin)	Anticholinergic
Biperidon	Akineton	Akineton	Anticholinergic
Bupropion	Wellbutrin, Wellbutrin-SR, Zyban	Zyban	Non-SSRI New Generation
Buspirone	Buspar, generic	Buspar, generic	Non-Benzodiazepine Anti-anxiety

Chemical (generic) name	USA brand name(s)	UK brand name(s)	Class of medication
Carbamazepine	Tegretol, generic	Tegretol, Teril, Timonil, generic	Mood Stabilizer
Chloral Hydrate	generic	Chloral Elixir, Welldorm	Sedative Hypnotic
Chlorazepate	Tranxene	Tranxene	Benzodiazepines
Chlordiazepoxide	Librium, generic	Tropium, Librium, generic	Benzodiazepines
Chlorpromazine	Thorazine, generic	Largactil, generic	Traditional Antipsychotic
Citalopram	Celexa	Cipramil	SSRI Antidepressant
Clobazam	NA	Clobazam	Benzodiazepines
Clomethiazole	NA	Heminevrin	Sedative Hypnotic
Clomipramine	(previously Anafranil), generic	Anafranil, Anafranil SR, generic	Tricyclic Antidepressant
Clonazepam	Klonopin, generic	Rivotril	Benzodiazepines
Clozapine	Clozaril, generic	Clozaril	Atypical Antipsychotic
Cyproheptadine	Periactin, generic	Periactin	Antihistamine
Desipramine	Norpramin, generic	Pertofrane	Tricyclic Antidepressant
Detroamphetamine and amphetamine	Adderall, Concordia	NA	Stimulant
Dexamphetamine	Dexedrine	Dexedrine	Stimulant
Dextroamphetamine	Dextrostat	NA	Stimulant
Diazepam	Valium, generic	Valium, Rimapam, Tensium	Benzodiazepines
Diphenhydramine	Benadryl, generic	generic	Antihistamine
Diphenoxylate and atropine	generic	Lomotil	Other medications
Disulfiram	Antabuse, generic	Antabuse	Medication for alcohol abuse
Docusate	Colace, Peri-Colace, generic	Dioctyl, Docusol	Other medications
Donepezil	Aricept	Aricept	Cholinestrase Inhibitor
Dothiepin/Dosulpein	NA	Prothiaden, generic	Tricyclic Antidepressant
Doxepin	Sinequan, generic	Sinequan	Tricyclic Antidepressant
Escitalopram	Lexapro	NA	SSRI Antidepressant
Estazolam	Prosom	NA	Benzodiazepines
Flunitrazepam	NA	Rohypnol	Benzodiazepines
Fluoxamine	previously Luvox, generic	Faverin, generic	SSRI Antidepressant
Fluoxetine	Prozac, Serafem, generic	Prozac, generic	SSRI Antidepressant
Flupentixol	NA	Depixol	Traditional Antipsychotic
Fluphenazine	generic (previously Prolixin)	Moditen, Modecate	Traditional Antipsychotic

Chemical (generic) name	USA brand name(s)	UK brand name(s)	Class of medication
Flurazepam	Flurazepam (previously Dalmane)	Flurazepam	Benzodiazepines
Gabapentin	Neurontin	Neurontin	Mood Stabilizer
Galantamine	Reminyl	Reminyl	Cholinestrase Inhibitor
Haloperidol	Haldol, generic	Haldol, Dozic, Serenace, generic	Traditional Antipsychotic
Hydroxyzine	Atarax, Vistaril, generic	Atarax, Cerax	Antihistamine
Imipramine	Tofranil, generic	Tofranil, generic	Tricyclic Antidepressant
Isocarboxazid	NA	generic	MAOI
Ispaghula husk	NA	Fybogel, Isogel, Ispagel, Konsyl, Regulan	Other medications
Lamotrigine	Lamictal	Lamictal	Mood Stabilizer
Levopromazine	NA	Nozinan	Traditional Antipsychotic
Levothyroxine	Levoxyl, Levothroid, Synthroid, Unithroid	Levothyroxine, Liothyronine, Terroxin	Other medications
Lithium Carbonate	Eskalith, Eskalith CR, Lithobid, generic	Liskonum, Camcolit	Mood Stabilizer
Lofepramine	NA	Gamanil, generic	Tricyclic Antidepressant
Loperamid	Immodium	Immodium, generic	Other medications
Loprazolam	NA	(previously Dormonoct)	Benzodiazepines
Lorazepam	Ativan, generic	Ativan, generic	Benzodiazepines
Lormetazepam	NA	generic	Benzodiazepines
Loxapine	Loxitane	Loxapac	Traditional Antipsychotic
L-Tryptophan	NA	Optimax	Other medications
Maprotiline	(previously Ludiomil), generic	Ludiomil	Heterocyclic Antidepressant
Meclobemide	NA	Manerix	MAOI
Meprobamate	Miltown, Equagesic, generic	Equagesic, generic	Other medications
Mesoridazine	Serentil	NA	Traditional Antipsychotic
Methamphetamine	Desoxyn	NA	Stimulant
Methylphenidate	Ritalin, Ritalin SR, Concerta, Concerta extended release, Metadate, Metadate ER, Methylin, Methylin ER, generic	Ritalin, Equasym	Stimulant

Chemical (generic) name	USA brand name(s)	UK brand name(s)	Class of medication
Mianserin	NA	generic	Heterocylic Antidepressant
Mirtazepine	Remeron	Zispin	Non-SSRI New Generation
Modafanil	Provigil	Provigil	Stimulant
Molindone	Moban	NA	Traditional Antipsychotic
Naltrexone	Depade	Nalorex	Medication for alcohol abuse
Nefazodone	Serzone	Dutonin	Non-SSRI New Generation
Nitrazepam	NA	Somnite, Mogadon	Benzodiazepines
Nortriptyline	(previously Pamelor), Aventyl, generic	Allegron, Motipress, Motival	Tricyclic Antidepressant
Olanzapine	Zyprexa	Zyprexa	Atypical Antipsychotic
Orlistat	Xenical	Xenical	Anti-obesity agent
Oxazepam	(previously Serax), generic	generic	Benzodiazepines
Oxcarbazepine	Trileptal	Trileptal	Mood Stabilizer
Oxypertine	NA	generic	Traditional Antipsychotic
Paroxetine	Paxil, Paxil CR	Seroxat	SSRI Antidepressant
Pemoline	Cylert	NA	Stimulant
Pericyazine	NA	Neulactil	Traditional Antipsychotic
Perphenazine	Trilafon, Etrafon, generic	Fentazin	Traditional Antipsychotic
Phenelzine	Nardil	Nardil	MAOI
Phentermine	Ionamin, Apidex	NA	Appetite Suppressant
Pimozide	Orap	Orap	Traditional Antipsychotic
Pindolol	generic	Viskin, Viskaldix	Beta Blocker
Procyclidine	NA	Arpicolin, Kemadrin, generic	Anticholinergic
Promazine	NA	generic	Traditional Antipsychotic
Propanolol	Inderal	Inderal, generic, Inderetic, Inderex	Beta Blocker
Protriptyline	Vivactil	Concordin, generic	Tricyclic Antidepressant
Psyllium husk	Metmucil, generic		Other medications
Quetiapine	Seroquel	Seroquel	Atypical Antipsychotic
Reboxetine	NA	Edronax	Non-SSRI New Generation
Risperidone	Risperdal	Risperdal	Atypical Antipsychotic

Chemical (generic) name	USA brand name(s)	UK brand name(s)	Class of medication
Rivastigmine	Exelon	Exelon	Cholinestrase Inhibitor
Senna	Senekot	Manevac, Senekot, generic	Other medications
Sertraline	Zoloft	Lustral	SSRI Antidepressant
Sibutramine	Meridia	Reductil	Appetite Suppressant
Sildenafil	Viagra		Other medications
Sulpiride	NA	Dolmatil, Clopixol, Sulpital, Sulpor, generic	Traditional Antipsychotic
Tacrine	Cognex	NA	Cholinestrase Inhibitor
Temazepam	Restoril	generic	Benzodiazepines
Thioridazine	generic (previously Mellaril)	Mellaril, generic	Traditional Antipsychotic
Thiothixene	Navane	NA	Traditional Antipsychotic
Topiramate	Topamax	Topamax	Mood Stabilizer
Tranylcypromine	Parnate	Parnate	MAOI
Trazodone	(previously Desyrel)	Molipaxin, generic	Heterocyclic Antidepressant
Triazolam	Halcion	N/A	Benzodiazepines
Trifluoperazine	Stelazine, generic	Stelazine, generic	Traditional Antipsychotic
Trihexyphenidyl	Artane, generic	Broflex, generic	Anticholinergic
Trimipramine	Surmontil	Surmontil	Tricyclic Antidepressant
Valproic Acid	Depakote, Depakote ER, Depakene, generic	Epilim, Convulex, Depakote, generic	Mood Stabilizer
Venlafaxine	Effexor-XR, Effexor	Efexor-XR, Efexor	Non-SSRI New Generation
Verapamil	Verelan, Calan, Isoptin, generic	Cordilox, Securon, Univer, Verapress, Vertab, generic	Mood Stabilizer
Zaleplon	Sonata	Sonata	Sedative Hypnotic
Ziprasidone	Geodon	NA	Atypical Antipsychotic
Zolpidem	Ambien	Stilnoct	Sedative Hypnotic
Zopiclone	N/A	Zimovane	Sedative Hypnotic
Zotepine	NA	Zoleptil	Atypical Antipsychotic
Zuclopenthixol	NA	Clopixol	Traditional Antipsychotic

Common psychotropic medications available in the USA, listed alphabetically by brand name

These drug categories list those compounds commonly used in mental health treatment or in amelioration of mental health medication side effects. They are not exhaustive of every medication in each category.

USA brand name(s)	Chemical (generic) name	Starting dose (mg) except as specified	Standard therapeutic dose (mg)	Useful blood levels
Abilify	Aripiprazole	10–15	10–30	No
Adderall	Detroamphetamine and amphetamine	2.5–5 BID	5–60	No
Akineton	Biperidon	1 BID	2–8	No
Ambien	Zolpidem	5	5–10	No
Anafranil	Clomipramine	25–100	25–250	100–250 ng/ml
Antabuse	Disulfiram	250	125–500	No
Apidex	Phentermine	37.5	18.75–37.5	No
Aricept	Donepezil	5	5–10	No
Artane	Trihexyphenidyl	1	2–15	No
Asendin	Amoxapine	50 BID	50–600	No
Atarax	Hydroxyzine	25	50–100	No
Ativan	Lorazepam	1–2	1–10	No
Aventyl	Nortriptyline	50–100	75–150	50–150 ng/ml
Benadryl	Diphenhydramine	25 BID	50–400	No
Buspar	Buspirone	5–10 TID	30–60	No
Calan	Verapamil	40 TID	80–120 TID	No
Celexa	Citalopram	20	20–60	No
Clozaril	Clozapine	12.5 BID	12.5–900	> 350 mg/ml
Cogentin	Benztropine	0.5–1	1–8	No
Cognex	Tacrine	10 QID	40–160	No
Colace	Docusate	50	50–200	No

USA brand name(s)	Chemical (generic) name	Starting dose (mg) except as specified	Standard therapeutic dose (mg)	Useful blood levels
Concerta	Methylphenidate	5–10 BID	10–60	No
Concerta extended release	Methylphenidate	5–10 BID	10–60	No
Concordia	Detroamphetamine and amphetamine	2.5–5 BID	5–60	No
Cylert	Pemoline	37.5	37.5–112.5	No
Depade	Naltrexone	25	50	No
Depakene	Valproic acid	250 TID	750–4200	50–100 μg/ml
Depakote	Valproic acid	250 TID	750–4200	50–100 μg/ml
Depakote ER	Valproic acid	250 TID	750–4200	50–100 μg/ml
Desoxyn	Methamphetamine	5 BID	5–25	No
Desyrel	Trazodone	50–100	150–600	No
Dexedrine	Dexamphetamine	10	10–60	No
Dextrostat	Dextroamphetamine	10	10–60	No
Effexor	Venlafaxine	37.5 BID (STD) 37.5–75 (-XR)	75–375 (STD) 75–225 (-XR)	No
Effexor-XR	Venlafaxine	37.5 BID (STD) 37.5–75 (-XR)	75–375 (STD) 75–225 (-XR)	No
Elavil	Amitriptyline	25–50	50–300	120–250 ng/ml
Equagesic	Meprobamate	400 TID	1200–1600	No
Eskalith	Lithium carbonate	300–600	600–1800	0.6–1.2 meq/l
Eskalith CR	Lithium carbonate	300–600	600–1800	0.6–1.2 meq/l
Etrafon	Amitriptyline + perphenazine	2–25 tab TID	2–25 tab BID–QID	No
Etrafon	Perphenazine	4 TID	12–64	No
Etrafon Forte	Amitriptyline + perphenazine	2–25 tab TID	2–25 tab BID–QID	No
Exelon	Rivastigmine	1.5 BID	6–12	No
Flurazepam	Flurazepam	15	15–30	No
Geodon	Ziprasidone	20–40	40–160	No
Halcion	Triazolam	0.125	0.125–0.5	No
Haldol	Haloperidol	1–3 BID	1–100	No
Immodium	Loperamid	4	6–16	No
Inderal	Propanolol	10–20 BID–TID	20–320	No
Ionamin	Phentermine	37.5	18.75–37.5	No
Isoptin	Verapamil	40 TID	80–120 TID	No
Klonopin	Clonazepam	1	1.5–20	No
Lamictal	Lamotrigine	25	100–400	No
Levothroid	Levothyroxine	12.5–50 μg	12.5–500 μg	No
Levoxyl	Levothyroxine	12.5–50 μg	12.5–500 μg	No
Lexapro	Escitalopram	10	10–20	No
Librium	Chlordiazepoxide	10 TID	15–100	No

USA brand name(s)	Chemical (generic) name	Starting dose (mg) except as specified	Standard therapeutic dose (mg)	Useful blood levels
Limbitrol	Amitriptyline + chlordiazepoxide	1 tab TID	1 tab–2 tabs TID	No
Lithobid	Lithium carbonate	300–600	600–1800	0.6–1.2 meq/l
Loxitane	Loxapine	10–25 BID	20–250	No
Ludiomil	Maprotiline	25 TID	75–225	No
Luvox	Fluoxamine	50	50–300	No
Mellaril	Thioridazine	50–300	20–600	No
Meridia	Sibutramine	10	5–15	No
Metadate	Methylphenidate	5–10 BID	10–60	No
Metadate ER	Methylphenidate	5–10 BID	10–60	No
Methylin	Methylphenidate	5–10 BID	10–60	No
Methylin ER	Methylphenidate	5–10 BID	10–60	No
Metmucil	Psyllium husk	1 tsp in water	1 tsp in water	No
Miltown	Meprobamate	400 TID	1200–1600	No
Moban	Molindone	50 TID	15–225	No
Nardil	Phenelzine	15	15–90	No
Navane	Thiothixene	2 TID	6–60	No
Neurontin	Gabapentin	300	1800–3600	No
Norpramin	Desipramine	25 TID	100–300	115–180 ng/ml
Orap	Pimozide	2	2–20	No
Pamelor	Nortriptyline	50–100	75–150	50–150 ng/ml
Parnate	Tranylcypromine	10	30–60	No
Paxil	Paroxetine	20	10–60	No
Paxil CR	Paroxetine	20	10–60	No
Periactin	Cyproheptadine	4 TID	4–32	No
Peri-Colace	Docusate	50	50–200	No
Prolixin	Fluphenazine	2.5–10	1–40	No
Prosom	Estazolam	0.5	0.5–2	No
Provigil	Modafanil	100–200	200–400	No
Prozac	Fluoxetine	20	20–80	No
Remeron	Mirtazepine	15	15–45	No
Reminyl	Galantamine	4 BID	16–32	No
Restoril	Temazepam	15	7.5–30	
Risperdal	Risperidone	0.5	0.5–16	No
Ritalin	Methylphenidate	5–10 BID	10–60	No
Ritalin SR	Methylphenidate	5–10 BID	10–60	No
Senekot	Senna	15	15–30	No
Serafem	Fluoxetine	20	20–80	No
Serax	Oxazepam	10	30–120	No
Serentil	Mesoridazine	50 TID	100–400	No
Seroquel	Quetiapine	25	50–750	No

USA brand name(s)	Chemical (generic) name	Starting dose (mg) except as specified	Standard therapeutic dose (mg)	Useful blood levels
Serzone	Nefazodone	100 QD–100 BID	200–600	No
Sinequan	Doxepin	25 TID	75–300	200–250 ng/ml Blood level of parent compound plus metabolite
Sonata	Zaleplon	5	5–20	No
Stelazine	Trifluoperazine	5 BID	2–40	No
Surmontil	Trimipramine	75	50–300	No
Synthroid	Levothyroxine	12.5–50 μg	12.5–500 μg	No
Tegretol	Carbamazepine	100–400	400–1600	4–12 μg/ml
Tenormin	Atenolol	50	50–100	No
Thorazine	Chlorpromazine	25 TID	30–800	No
Tofranil	Imipramine	25 TID	75–300	200–250 ng/ml Blood level of parent compound plus metabolite
Topamax	Topiramate	25	200–400	No
Tranxene	Chlorazepate	7.5	7.5–60	No
Trilafon	Perphenazine	4 TID	12–64	No
Trileptal	Oxcarbazepine	300 BID	600–2400	No
Unithroid	Levothyroxine (Tx synthetic)	12.5–50 μg	12.5–500 μg	No
Valium	Diazepam	2 TID	4–40	No
Verelan	Verapamil	40 TID	80–120 TID	No
Viagra	Sildenafil	50	25–100	No
Vistaril	Hydroxyzine	25	50–100	No
Vivactil	Protriptyline	15	15–60	70–250 ng/ml
Wellbutrin	Bupropion	100 QD (STD) 150mg QD (-SR)	200–450 (STD) 150–400 (-SR)	No
Wellbutrin-SR	Bupropion	100 QD (STD) 150mg QD (-SR)	200–450 (STD) 150–400 (-SR)	No
Xanax	Alprazolam	0.25 TID	0.25–10	No
Xenical	Orlistat	120 TID	120 TID	No
Zoloft	Sertraline	50	50–200	No
Zyban	Bupropion	100 QD (STD) 150mg QD (-SR)	200–450 (STD) 150–400 (-SR)	No
Zyprexa	Olanzapine	2.5–10	2.5–20	No

Appendix 5

Common psychotropic medications available in the UK, listed alphabetically by brand name

These drug categories list those compounds commonly used in mental health treatment or in amelioration of mental health medication side effects. They are not exhaustive of every medication in each category.

UK brand name(s)	Chemical (generic) name	Starting dose (mg) except as specified	Standard therapeutic dose (mg)	Useful blood levels
Akineton	Biperidon	1 BID	2–8	No
Allegron	Nortriptyline	50–100	75–150	50–150 ng/ml
Anafranil	Clomipramine	25–100	25–250	100–250 ng/ml
Anafranil SR	Clomipramine	25–100	25–250	100–250 ng/ml
Anquil	Benperidol	0.25–1.5	0.25–1.5	No
Antabuse	Disulfiram	250	125–500	No
Aricept	Donepezil	5	5–10	No
Arpicolin	Procyclidine	2.5 TID	7.5–20	No
Asendis	Amoxapine	50 BID	50–600	No
Atarax	Hydroxyzine	25	50–100	No
Ativan	Lorazepam	1–2	1–10	No
Broflex	Trihexyphenidyl	1	2–15	No
Buspar	Buspirone	5–10 TID	30–60	No
Camcolit	Lithium carbonate	300–600	600–1800	0.6–1.2 meq/l
Campral EC	Acamprosate	666 BID	2000	No
Cerax	Hydroxyzine	25	50–100	No
Chloral Elixir	Chloral hydrate	500	500–2000	No
Cipramil	Citalopram	20	20–60	No
Clobazam	Clobazam	20	20–60	
Clopixol	Sulpiride	200–400	400–2400	No
Clopixol	Zuclopenthixol	20–30	20–150	No

UK brand name(s)	Chemical (generic) name	Starting dose (mg) except as specified	Standard therapeutic dose (mg)	Useful blood levels
Clozaril	Clozapine	12.5 BID	12.5–900	> 350 mg/ml
Cogentin	Benztropine	0.5–1	1–8	No
Concordin	Protriptyline	15	15–60	70–250 ng/ml
Convulex	Valproic acid	250 TID	750–4200	50–100 μg/ml
Cordilox	Verapamil	40 TID	80–120 TID	No
Depakote	Valproic acid	250 TID	750–4200	50–100 μg/ml
Depixol	Flupentixol	3–9 BID	6–18	No
Dexedrine	Dexamphetamine	10	10–60	No
Dioctyl	Docusate	50	50–200	No
Docusol	Docusate	50	50–200	No
Dolmatil	Sulpiride	200–400	400–2400	No
Dozic	Haloperidol	1–3 BID	1–100	No
Dutonin	Nefazodone	100 QD–100 BID	200–600	No
Edronax	Reboxetine	4 BID	8–12	No
Efexor	Venlafaxine	37.5 BID (STD) 37.5–75 (-XR)	75–375 (STD) 75–225 (-XR)	No
Efexor-XR	Venlafaxine	37.5 BID (STD) 37.5-75 (-XR)	75–375 (STD) 75–225 (-XR)	No
Epilim	Valproic acid	250 TID	750–4200	50–100 μg/ml
Equagesic	Meprobamate	400 TID	1200–1600	No
Equasym	Methylphenidate	5–10 BID	10–60	No
Exelon	Rivastigmine	1.5 BID	6–12	No
Faverin	Fluoxamine	50	50–300	No
Fentazin	Perphenazine	4 TID	12–64	No
Flurazepam	Flurazepam	15	15–30	No
Fybogel	Ispaghula husk	1 packet BID	1 packet QD–TID	No
Gamanil	Lofepramine	70	40–210	No
Haldol	Haloperidol	1–3 BID	1–100	No
Heminevrin	Clomethiazole	1 capsule	1–2 capsules	No
Immodium	Loperamid	4	6–16	No
Inderal	Propanolol	10–20 BID–TID	20–320	No
Inderetic	Propanolol	10–20 BID–TID	20–320	No
Inderex	Propanolol	10–20 BID–TID	20–320	No
Isogel	Ispaghula husk	1 packet BID	1 packet QD–TID	No
Ispagel	Ispaghula husk	1 packet BID	1 packet QD–TID	No
Kemadrin	Procyclidine	2.5 TID	7.5–20	No
Konsyl	Ispaghula husk	1 packet BID	1 packet QD–TID	No

UK brand name(s)	Chemical (generic) name	Starting dose (mg) except as specified	Standard therapeutic dose (mg)	Useful blood levels
Lamictal	Lamotrigine	25	100–400	No
Largactil	Chlorpromazine	25 TID	30–800	No
Lentizol	Amitriptyline	25–50	50–300	120–250 ng/ml
Levothyroxine	Levothyroxine	12.5–50 μg	12.5–500 μg	No
Librium	Chlordiazepoxide	10 TID	15–100	No
Liothyronine	Levothyroxine	12.5–50 μg	12.5–500 μg	No
Liskonum	Lithium carbonate	300–600	600–1800	0.6–1.2 meq/l
Lomotil	Diphenoxylate and atropine	1 tab QID	2 tabs Q 6 hours	No
Loxapac	Loxapine	10–25 BID	20–250	No
Ludiomil	Maprotiline	25 TID	75–225	No
Lustral	Sertraline	50	50–200	No
Manerix	Meclobemide	100–300	300–600	No
Manevac	Senna	15	15–30	No
Mellaril	Thioridazine	50–300	20–600	No
Modecate	Fluphenazine	2.5–10	1–40	No
Moditen	Fluphenazine	2.5–10	1–40	No
Mogadon	Nitrazepam	5	5–10	No
Molipaxin	Trazodone	50–100	150–600	No
Motipress	Nortriptyline	50–100	75–150	50–150 ng/ml
Motival	Nortriptyline	50–100	75–150	50–150 ng/ml
Nalorex	Naltrexone	25	50	No
Nardil	Phenelzine	15	15–90	No
Neulactil	Pericyazine	25 TID	75–300	No
Neurontin	Gabapentin	300	1800–3600	No
Nozinan	Levopromazine	25–50	100–200	No
Optimax	L-Tryptophan	1 TID	6	No
Orap	Pimozide	2	2–20	No
Parnate	Tranylcypromine	10	30–60	No
Periactin	Cyproheptadine	4 TID	4–32	No
Pertofrane	Desipramine	25 TID	100–300	115–180 ng/ml
Prothiaden	Dothiepin/dosulpein	75	150–225	No
Provigil	Modafinil	100–200	200–400	No
Prozac	Fluoxetine	20	20–80	No
Reductil	Sibutramine	10	5–15	No
Regulan	Ispaghula husk	1 packet BID	1 packet QD–TID	No
Reminyl	Galantamine	4 BID	16–32	No
Rimapam	Diazepam	2 TID	4–40	No
Risperdal	Risperidone	0.5	0.5–16	No
Ritalin	Methylphenidate	5–10 BID	10–60	No
Rivotril	Clonazepam	1	1.5–20	No

UK brand name(s)	Chemical (generic) name	Starting dose (mg) except as specified	Standard therapeutic dose (mg)	Useful blood levels
Rohypnol	Flunitrazepam	0.5–1	0.5–2	No
Securon	Verapamil	40 TID	80–120 TID	No
Senekot	Senna	15	15–30	No
Serenace	Haloperidol	1–3 BID	1–100	No
Seroquel	Quetiapine	25	50–750	No
Seroxat	Paroxetine	20	10–60	No
Sinequan	Doxepin	25 TID	75–300	200–250 ng/ml Blood level of parent compound plus metabolite
Solian	Amisulpride	50–100	50–1200	No
Somnite	Nitrazepam	5	5–10	No
Sonata	Zaleplon	5	5–20	No
Stelazine	Trifluoperazine	5 BID	2–40	No
Stilnoct	Zolpidem	5	5–10	No
Sulpital	Sulpiride	200–400	400–2400	No
Sulpor	Sulpiride	200–400	400–2400	No
Surmontil	Trimipramine	75	50–300	No
Tegretol	Carbamazepine	100–400	400–1600	4–12 µg/ml
Tenormin	Atenolol	50	50–100	No
Tensium	Diazepam	2 TID	4–40	No
Teril	Carbamazepine	100–400	400–1600	4–12 µg/ml
Terroxin	Levothyroxine	12.5–50 µg	12.5–500 µg	No
Timonil	Carbamazepine	100–400	400–1600	4–12 µg/ml
Tofranil	Imipramine	25 TID	75–300	200–250 ng/ml Blood level of parent compound plus metabolite
Topamax	Topiramate	25	200–400	No
Tranxene	Chlorazepate	7.5	7.5–60	No
Trileptal	Oxcarbazepine	300 BID	600–2400	No
Triptafen	Amitriptyline	25–50	50–300	120–250 ng/ml
Tropium	Chlordiazepoxide	10 TID	15–100	No
Univer	Verapamil	40 TID	80–120 TID	No
Valium	Diazepam	2 TID	4–40	No
Verapress	Verapamil	40 TID	80–120 TID	No
Vertab	Verapamil	40 TID	80–120 TID	No
Viskaldix	Pindolol	5 BID	15–45	No
Viskin	Pindolol	5 BID	15–45	No
Welldorm	Chloral Hydrate	500	500–2000	No
Xanax	Alprazolam	0.25 TID	0.25–10	No
Xenical	Orlistat	120 TID	120 TID	No

UK brand name(s)	Chemical (generic) name	Starting dose (mg) except as specified	Standard therapeutic dose (mg)	Useful blood levels
Zimovane	Zopiclone	3.75	3.75–7.5	No
Zispin	Mirtazepine	15	15–45	No
Zoleptil	Zotepine	25 TID	50–300	No
Zyban	Bupropion	100 QD (STD) 150mg QD (-SR)	200–450 (STD) 150–400 (-SR)	No
Zyprexa	Olanzapine	2.5–10	2.5–20	No

Appendix 6

The National Institute of Mental Health Abnormal Involuntary Movement Scale (AIMS)

Examination procedure

Either before or after completing the examination procedure, observe the patient unobtrusively, at rest (e.g. in waiting room). The chair to be used in this examination should be a hard firm one without arms.

1   Ask patient to remove shoes and socks.
2   Ask patient if there is anything in his mouth (e.g. gum, candy), and if there is, to remove it.
3   Ask patient about the current condition of his teeth. Ask patient if he wears dentures. Do teeth or dentures bother the patient now?
4   Ask patient whether he notices any movements in mouth, face, hands, or feet. If yes, ask him/her to describe these and to what extent they currently bother patient or interfere with his/her activities.
5   Have patient sit in a chair with hands on knees, legs slightly apart and feet flat on floor. (Look at entire body for movements while in this position.)
6   Ask patient to sit with hands hanging unsupported – if male, between legs, if female and wearing a dress, hanging over knees. (Observe hands and other body areas.)
7   Ask patient to open mouth. (Observe tongue at rest in mouth.) Do this twice.
8   Ask patient to protrude tongue. (Observe abnormalities of tongue movement.) Do this twice.
9   Ask patient to tap thumb with each finger, as rapidly as possible for 10–15 seconds; separately with right hand, then with left hand. (Observe facial and leg movements.)
10 Flex and extend patient's left and right arms (one at a time). (Note any rigidity.)

11 Ask patient to stand up. (Observe in profile. Observe all body areas again, hips included.)

12 Ask patient to extend both arms outstretched in front with palms down. (Observe trunk, legs and mouth.)

13 Have patient walk a few paces, turn and walk back to chair. (Observe hands and gait.) Do this twice.

Rating sheet

Patient name		Rater name	
Patient #	Data group: AIMS		Evaluation date
Instructions: Complete the above examination procedure before making ratings. For movement ratings, circle the highest severity observed.		**Code:** 0: None 1: Minimal, may be extreme normal 2: Mild 3: Moderate 4: Severe	

Facial and oral movements	**1 Muscles of facial expression** • e.g. movements of forehead, eyebrows, periorbital area, cheeks • Include frowning, blinking, smiling, and grimacing	0 1 2 3 4
	2 Lips and perioral area e.g. puckering, pouting, smacking	0 1 2 3 4
	3 Jaw e.g. biting, clenching, chewing, mouth opening, lateral movement	0 1 2 3 4
	4 Tongue Rate only increase in movements both in and out of mouth, NOT the inability to sustain movement	0 1 2 3 4
Extremity movements	**5 Upper** (*arms, wrists, hands, fingers*) • Include choreic movements (i.e. rapid, objectively purposeless, irregular, spontaneous), athetoid movements (i.e. slow, irregular, complex, serpentine) • Do NOT include tremor (i.e. repetitive, regular, rhythmic)	0 1 2 3 4
	6 Lower (*legs, knees, ankles, toes*) e.g. lateral knee movement, foot tapping, heel dropping, foot squirming, inversion and eversion of the foot	0 1 2 3 4
Trunk movements	**7 Neck, shoulders, hips** e.g. rocking, twisting, squirming, pelvic gyrations	0 1 2 3 4
	8 Severity of abnormal movements	0 1 2 3 4
Global judgments	**9 Incapacitation due to abnormal movements**	0 1 2 3 4
	10 Patient's awareness of abnormal movements Rate only patient's report	0 1 2 3 4
Dental status	**11 Current problems with teeth and/or dentures**	0: No 1: Yes
	12 Does patient usually wear dentures?	0: No 1: Yes

Appendix 7

The American Medical Association recommendations on gifts to physicians

Issued June 1992, based on the report, "Gifts to Physicians from Industry," adopted December 1990 (*JAMA*, 1991;265:501 and *Food and Drug Law Journal* 1992;47:445-458).

Opinion 8.061

Many gifts given to physicians by companies in the pharmaceutical, device, and medical equipment industries serve an important and socially beneficial function. For example, companies have long provided funds for educational seminars and conferences. However, there has been growing concern about certain gifts from industry to physicians. Some gifts that reflect customary practices of industry may not be consistent with the Principles of Medical Ethics. To avoid the acceptance of inappropriate gifts, physicians should observe the following guidelines:

- Any gifts accepted by physicians individually should primarily entail a benefit to patients and should not be of substantial value. Accordingly, textbooks, modest meals, and other gifts are appropriate if they serve a genuine educational function. Cash payments should not be accepted. The use of drug samples for personal or family use is permissible as long as these practices do not interfere with patient access to drug samples. It would not be acceptable for non-retired physicians to request free pharmaceuticals for personal use or use by family members.
- Individual gifts of minimal value are permissible as long as the gifts are related to the physician's work (e.g. pens and notepads).
- The Council on Ethical and Judicial Affairs defines a legitimate "conference" or "meeting" as any activity, held at an appropriate location, where:
    The gathering is primarily dedicated, in both time and effort, to promoting objective scientific and educational activities and discourse (one or

more educational presentation(s) should be the highlight of the gathering, and

The main incentive for bringing attendees together is to further their knowledge on the topic(s) being presented. An appropriate disclosure of financial support or conflict of interest should be made.

■ Subsidies to underwrite the costs of continuing medical education conferences or professional meetings can contribute to the improvement of patient care and therefore are permissible. Since the giving of a subsidy directly to a physician by a company's representative may create a relationship that could influence the use of the company's products, any subsidy should be accepted by the conference's sponsor, who in turn can use the money to reduce the conference's registration fee. Payments to defray the costs of a conference should not be accepted directly from the company by the physicians attending the conference.

■ Subsidies from industry should not be accepted directly or indirectly to pay for the costs of travel, lodging, or other personal expenses of physicians attending conferences or meetings, nor should subsidies be accepted to compensate for the physicians' time. Subsidies for hospitality should not be accepted outside of modest meals or social events held as a part of a conference or meeting. It is appropriate for faculty at conferences or meetings to accept reasonable honoraria and to accept reimbursement for reasonable travel, lodging, and meal expenses. It is also appropriate for consultants who provide genuine services to receive reasonable compensation and to accept reimbursement for reasonable travel, lodging, and meal expenses. Token consulting or advisory arrangements cannot be used to justify the compensation of physicians for their time or their travel, lodging, and other out-of-pocket expenses.

■ Scholarship or other special funds to permit medical students, residents, and fellows to attend carefully selected educational conferences may be permissible as long as the selection of students, residents, or fellows who will receive the funds is made by the academic or training institution. Carefully selected educational conferences are generally defined as the major educational, scientific or policymaking meetings of national, regional or specialty medical associations.

■ No gifts should be accepted if there are strings attached. For example, physicians should not accept gifts if they are given in relation to the physician's prescribing practices. In addition, when companies underwrite medical conferences or lectures other than their own, responsibility for and control over the selection of content, faculty, educational methods, and materials should belong to the organizers of the conferences or lectures.

Appendix 8

Pharmaceutical Research and Manufacturers of America (PhRMA)

Code of Interactions with Healthcare Professionals

1 BASIS OF INTERACTIONS

Our relationships with healthcare professionals are intended to benefit patients and to enhance the practice of medicine. Interactions should be focused on informing healthcare professionals about products, providing scientific and educational information, and supporting medical research and education.

2 INFORMATIONAL PRESENTATIONS BY OR ON BEHALF OF A PHARMACEUTICAL COMPANY

Informational presentations and discussions by industry representatives and others speaking on behalf of a company provide valuable scientific and educational benefits. In connection with such presentations or discussions, occasional meals (but no entertainment/recreational events) may be offered so long as they: (a) are modest as judged by local standards; and (b) occur in a venue and manner conducive to informational communication and provide scientific or educational value. Inclusion of a healthcare professional's spouse or other guests is not appropriate. Offering "take-out" meals or meals to be eaten without a company representative being present (such as "dine & dash" programs) is not appropriate.

3 THIRD-PARTY EDUCATIONAL OR PROFESSIONAL MEETINGS

a Continuing medical education (CME) or other third-party scientific and educational conferences or professional meetings can contribute to the improvement of patient care and therefore, financial support from companies is permissible. Since the giving of any subsidy directly to a healthcare professional by a company may be viewed as an inappropriate cash gift, any financial support should be given to the conference's sponsor which, in turn, can use the money to reduce the overall conference registration fee for all attendees. In addition, when companies underwrite medical conferences or meetings other than their own, responsibility for any control over the selection of content, faculty, educational methods, materials, and venue belongs to the organizers of the conferences or meetings in accordance with their guidelines.

b   Financial support should not be offered for the costs of travel, lodging, or other personal expenses of non-faculty healthcare professionals attending CME or other third-party scientific or educational conferences or professional meetings, either directly to the individuals attending the conference or indirectly to the conference's sponsor (except as set out in section 6 below). Similarly, funding should not be offered to compensate for the time spent by healthcare professionals attending the conference or meeting.

c   Financial support for meals or receptions may be provided to the CME sponsors who in turn can provide meals or receptions for all attendees. A company also may provide meals or receptions directly at such events if it complies with the sponsoring organization's guidelines. In either of the above situations, the meals or receptions should be modest and be conducive to discussion among faculty and attendees, and the amount of time at the meals or receptions should be clearly subordinate to the amount of time spent at the educational activities of the meeting.

d   A conference or meeting shall mean any activity, held at an appropriate location, where (a) the gathering is primarily dedicated, in both time and effort, to promoting objective scientific and educational activities and discourse (one or more educational presentation(s) should be the highlight of the gathering), and (b) the main incentive for bringing attendees together is to further their knowledge on the topic(s) being presented.

4   CONSULTANTS

a   It is appropriate for consultants who provide services to be offered reasonable compensation for those services and to be offered reimbursement for reasonable travel, lodging, and meal expenses incurred as part of providing those services. Compensation and reimbursement that would be inappropriate in other contexts can be acceptable for *bona fide* consultants in connection with their consulting arrangements. Token consulting or advisory arrangements should not be used to justify compensating healthcare professionals for their time or their travel, lodging, or other out-of-pocket expenses. The following factors support the existence of a *bona fide* consulting arrangement (not all factors may be relevant to any particular arrangement):

■   A written contract specified the nature of the services to be provided and the basis for payment of those services;

■   A legitimate need for the services has been clearly identified in advance of requesting the services and entering into arrangements with the prospective consultants;

- The criteria for selecting consultants are directly related to the identified purpose and the persons responsible for selecting the consultants have the expertise necessary to evaluate whether the particular healthcare professionals meet those criteria;
- The number of healthcare professionals retained is not greater than the number reasonably necessary to achieve the identified purpose;
- The venue and circumstances of any meeting with consultants are conducive to the consulting services and activities related to the services are the primary focus of the meeting, and any social or entertainment events are clearly subordinate in terms of time and emphasis.

b It is not appropriate to pay honoraria or travel or lodging expenses to non-faculty and non-consultant attendees at company-sponsored meetings, including attendees who participate in interactive sessions.

5 SPEAKER TRAINING MEETINGS

It is appropriate for healthcare professionals who participate in programs intended to recruit and train speakers for company sponsored speaker bureaus to be offered reasonable compensation for their time, considering the value of the type of services provided, and to be offered reimbursement for reasonable travel, lodging, and meal expenses, when (1) the participants receive extensive training on the company's drug products and on compliance with FDA regulatory requirements for communications about such products, (2) this training will result in the participants providing a valuable service to the company, and (3) the participants meet the criteria for consultants (as discussed in part 4.a. above).

6 SCHOLARSHIPS AND EDUCATIONAL FUNDS

Financial assistance for scholarships or other educational funds to permit medical students, residents, fellows, and other healthcare professionals in training to attend carefully selected educational conferences may be offered so long as the selection of individuals who receive the funds is made by the academic or training institution. "Carefully selected educational conferences" are generally defined as the major educational, scientific, or policy-making meetings of national, regional, or specialty medical associations.

7 EDUCATIONAL AND PRACTICE-RELATED ITEMS

a Items primarily for the benefit of patients may be offered to healthcare professionals if they are not of substantial value ($100 or less). For example, an anatomical model for use in an examination room primarily involves a patient benefit, whereas a VCR or CD player does not. Items should not be offered on more than an occasional basis, even if each individual item is appropriate. Providing product samples for patient use in accordance with the Prescription Drug Marketing Act is acceptable.

b Items of minimal value may be offered if they are primarily associated with a healthcare professional's practice (such as pens, notepads, and similar "reminder" items with company or product logos).

c Items intended for the personal benefit of healthcare professionals (such as floral arrangements, artwork, music CDs or tickets to a sporting event) should not be offered.

d Payments in cash or cash equivalents (such as gift certificates) should not be offered to healthcare professionals either directly or indirectly, except as compensation for *bona fide* services (as described in parts 4 and 5). Cash or equivalent payments of any kind create a potential appearance of impropriety or conflict of interest.

8 INDEPENDENCE OF DECISION MAKING

No grants, scholarships, subsidies, support, consulting contracts, or educational or practice-related items should be provided or offered to a healthcare professional in exchange for prescribing products or for a commitment to continue prescribing products. Nothing should be offered or provided in a manner or condition that would interfere with the independence of a healthcare professional's prescribing practices.

9 ADHERENCE TO CODE

Each member company is strongly encouraged to adopt procedures to assure adherence to this Code.

Index